D1573093

Bonney's Gynaecological Surgery

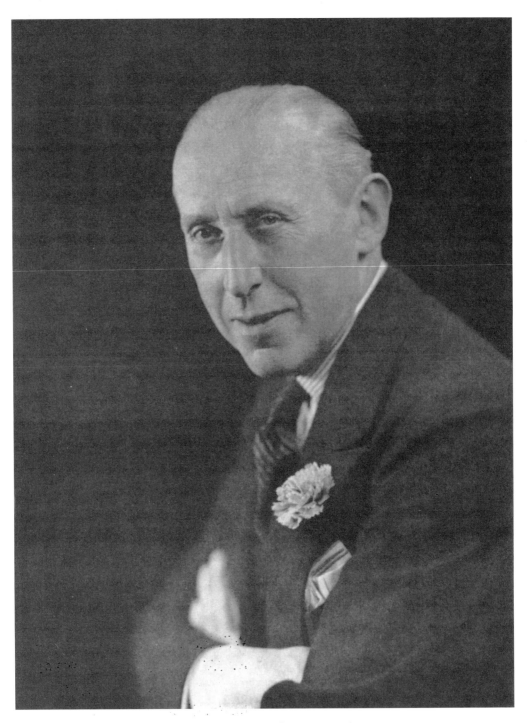

This book is dedicated to the memory of Victor Bonney.
It is also dedicated to our wives Maggie, Jane and Rupal for their support,
understanding, patience and love which they have shown us in our lives together

Bonney's Gynaecological Surgery

John M. Monaghan
MB ChB, FRCS(Ed), FRCOG
Consultant Surgeon
Whitton Grange
Whitton
Northumberland
England

Alberto (Tito) de Barros Lopes
Consultant Gynaecological Oncologist
Northern Gynaecological Oncology Centre
Queen Elizabeth Hospital
Sheriff Hill
Gateshead

Raj Naik
Consultant Gynaecological Oncologist
Northern Gynaecological Oncology Centre
Queen Elizabeth Hospital
Sheriff Hill
Gateshead

TENTH EDITION

Blackwell
Science

© 2004 by Blackwell Science Ltd
a Blackwell Publishing Company
Blackwell Science, Inc., 350 Main Street, Malden, MA 02148-5020, USA
Blackwell Publishing Ltd, 9600 Garsington Road, Oxford OX4 2DQ, UK
Blackwell Science Asia Pty, 550 Swanson Street, Carlton, Victoria 3053, Australia

First published 1911
Eighth edition 1974 (Baillière Tindall)
Ninth edition 1986 (Baillière Tindall)
Tenth edition 2004 Blackwell Science Ltd

Library of Congress Cataloging-in-Publication Data
Monaghan, John M.
    Bonney's gynaecological surgery. — 10th ed. / John M. Monaghan,
Tito Lopes, Raj Naik.
        p. ; cm.
Includes bibliographical references and index.
    ISBN 0-632-05419-0
    1. Generative organs, Female — Surgery.
    [DNLM: 1. Gynaecologic Surgical Procedures.   2. Genitalia,
Female — surgery. WP 660 M734b 2004]   I. Title: Gynaecological surgery.
II. Lopes, Tito.   III. Naik, Raj.   IV. Bonney, Victor, 1872–1953.
Gynaecological surgery.   V. Title.
    RG104.B65 2004
    618.1′059 — dc22

                                                          2004020780

ISBN 0-632-05419-0

A catalogue record for this title is available from the British Library

Set in 9 on 11.5 Sabon by SNP Best-set Typesetter Ltd., Hong Kong
Printed and bound in India by Gopsons Papers Ltd, Noida

Production Editor: Rebecca Huxley
Commissioning Editor: Stuart Taylor
Editorial Assistant: Katrina Chandler
Production Controller: Mirjana Misina

For further information on Blackwell Publishing, visit our website:
http://www.blackwellpublishing.com

Contents

Preface to the tenth edition

Unfortunately the tenth edition of this famous text has been a little slow in arriving. The pressures on a surgeon in modern clinical practice have reduced markedly the time available for 'extra' work. As the senior editor I am extremely grateful for the contributions made to this edition by my colleagues Tito Lopes and Raj Naik, without their assistance this edition would have been even longer in the gestation.

Surgery remains an art form with a tinge of science to leaven the advances. Even though we have seen enormous advances in the medical treatment of a number of conditions previously diagnosed or treated by surgical means, the role of surgery remains vitally important. In many circumstances, particularly in gynaecological oncology, gynaecological urology, the management of the disordered pelvic floor and of advanced endometriosis, surgery continues to be the mainstay of treatment.

The need to teach surgery remains a high priority but with a significant reduction in working hours, an increase in the numbers of junior doctors and pressures from patients not to be treated as 'guinea pigs'; gaining a weight of surgical experience has become increasingly difficult. There are now very few countries where the teacher can utilise live animals for training. Cadaver experience is also becoming increasingly complex to access due to changes in consent rules and personal privacy laws.

However in spite of all these setbacks, some of which are almost medieval in their arbitrariness, surgeons around the world continue to innovate, inspire and develop this exciting field for the benefit of their patients. Much of the change reflected in the tenth edition is a combination of innovation from surgeons working closely with the surgical instrument industry. This combination has encouraged change and advancement and out of the difficulties identified above have developed new method of teaching with live demonstrations, animal work where possible and the use of simulators of increasing sophistication. The surgeon continues to demonstrate that eternal desire to improve. Like all art, surgery is going through another difficult phase which we hope can be alleviated by the production of this tenth edition which continues to extol the virtues of simple minimalistic surgery.

I am also grateful for the contribution from Stuart Stanton and John Newton. My thanks to Jane Fallows and Roger Hulley for their contribution to the artwork. Rebecca Huxley has kept my nose firmly to the grindstone once we started to move, she certainly has made the difficult phases of this book much easier to negotiate; many thanks.

John M. Monaghan
Whitton Grange
2004

Preface to the ninth edition

The influence of Victor Bonney and his pupils upon gynaecological surgery has developed from the publication of the first edition of *A Textbook of Gynaecological Surgery* in 1911. The first to the fourth editions were the results of the collaboration of Bonney with Sir Comynus Berkeley. Following the death of the latter, Victor Bonney produced the fifth and sixth editions alone. Bonney's pupils Howkins and Macleod then produced the seventh edition. The death of Macleod signalled virtually the end of those practising surgeons who had been trained by Victor Bonney. The very successful eighth edition was prepared by John Howkins and Sir John Stallworthy. These two great figures of Commonwealth Gynaecology had worked together as junior colleagues during the last years of Bonney's clinical career.

When the eighth edition was published in 1974 many changes were incorporated into the text. However, in the next 10 years, an enormous number of new developments have occurred, possibly the greatest being a resurgence of interest in gynaecological surgery and the growth and establishment of gynaecological oncology as a recognized subspecialty. The present editor has only a tenuous link with Victor Bonney in that he has been greatly influenced in his career by the late Dr A.F. Anderson of Edinburgh and by Mr Stanley Way, both of whom spoke frequently with great affection and reverence of the master surgeon. Indeed it was Way who introduced me to the Bonney scissors, which instruments the reader will see referred to throughout this edition.

When asked by the medical editor of Baillière Tindall for my opinion of the eighth edition of *Bonney's Gynaecological Surgery* some 2 years ago, I replied that I thought that it was undoubtedly the leading textbook of gynaecological surgery in the world, but would nevertheless benefit from a major revision. I also jokingly said 'Give me five years and I will do it for you'. The prompt rejoinder was 'We will give you two years if you will take it on'. Little did I know at the time that I had been 'set up', as the Americans say. I felt hesitant at the prospect of making major changes to such a well-established book but realized that large-scale changes were necessary and also that if modern materials and instruments were to be incorporated, most of the drawings would require reworking.

It was also clear that no single surgeon could encompass all the skills of modern gynaecological surgery and that I would need assistance with three major sections. I have been delighted with the response and the quality of the contributions from Sir Rustam Feroze, Stuart L. Stanton and Professor John R. Newton. I am indebted to them.

Victor Bonney had skills far beyond those of mere mortals; to be able to operate to the highest level and then to be capable of transferring those ideas to paper as the most clear and concise drawings was an amazing talent. I have been especially fortunate in obtaining the services of Mr Douglas Hammersley, once head of graphics at the University of Newcastle upon Tyne, to illustrate all the chapters which have been rewritten. Doug has now moved to Norfolk to be a little closer to his chief interest, that of observing and drawing butterflies. I am sure that the reader will appreciate the outstanding quality of the drawings in this new edition, in particular the way in which they have captured the movement and dynamism of surgery. I am totally indebted to Doug for bringing to life my attempts at surgery.

This book is very much my own; the philosophy of the surgery is entirely mine and the responsibility for making such drastic alterations to this classic text are also mine. I do not make apologies as I feel that Bonney would have approved because I have attempted to keep his beloved gynaecological surgery moving forward. Indeed, even between the beginning and end of the 2-year writing period, new developments have occurred which have had to be incorporated into the text.

I have attempted to show that by adopting an economy of movement in surgery as well as in the text, operations can be performed cleanly and neatly, without ritual. Operations should flow with a style and a natural pace, rather like a well-choreographed dance. There should be no great crises and the procedure should not be performed to the point of total exhaustion for the surgeon and his staff. I have tried to show the enormous enthusiasm which I have for gynaecological surgery and the way in which I feel that it can become a source of great satisfaction and pride. I hope that a little of this enthusiasm is transmitted to the reader and that this book will bring forth new energies for the development of our fascinating subject.

The updating of this text has been for me an enormous honour and a great pleasure. I have had to clarify my thoughts on many aspects of surgery and take bold decisions to cut out large quantities of the previous edition, particularly the results and complications sections, which although historically interesting are not relevant to modern-day practice except as records of the past. Their repetition would simply occupy space.

This ninth edition hopefully reflects the most modern aspects of gynaecological surgery as well as retaining all that is still valuable and relevant from past editions. It also emphasizes the continuing role of gynaecological surgery in the management of a multitude of gynaecological conditions, particularly highlighting the place of surgery in cancer care and the newer surgical technique relating to the infertile woman. The place of new tools such as the laser and staples has been added to the more standard instrumentation.

I would like to thank Baillière Tindall and in particular Dr Geoffrey Smaldon for his constant support. To all those who have assisted, guided and encouraged me during my career, occasionally allowing this stubborn, single-minded Yorkshireman to have his way, I am grateful.

Very special thanks must go to Mr Alan Evans who, as my senior registrar, painstakingly read all my first drafts and attempted to bring a Welsh view of the English language to bear upon my efforts.

I stand in great awe at the end of a long line of illustrious names in gynaecological surgery. I hope that I have done them justice in this the ninth edition of *Bonney's Gynaecological Surgery*.

John M. Monaghan   *Newcastle upon Tyne*
April 1986

1 Introduction and prologue

Introduction

As with the last edition of this famous text I have felt the need to retain the basic Bonney philosophy as it contains all that I feel is important in the development of the surgeon. This first chapter is virtually as Bonney wrote it because it remains relevant and vital for today's practising surgeon. It is also a tribute to the great skill and understanding shown by the father figure of British gynaecological surgery. I have spent over half my life working in gynaecological surgery and owe a great debt to my predecessors, many of whom can claim a direct link to Bonney and his colleagues. I now feel a solid part of that link and hope that I can pass on to my pupils the importance of a clear recognition of where we have come from but at the same time, encourage a searching desire to take the subject forward and constantly to question dogma by applying rigorous analysis to our entire practice.

This new text takes a lot from the old but is generated out of the need to recognize the enormous changes in technology and practice which have occurred in the last 10 years.

Surgical discipline is learned in three broad phases.
1 Learning to assist and appreciate the importance of teamwork.
2 Learning the detail of the steps in the operation and building up the skills to deal confidently with each step.
3 Learning to direct the assistants so that the operation flows in an efficient and timely manner.
As these three phases are being learned the surgeon will go on to develop the art and the science of surgery. Although it is understandable to try to emulate the facility and smoothness of one's teacher, the junior surgeon should soon realize that speed and ease of operating are the product of accuracy and safety. Accuracy and skill arise from assiduous practice and analysis of technique. This analysis will often take the form of 'playing back' procedures in the mind so that all steps can be assessed and evaluated. Unfortunately the most common drive to reassess surgical procedures is when 'things go wrong'; I would recommend to all surgeons that an ability to recall every tiny step in a procedure is vital. As this analytical process develops, the surgeon will realize that speed and ease of operating arise from a striving for perfection both in decision-making and technical skills. Surgery should be one continuous flowing movement, without undue stops and starts or alarms and excursions.

The most accomplished surgeon appears to be deliberate, making no unnecessary movement and directing both the instruments and assistants accurately. Communication of instrumental requirements to the scrub nurse should be in advance of the moment of need so that the surgery can flow without either significant pause or the stress generated by the urgency of immediate need. It is vitally important that the tyro should not regard the time spent as a junior as the sole period of learning of new techniques and observance of other surgeons working. Unfortunately, from the time appointed to independent practice, the majority of surgeons will rarely see other colleagues work. This is especially common in departments where the organization of clinic and operating lists are such that it is difficult or impossible for colleagues to come together in the operating theatre. In recent times the resurrection of the 'live' theatre demonstration has to some extent assisted the promulgation of new techniques and ideas.

The need for adequate continuing medical education (CME) has been recognized by clinicians and governing bodies alike with the result that there are now a plethora of live teaching and hands-on training courses available. The availability of cadavers and animals for surgical practice is severely limited and dependent upon the particular regulations of the countries involved. Where such facilities are available or the opportunities arise to visit such centres, both the established and the trainee surgeon should jump at the chance.

There are increasing pressures on all clinicians to be 'cost effective' and to practise 'evidence-based' medicine within the overarching ambience of 'clinical governance'. Although the words may be novel within the bounds of traditional medical practice, if the surgeon can step back from the fashionable and novel jargon for a moment they will see that the high-quality surgeon need modify little in their practice. The stimulation of a never-ending desire to improve one's practice linked to rigorous audit and research will provide a constant framework which will stand the test of time.

Prologue — after Victor Bonney

The surgeon

A surgeon should always remember that the work of his subordinates is influenced by his own behaviour. It is impossible to lay down rules for all temperaments but there are certain considerations which may prove useful to those embarking on a surgical career. Anyone who cares to observe the work of other operators cannot fail to see how variously the stress and strain of operating are borne by different individuals and will deduce from a consideration of the strong and weak points of each operator some conception of the ideal.

The thoughtful surgeon, influenced by this study, will endeavour so to discipline himself so that he will strive constantly to achieve the ideal. By so doing, he will encourage all who work in the wards and theatres with him — young colleagues in training, anaesthetists, nurses, theatre assistants and orderlies — to appreciate the privileges and responsibilities of their common task. Expert coordinated teamwork is essential to the success of modern surgery. This teamwork has resulted in a significant lowering of operative morbidity and mortality.

However, it is important to recognize the enormous contribution to the safety of modern surgery made by other disciplines, especially anaesthesiology. The preoperative assessment and the postoperative care carried out by the anaesthetist has rendered surgery safer and has also allowed patients who would not in the past have been considered eligible for surgery to have their procedures performed successfully. The role of specialties such as haematology, biochemistry, microbiology, radiology, pathology and physiotherapy are also well recognized.

Bonney maintained that the keystone of a surgeon's bearing should be his self control; and whilst it is his duty to keep a general eye on all that takes place in the operating theatre and without hesitation correct mistakes, he should guard against becoming irritable or losing temper. The surgeon who when faced with difficulties loses control has mistaken his vocation, however dextrous he may be, or however learned in the technical details of the art. The habit of abusing the assistants, the instruments or the anaesthetist, so easy to acquire and so hard to lose, is not one to be commended; the lack of personal confidence from which such behaviour stems will inevitably spread to other members of staff, so that at the very time the surgeon needs effective help it is likely to be found wanting. However, the converse of accepting poor standards of care and behaviour is not to be condoned. The continual presentation of inadequately prepared instrumentation should not be accepted. There is little excuse for staff or equipment to arrive in theatre in a state ill prepared for the task ahead.

The whole team should look forward to a theatre session as a period of pleasure, stimulation and achievement, not as a chore and a period of misery to be suffered. The surgeon should also remember that he is on 'display' and his ability to cope with adversity as well as his manner when the surgery is going well will be keenly observed. The surgeon should teach continuously, point out to assistants and observers the small points of technique as well as related facts to the case in hand.

Bonney enjoined that the surgeon should not gossip; the present editor feels that day-to-day chit chat is not out of place in the operating theatre and is to be preferred to the media view of an operating theatre as a place of knife-like tension fraught with grave interpersonal relationships. However, the mark of the good surgeon and his team is that at the time of stress, the noise level in theatre should fall rather than rise, as each member of the team goes about his or her task with speed and efficiency.

It is inevitable that at some point the surgeon will come face to face with imminent disaster; even the most stalwart individual will feel his heart sink at such a moment. The operator should always remember that at such moments if basic surgical principles are applied quickly and accurately the situation will be rapidly rescued. Hesitation and uncertainty will all too often terminate in disaster. A sturdy belief in his own powers and a refusal to accept defeat are the best assets of a calling which pre-eminently demands moral courage.

Before operating the surgeon should prepare by going over in his own mind the various possibilities in the projected procedure, so that there may be no surprises and he may all the better meet any eventuality. Likewise, following the procedure, it is valuable to go over in one's mind every step in the operation in order to analyse any deficiencies and difficulties experienced; it is only by this continuous self-assessment and analysis that the surgeon can from his own efforts improve his practice.

It is of increasing importance that the surgeon understands the need for meticulous record keeping in order to build a comprehensive database for future analysis. The modern surgeon has to examine continually his and other's work in order to practise to the highest possible standards. More and more guidelines are being generated; the surgeon has to be sure that his work meets the quality requirements of modern practice. Patients, purchasers and professional bodies wish to be able to access the best possible practices. Transparency of standards is essential to modern medical practice. The high-quality surgeon has little to fear from the implementation of guidelines and should look upon these times as opportunities for developing the highest quality of care.

Surgery is physically and mentally tiring. The surgeon should be sure to be adequately equipped in both these areas to meet the demands of theatre. It is important to remember that driving the staff on for long, tiring sessions is counterproductive; there is little merit in performing long procedures with an already exhausted staff. The surgeon's hands and mind become less steady, his assistants less attentive and the nurses tired and disillusioned. It is under these circumstances that mistakes occur. It is important, however, not to be dogmatic about the ideal length of either individual operations or of operating lists. A full day in the operating theatre may suit one surgical team but be anathema to another.

Speed in operating

Speed, as the outcome of perfect operating technique, is as characteristic of a fine surgeon as striving for effect is the stock-in-trade of the showman. An operation rapidly yet correctly performed has many advantages over one technically as correct yet laboriously and tediously accomplished. The period over which haemorrhage may occur is shortened, the tissues are handled less and are therefore less bruised, the time the peritoneum is open and exposed is shortened, the amount and length of anaesthesia is shortened and the impact of the operative shock, which is an accumulation of all these factors, is reduced. Moreover, less strain is put upon the legs and temper of the operator and the assistants with the result that the interest of the latter and the onlookers is maintained at the highest level.

However, this speed must be tempered with attention to detail, particularly of haemostasis and by a conscious effort not to handle tissue unnecessarily.

Operative manipulation

Minimizing trauma is of fundamental importance for uncomplicated wound healing. *The art of gentle surgery must be developed* (Moynihan). Sadly, many surgeons achieve speed by being rough with tissue, particularly by direct handling. This must be avoided at all costs and the temptation to tear tissue with the hands rather than to incise and dissect delicately with instruments is to be eschewed. All operative manipulations should be gentle; force is occasionally essential but should be applied with accuracy, only to the tissue to be removed, and for limited periods of time. The surgeon who tears and traumatizes tissue will see the error of his ways in the long recovery periods that his patients require and in the high complication rate.

Minimalistic surgery

Moynihan spoke in 1920 at the inaugural meeting of the British Association of Surgeons on 'the Ritual of a Surgical Operation', stating, 'he [the surgeon] must set endeavour in continual motion, and seek always and earnestly for simpler methods and a better way. In the craft of surgery the master word is *simplicity*'.

The author has often been described as minimalistic, a description received gratefully, endorsing the words of Moynihan of long ago.

The surgeon should continually endeavour to reduce the number of manipulations involved in a procedure to the absolute minimum consistent with sound performance. If an operation is observed critically, one is struck by the vast number of unnecessary movements performed, the majority of which are due to the uncertainty and inexperience of the operator. In older surgeons unless care is taken to analyse these movements and eliminate them they will become part of the habits and ritual of the procedure. The editor has found the discipline of making video films of operative procedures a salutary experience, highlighting repetitive and pointless movements. In more recent times the advent of digital recording, mixing still photographs with video, is an invaluable development. The group analysis of procedures by the 'team' can be extremely instructive, often generating change in habits and technique by example and questioning of traditional dogma. Often new research and audit projects are generated from these constructive meetings.

Further reading

Textbooks

It is difficult to bring the reader's attention to further reading following a general introductory chapter; however, there are one or two texts which the editor feels the aspiring surgeon should acquire and the trained practitioner should dip into from time to time.

First, he would recommend the reader to look back to his training days and make regular reference to a first class text of general gynaecological pathology. The one he would recommend is *Pathology of the Female Genital Tract* by Ancel Blaustein. It is published by Springer-Verlag, New York, and although weighty and a little expensive it is very readable with an extensive list of references for each chapter.

The second book the editor would recommend reading and, ideally, obtaining is *Lymphatic System of the Female Genitalia* by Plentl and Friedman, published by W.B. Saunders, Philadelphia. Sadly, it is now out of print but well worth seeking out. Although the book is subtitled *The morphologic basis of oncologic diagnosis and therapy* its contents apply to the whole of gynaecological surgery and brings a wider understanding of the pelvic anatomy and its function.

In a more relaxed vein, the editor would recommend a small volume which is a gem; it is entitled *Classical Contributions to Obstetrics and Gynecology* by Herbert Thoms, Associate Professor of Obstetrics and Gynaecology at Yale University, with a foreword by Howard A. Kelly of the 'bladder buttressing stitch' fame. This small volume consists of brief monographs, each dedicated to one of the great names in obstetrics and gynaecology. Sadly, Bonney is not among the illustrious list mainly because the list stops in the early part of the twentieth century but also because it is a little light on gynaecologists. It will, however, demonstrate to the reader that there is very little truly new and also impress him with the enormous strides made by some of our predecessors in the face of the most amazing adversity.

The text *Victor Bonney: The Gynaecological Surgeon of the Twentieth Century*, edited by Geoffrey Chamberlain, published by Panthenon Publishing (2000) is a 'must read' for all students of great surgery and surgeons.

2 Instruments, operative materials and basic surgical techniques

In virtually all modern operating theatres, instruments and drapes are prepacked and sterilized in 'sets' for individual or generic procedures in a central sterile supply department (CSSD). This clearly has major advantages in terms of high standards of sterility over selecting instruments for a specific procedure and sterilizing them immediately prior to an operation in or close to the operating theatre. However, as with all things the need for much specialized instrumentation has resulted in two developments.

The first is the introduction of a wide range of prepacked and sterile disposable instruments of amazing complexity, including much of the equipment used in minimal access surgery.

The second is a recognition that from time to time an 'immediate' sterilizing facility is required so that in many operating theatres on-the-spot sterilization is available for a small number of specialized pieces of equipment.

The generic tray system, however, remains the central plank of instrument provision for the majority of gynaecological procedures.

The content of the trays must represent the actual requirements of the surgeons involved, this means that the instrument choice must be the surgeon's and not that of a manager of a CSSD who may never handle the equipment and has no concept of the surgeon's requirements. Good communication of the surgeon's need to those in control of the budget is essential. It is important that a surgeon does not develop a reputation for desiring every minor new development seen at surgical meetings, but should instead insist on a broad range of high-quality functioning equipment that does not continually irritate by failing to work, whether this be a simple pair of scissors or the most sophisticated minimal access equipment.

Instruments for major gynaecological procedures

The instruments currently used in the editor's gynaecological general operating set are listed in Table 2.1.

The instruments used in the gynaecological minor procedures set are shown in Table 2.2. Some of the instruments mentioned warrant special comment.

Scissors

Bonney's dissecting scissors (Fig. 2.1) are often marketed as Mayo scissors. They are heavy, but have a sureness about them, which allows for accurate gentle dissection, particularly of the 'separate and cut' type. The ends of the scissors are relatively blunt and will do little damage when separating tissue, whereas the blades are powerful enough when coupled with the long levers of the 10″ handles to cope with the toughest of scar tissue. This latter characteristic is especially important in cancer work when operating on tissues previously treated with radiotherapy.

Monaghan's dissecting scissors (Fig. 2.2) developed out of a need for a lighter pair of dissecting scissors which retained the wonderful 'feel' of the Bonney scissor without the weight. This instrument has allowed the scissor dissection technique taught by the editor to reach the level of anatomical dissection required to meet the most stringent standards of cancer surgery. The tips of the instrument remain relatively blunt but

Table 2.1 Gynaecological general set

4 Sponge handles forceps	1 Packing forceps
5 Towel clips	1 Volsellum, toothed
2 Bard Parker knife handles, no. 4	1 Amreich retractor
1 Bard Parker knife handle, no. 3	1 Balfour self-retaining retractor
1 Debakey dissecting forceps	1 Large Kelly's retractor
2 Lane's dissecting forceps, toothed	1 Small Kelly's retractor
1 Small dissecting forceps, non-toothed	2 Large Morris retractor
2 Scissors, tungsten carbide, 6″ straight	2 Langenbeck retractors
1 Scissors, 8″ straight	1 Cushing's vessel retractor
1 Monaghan's dissecting scissors, 8″	1 Aneurysm needle
1 Bonney's dissecting scissors	1 Sinus forceps
1 Dressing scissors	1 Brodies' probe and 1 malleable probe
2 Lloyd-Davis needle holders	1 Graduated metal ruler, inches and centimetres
2 Medium needle holders	1 Raytec intra-abdominal pack (18″ × 18″)
15 Grey Turner artery forceps, straight	1 Receiver
10 Medium Spencer Wells forceps, straight	2 Gallipots
5 Long Spencer Wells forceps	1 Sanitary towel
5 Long Meigs' (Navratil) artery forceps	
5 Littlewood's tissue forceps	
5 Lane's tissue forceps	
6 Zeppelin tissue clamps	

Table 2.2 Gynaecological minor procedure set

1 Auvard's vaginal speculum	1 Set of cervical dilatators
1 Sims' vaginal speculum	1 Bard Parker blade handle, no. 3
2 Sponge handles	2 Small Spencer Wells artery forceps
1 Endometrial polyp forceps	3 Sharp uterine curettes; small, medium and large
1 Single-toothed tenaculum	1 Medium, toothed dissecting forceps
1 Vulsellum, toothed	1 Scissors, 6″ straight
1 Uterine sound	1 Medium needle holder

do allow for accurate point dissection without the risk of trauma to tissues that need to be preserved. For example, the dissection of all nodal material from blood vessels can be achieved without any trauma to the vessels themselves.

Artery forceps

The forceps included in the set are almost all straight, merely reflecting the editor's personal preferences. The only exceptions to this general rule are the Meigs' (Navratil) forceps (Fig. 2.3) which is of great value in dealing with vessels deep in the pelvis; the right angle of the small head of the instrument allows ties to be accu-

rately placed. The throw of the suture material or tie can be placed around either the points or the heel of the forcep, and if the assistant then rotates the forceps, the opposite end automatically loops around the tie, allowing the surgeon to deal with vessels surely and confidently. As with many instruments in the set, the Meigs/Navratil is long and reaches easily into the depths of the pelvis.

Tissue forceps

The two forceps favoured by the editor for gentle manipulation of tissues are the Lane's (Fig. 2.4) for grasping large blocks of tissue which will be removed as a

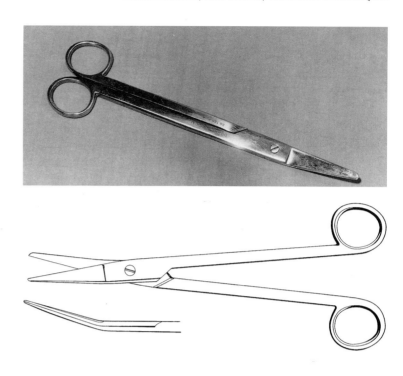

Fig. 2.1 Bonney's gynaecological scissors.

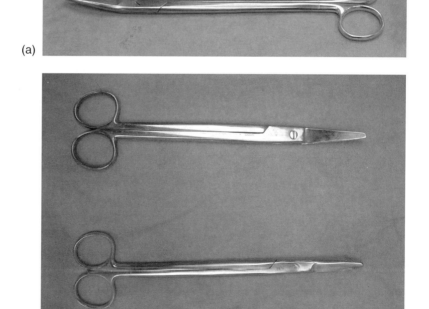

(a)

(b)

Fig. 2.2 (a) Monaghan's gynaecological dissecting scissors. (b) Comparison of Bonney's scissors (top) and Monaghan's scissors (bottom).

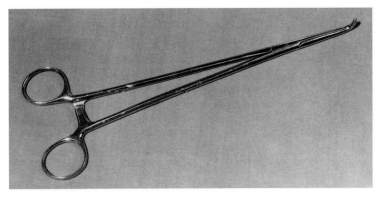

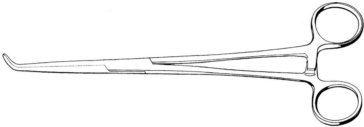

Fig. 2.3 Meig's (Navratil's) tissue forceps.

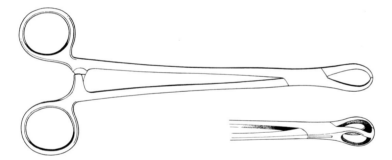

Fig. 2.4 Lane's tissue forceps.

specimen, and the Littlewood's (Fig. 2.5) which is gentler and used on tissue which is to be preserved. These two forceps are occasionally augmented with Allis', both short and long, and Babcock's tissue forcep which is used exclusively for holding bowel.

Tissue clamps

On many occasions in gynaecological surgery, it is necessary to clamp discrete blocks of tissue firmly and then suture the block to occlude the vessels contained with it. It is important that these clamps are strong, that the jaws appose accurately and that tissue does not slide out from between the jaws. Many different varieties have been designed and produced probably because these requirements are difficult to achieve.

As a general principle, it appears that those designs with longitudinal ridging of the jaws have an advantage over those with transverse. In addition, a single tooth interdigitating with a double tooth at the tips of the jaws assists correct apposition. Currently the editor uses Zeppelin slightly curved tissue clamps (Fig. 2.6). These clamps have been used for many years and meet the requirements mentioned above. The markedly angled Zeppelin clamps are particularly useful when incision of a pedicle is required at right angles to the line of

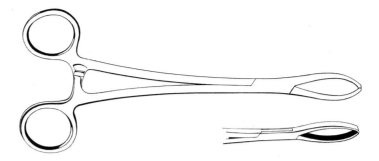

Fig. 2.5 Littlewood's tissue forceps.

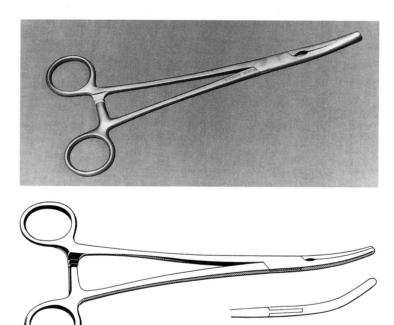

Fig. 2.6 Zeppelin tissue clamps.

application of the clamps (for example, when clamping the paracolpos during a Wertheim hysterectomy).

Suture needles

There is virtually no place in modern gynaecological surgery for the use of eyed needles. Modern swaging techniques produce a powerful bond between the needle and the suture material with little if any change in diameter from the needle through to the suture, resulting in the smallest necessary hole in the tissues. Sutures can be placed extremely accurately allowing use of smaller pedicles and causing little if any trauma to tissues alongside the needle track.

Suture materials

It is important to understand that there is no ideal, universal, suture material. The purpose of a suture material is to hold a tissue in apposition until such time that the tissues have achieved enough tensile strength to maintain the apposition. Although this statement is clearly true, it is interesting that sutures are commonly removed from the skin at intervals of between 5 and 7 days when the skin has only recovered approximately 10% of its tensile strength. Clearly, other factors than tensile strength maintain the integrity of the tissue at this time.

9

Ideal suture characteristics

These will include good knot security, inertness, adequate tensile strength, flexibility, ease of handling, non-allergenic nature, resistance to infection, smooth passage through the tissues and absorbability.

Although traditional materials such as silk and catgut have continued to be used on a surprisingly large scale, the recent decision by one of the major suture manufacturers to cease producing catgut will bring a lot of surgical practice into the modern age.

The great advantages of using strong, slowly absorbable synthetic sutures, such as Vicryl (introduced in the early 1970s) and Dexon (introduced in 1970), have been known for three decades. These materials have similar characteristics with tensile strength lasting for up to 14 days and all material being absorbed between 70 and 90 days, leaving virtually no tissue reaction. Newer materials such as Monocryl (dyed) has only 30% of its strength at 14 days, whereas Panacryl still has 80% at 90 days and 60% at 180 days. It is still surprising that so many surgeons remain wedded to catgut and silk, which are clearly poorer surgical suture materials in terms of reaction but may have reassuring handling properties which maintain the surgeon's desire to use them.

The increased strength, on a weight-for-weight basis, of the synthetic materials means that smaller diameter materials can be used with less tissue trauma and weight of material to be absorbed.

As the diameter and therefore strength of the synthetic materials is constant when compared to the variability of catgut, the surgeon finds that a standard 'pull' does not generate those embarrassing moments of breakage which have to be accepted when using catgut. Probably the most important element, which has influenced transfer to the synthetic materials, is that the tissue reaction involved in absorption is considerably less. In more recent times newer suture materials such as PDS, Maxon, Panacril and Monocril have further enhanced the range of synthetic materials available.

Modern suture materials tend be very hard and can traumatize the surgeon's hands. However, this slight disadvantage is markedly outweighed by the sureness of suture holding. Criticism of the knot-holding properties of these modern materials is unfounded once it is understood that the first knot must be tied firmly and accurately to the final required tension, i.e. it is not possible to run down the second knot so as to increase tension on the first.

The use of permanent suture material such as nylon has to be carefully considered and applied in selected cases. Skin closure has now almost entirely been taken over by stapling devices that simply grip the skin edges rather than provide a route for the ingress of infection.

The maxim of never using a braided material for skin must always be adhered to, as the risk of ingress of bacteria along the braiding is significant compared to the risk with monofilament sutures.

Staples

The use of staples in general surgery began in Hungary in the early part of the 20th century. The initial development was carried out by a surgeon named Huntl who designed staples, which closed into a 'B' shape, setting the standard pattern for the remainder of the century.

In general gynaecology stapling has not enjoyed a significant role except for skin closure. However, in recent times the increased interest in minimal access surgery (MAS) and the growth of the subspecialty of gynaecological oncology has resulted in a massive expansion of the use of stapling devices. The range of staplers used is identified in the chapters dealing with MAS and oncological procedures.

The skin staples are very popular with many variations of the original Michel Clips now available (Fig. 2.7 shows a typical example).

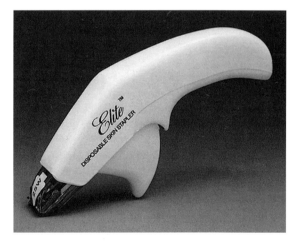

Fig. 2.7 Elite skin stapler (by kind permission of Autosuture UK Ltd; the artwork was originally prepared for the United States Surgical Corporation's General Atlas and for publication by Professors Mark Ravitch MD and Felicien Steichen MD, ©USC 1981).

Suture techniques

In previous editions of this textbook a large variety of suture techniques was shown. The current editor has selected those that are of most value to the gynaecologist and, where possible, has retained some of Bonney's original drawings.

As modern suture materials have completely replaced the need for eyed needles, the major choice left to the clinician is the choice of needle tip. Round-bodied needles are of value in suturing relatively thin or soft materials, whereas cutting needles are essential for use on strong or thicker materials such as cervix or skin. The combination trochar cutting needle is of value for a broad range of use and has the advantage of minimal tissue trauma.

Interrupted sutures

Interrupted suture are used where it is necessary to remove individual sutures or where there is a risk of infection such as in skin closure. The interrupted suture is of particular value where there is a risk of serous or bloody ooze, which should not be allowed to develop further in deep tissues; drainage will easily occur between the individual sutures.

The interrupted suture may be simple (Fig. 2.8) or mattress (Fig. 2.9); the editor does not favour sutures which 'roll in' the edge of the material to be sutured since this may hide bleeding points inside the wound and compromise the healing of the area. The mattress suture has the added advantage that haemostasis will be further improved by an increased area of local pressure on fine bleeding points. However, it is important to note that the suture should be used to *appose* the tissues not to *necrose* them; excessive force must not be used. Following all surgery the tissue thickness will increase markedly, so the suture can be placed relatively lightly to achieve apposition and haemostasis.

In areas where a significant amount of small vessel oozing commonly occurs, such as the vulva, around the clitoral base, the use of a horizontal mattress or crossed mattress suture is frequently of value (Fig. 2.10).

Continuous sutures

Continuous sutures can produce a near perfect closure and apposition of two surfaces with excellent haemostasis. They are more rapidly performed than

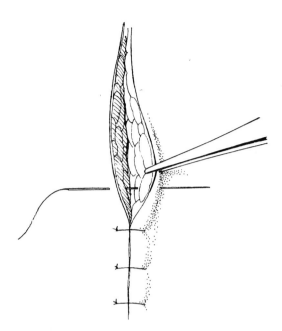

Fig. 2.8 Simple interrupted suture.

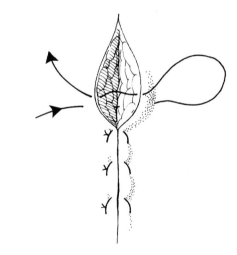

Fig. 2.9 Vertical mattress suture.

interrupted sutures and obviously require fewer knots. Their major disadvantage is that the whole stitch has to be removed if there is infection, and serous and bloody ooze cannot escape from below the suture line. Simple continuous suturing is used for peritoneum and sheaths of muscles, but it is not generally used for skin.

Lembert sutures (Fig. 2.11) are used for water- and

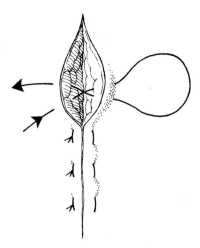

Fig. 2.10 Crossed or horizontal mattress suture.

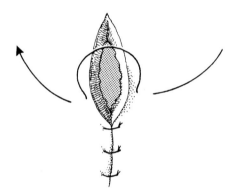

Fig. 2.11 Lembert sutures.

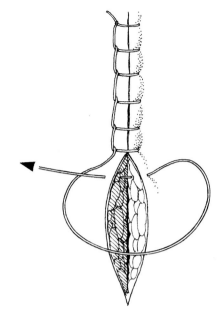

Fig. 2.12 Locked or blanket sutures.

gas-tight closure of bowel and bladder, but are often re-placed in the former by simple continuous suture, sta-pling devices or mass closure with interrupted sutures in large bowel.

Subcuticular sutures are popular for skin closure as they give an immediate attractive cosmetic effect. They do however have the same disadvantages as the other continuous sutures and often generate a dense scar pos-sibly related to the larger amount of suture material, which has to be absorbed. The editor would recom-mend that if a subcuticular suture is to be used it should be of a fine non-absorbable monofilament type and should be removed at approximately 5 days after skin closure.

Locked or blanket stitches are of great value in achieving haemostasis; the editor uses this stitch to oversew the vaginal edge at the completion of the hysterectomy procedure (Fig. 2.12).

Puckering sutures are used for shortening tissues and where there are series of small vessels in a tissue edge which cannot be easily dealt with individually (Fig. 2.13).

Purse string sutures (Fig. 2.14) are of value in closing gaps such as in peritoneum and for burying pedicles. Purse string inverting sutures are used for burying the stump of the appendix (Fig. 2.15), or closing very small holes in the bladder.

Some suture techniques can be combined to provide multiple functions: the editor uses a combined figure-of-eight sutures and simple continuous technique (Fig. 2.16) for closing the posterior vaginal skin and at the same time closing the subcutaneous tissue, thus elimi-nating dead space and removing the risk of haematoma formation during perineorrhaphy.

Surgical knots and methods of tying

Facility in tying knots is an important part of the surgi-cal technique in which all young surgeons should attempt to excel. They must also remember that it is not adequate to be competent to tie one knot—they should

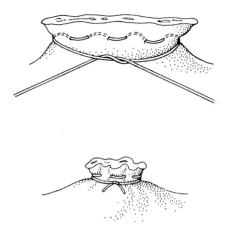

Fig. 2.13 Puckering sutures.

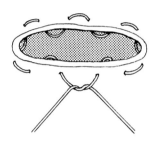

Fig. 2.14 Purse-string sutures.

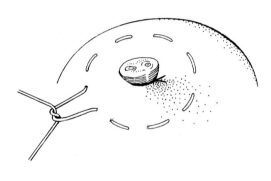

Fig. 2.15 Purse-string inverting sutures.

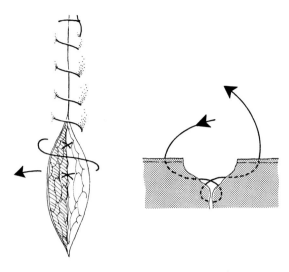

Fig. 2.16 Continuous locked figure-of-eight sutures.

practise a wide variety, learning the indication for their uses as skills improve. As an assistant, the young surgeon learns to cut the tails of sutures accurately and quickly, taking care to leave a short but adequate length. The cut should be made with the scissors stationary and with due regard to the position of the tips of the blades at the end of the cutting stroke. Equally, the surgeon should present the suture in such a way that the assistant could easily see and safely cut without hazarding adjacent tissues or organs.

It is often tempting to try to use very short lengths of suture material in difficult places: this practice must be eschewed. The suture material for knot tying must be presented to the surgeon in at least 'half lengths', and, ideally, on the reel so that the surgeon can efficiently continue to tie without asking for more suture. This mode of presentation is also more economical in the long term.

The granny knot

This is the simplest and quickest knot to make, consisting of two identical hitches. It has the advantage that the first hitch is easily held tight while the second is being made and that should the first tie slip the second will tighten it up again. This only applies to suture materials which slide, such as Nylon, PDS, Monocril and catgut. If the surgeon uses Dexon, Vicryl or equivalents he must learn to tie all knots as he wishes them to end up—the tension on the first knot must be exactly as it is wished to be, as there is no possibility of 'snugging' down the second throw. This facility of catgut to 'snug down' has generated some very sloppy surgical practices, which must be eliminated before being able to competently use materials that are more modern. When the granny knot is used, a third throw is an important safety feature. Figure 2.17 (1–3) shows the technique of tying as described by Bonney.

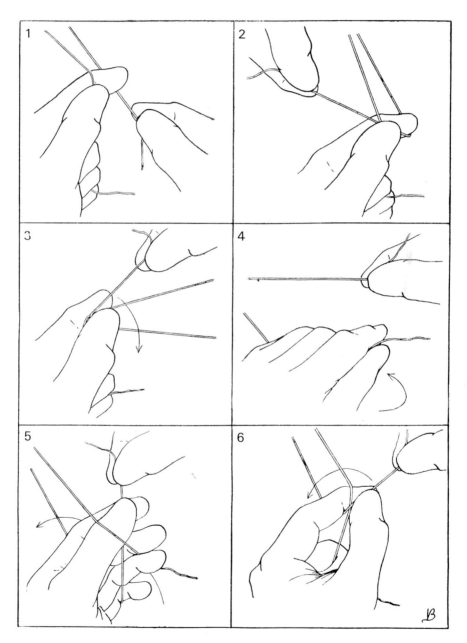

Fig. 2.17 Two-handed technique for tying knots (after Bonney).

The reef knot

This knot consists of two hitches, one tied with one end of the ligature and one tied with the other end (Fig. 2.17 4–6). This two-handed technique produces a firm knot but it is possible by crossing the hands to perform a reef knot using the one-handed technique. The safest technique of all, which the editor uses constantly, is to throw two granny knots followed by a reef knot, which completely locks the whole knot firmly.

It is important to remember that any cord with a knot in it is significantly less strong than one without. Do not therefore be surprised to find suture material breaking at the knot when excess tension is applied.

The single-handed knot

This fast, elegant and simple technique allows the surgeon to operate dexterously and rapidly without putting down the instruments or requiring special tools for tying knots. The technique is shown in Fig. 2.18 (1–4).

The forceps knot

This elegant method of tying is shown in Fig. 2.18 (5 & 6). It is particularly useful when there is only a short piece of suture material available.

Knot tying in deep holes

It has been recommended that the lasso technique be used when a bleeding point occurs in a deep or inaccessible spot. The editor would instead recommend the use of a long angled clamp such as the Meigs/Navratil (see Fig. 2.3). This type of clamp, which has attributes of gall-bladder forceps, will allow the tie to be hooked either around the heel or the tip of the clamp so that it is firmly held while the knot is being made (Fig. 2.19). If the bleeding point is extremely difficult to reach the use of small metal artery clips such as liga clips or the preloaded variety (Ethicon) is of enormous value (Fig. 2.20).

Ligatures

Ligatures should always be tied where possible so that complete haemostasis is achieved. The material to be ligated is held in a clamp, which is placed so that a small part of the tip projects beyond the tissue to be tied. This allows the suture material to be firmly held by hooking it around the projecting tip while the knot is tied (Fig. 2.21).

Simple pedicle ties

The ligature may be simple, carrying the entire throw around the mass of tissue to be ligated. The major drawback of this method is the potential for slipping: this risk is reduced if the tension is adequate and if the tissue beyond the tie is of a reasonable amount.

It is important to remember not to be too ambitious and try to include so large a mass that the edges slip out and produce haemorrhage which may be difficult to control.

Remember the simple loop pedicle ligature should never be used if there is tension on the pedicle. Double tying of pedicles is now rarely used. The editor feels that with modern suture materials there is virtually no place for this technique. The amount of material included in a double-tied pedicle is considerable, generating a large amount of necrotic material which has to be removed.

Transfixion stitch

The mass of material to be ligated can be transfixed at one or both ends so that the ligature will not slip and material escape. The transfixion stitch should be used with great care in pedicles which are known to contain significant blood vessels. The risk of damage to vessels is greatest when suturing the ovarian or uterine pedicles during a total hysterectomy. The ovarian vessels in the infundibulopelvic ligament are thin and wide. It is the editor's practice to use a simple tie on this pedicle and not to put any tension upon it. The uterine artery or a large vein is easily pierced when stitch ligaturing the lower pedicles alongside the uterus during a hysterectomy. When this occurs a rapidly developing haematoma grows into the soft tissues of the broad ligament behind the pedicle, discolouring the tissues and making identification of bleeding points extremely difficult. It is not usually safe simply to reclamp the bleeding area as the vein or artery often retracts once it is cut.

There is also considerable danger in blindly clamping alongside the uterus and cervix, as the ureter is not far away. It is better to open up the pelvic side wall, identify the uterine artery at its origin, tie it and then follow it through to the uterus over the top of the ureter. This

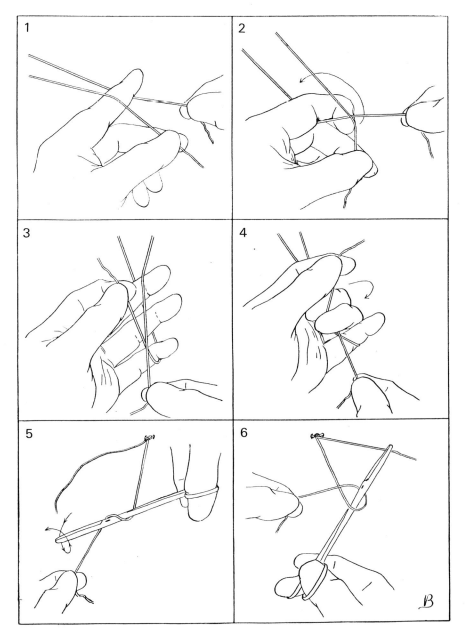

Fig. 2.18 Single-handed technique for tying knots and the forceps knot (after Bonney).

simple demonstration of the ureter in its lower course is immensely reassuring.

Burying the stumps of ligatures

In recent editions of this text, a paragraph dealing with burying the stumps of ligatures and reperitonealization of the pelvis was included (Fig. 2.22). It is now generally accepted that attempts to reperitonealize the pelvis by closure of the peritoneum is at best superfluous and at worst may be causative in the development of lymphocysts and possibly incriminated in small bowel obstruction. It is now felt that with the exception of po-stirradiation surgery no attempt to cover 'raw' areas should be made, as the body is able to generate a covering of a sheet of peritoneal cells within days of surgery. Simply drawing the sigmoid colon down into the pelvis is all that is required.

Drainage

In modern gynaecological practice, the indications for drainage of the pelvis/abdomen are very few. The widespread use of intraoperative antibiotic has probably contributed to this situation, and reduced the indications to the following:

1 Any procedure where it has been impossible to achieve perfect haemostasis or where a significant post-operative serous ooze is anticipated. This latter indication used to be linked to radical cancer surgery, but drains are now rarely used in even the most radical procedures.
2 Where there is a danger of urine leakage such as following repair to a damaged bladder or ureter or following elective surgery on these structures.
3 Where there has been widespread contamination of the peritoneal cavity with infected material.
NB: drains should not be put in place following ovarian cancer surgery or the treatment of *Pseudomyxoma peritonei*.

Drainage route

After many years of utilizing drainage by the vaginal route, the last two decades have demonstrated the superiority of transabdominal suction drainage. The disposable prevacuumed systems now available are efficient and leave little scarring at the drainage exit site. Where there has been gross soiling of the peritoneal cavity, such as following bowel opening, a larger

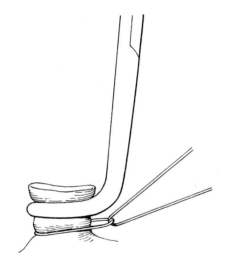

Fig. 2.19 Tying a pedicle around a Meig's forcep.

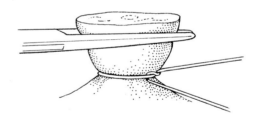

Fig. 2.21 Ligating a pedicle.

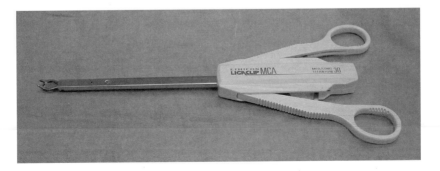

Fig. 2.20 A commonly used automatic clip dispenser.

17

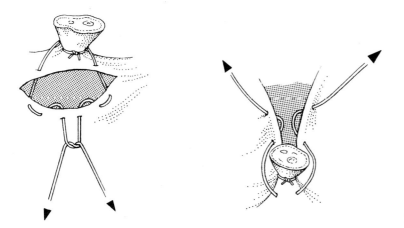

Fig. 2.22 Burying the stump.

bore drain coupled with meticulous peritoneal lavage may be necessary (Jackson-Pratt, pencil, etc.).

Wound drainage may be necessary where wounds are extensive, the operation is a repeat procedure or the patient is on heparin. Wound drains can be very small, should be placed down to the rectus sheath and are usually removed within 48 hours of surgery as drainage resolves.

Management of drains

Drains should be removed when they have ceased to function or drainage has stabilized at a low level. It is important that they be anchored carefully by adequate fixation in theatre. Suction drains can be fixed by a simple multiple loop tie with nylon around the plastic drain and attached to the abdominal wall. Larger bore drains may be marked with a large safety pin so that they may be shortened at regular intervals.

The presence and type of drain must be accurately recorded in the operation note and clear instructions for drain care included in the postoperative instructions. Decisions for removal are usually made and recorded during the postoperative ward rounds.

Further reading

The editor's recommendations for further reading following a chapter covering general instrumentation and basic techniques may seem a little strange but he would heartily recommend the habit of reading instrument catalogues from cover to cover. It is amazing how frequently an instrument used in a dif-ferent surgical discipline will be seen to have valuable applications in another, the classic example in the editor's own practice being the use of the McGill's endotracheal forceps in inserting a vaginal drain deep in the pelvis at the end of a Wertheim's hysterectomy. This technique was introduced to the department by the editor's predecessor Mr Stanley Way. As vaginal drains are not used any more, the instrument is rarely used but still resides on the tray for the time being. For more on modern approaches to drainage, see Lopes A de B, Hall JR, Monaghan JM. Drainage following radical hysterectomy and pelvic lymphadenectomy: dogma or need? *Obstet Gynecol* 1995;86(6):1–4.

Textbooks

For the more enterprising trainee or surgeon, the textbook *Stapling in Surgery* by Felicien Steichen and Mark Ravitch, published in 1983 by Year Book Medical Publishers, Chicago, will give a marvellous view of the history and the role of staples in all forms of surgery. A number of the techniques demonstrated in the book have been incorporated into this the tenth edition of *Bonney's Gynaecological Surgery*, particularly in the oncology sections. For the surgeon who is able to read German, the recently published text *Nahtmaterialien und Nahttechniken in der operativen Gynakologie* by Professors Hepp and Scheidel and published by Urban and Schwarzenberg, Munich, is recommended. The text comprehensively covers the use of all modern suture and stapling materials in gynaecological surgery, including an appendix with recommendations for the various weights of suture required for different procedures.

There are a multitude of articles and textbooks on different suture materials and their various applications in surgery; the surgeon should always be prepared to read them but should not expect too many totally new comments.

3 Patient assessment, consent and preparation for surgery

Before major surgery . . . Submit yourself to your God, your love to your beloved and friends and your trust in your doctor.
Lord Gowrie, 1999

Most gynaecological surgery is elective. Consequently, for most patients, preoperative assessment and preparation for surgery can be comprehensive. Most patients will be first seen in the outpatient department or private practice office where a preliminary assessment and provisional diagnosis will be made. At this first visit, the clinician will be able to examine the patient fully including the pelvis and abdomen and to organize the next series of steps in the diagnostic process.

These next steps will involve procedures such as radiology, including ultrasound assessments. Blood tests such as those for tumour markers and hormonal status, and possibly local biopsies, are carried out in the outpatient department to confirm the clinical impressions. Once this information is collated, a provisional diagnosis is made and admission dates for surgery if appropriate are organized.

Referral

The traditional route of referral for a consultant opinion in British practice has been from the patient's general practitioner to a consultant of their choice at the local hospital. For the majority of patients this will continue. However, with the steady growth and development of subspecialization, it is becoming increasingly common for referral to occur outside the local area to clinicians with special skills. This applies particularly to gynaeco-logical oncology, urogynaecology and specialist infertility services including IVF. This practice is growing rapidly to cope with the increased aspirations of patients to receive 'best care', the shortage of highly specialized skills and the need to work in large multidisciplinary teams (MDTs).

Such arrangements may seem unnecessarily cumbersome, but they do allow the maximum number of patients to be treated by the best clinicians working in environments with the best diagnostic and treatment facilities.

This recognition of the need for a significant degree of centralization of clinical care has been outlined in the documents generated during the 1990s.

Rapid access clinics

Increasingly there is a pressure on clinicians to see patients rapidly and to come to definitive diagnoses as quickly as possible. This pressure is most frequently seen to be applied in the diagnosis and management of cancer. It is often difficult to balance the desire for speed in diagnosis and treatment in cancer care with the relative slowness and testing of a variety of conservative management options in 'benign' gynaecology.

The rapid access clinic system sets time limits of 2 weeks for the patient to be seen and started on management of the problem. In order to reach such targets the clinics have to be so structured that referral can be made by telephone or fax, that the clinics are run on a number of days in the week and that all diagnostic facilities — including colposcopy, endometrial sampling and vaginal/abdominal ultrasound — can be obtained at the one visit. In some centres, the diagnosis or plan of management is given at the end on the clinic visit. Other philosophies consider that the patient should be asked to return to the clinic where a relaxed environment can be generated in order to go through the results of the investigations and to communicate the plan of management, this is thought to be particularly appropriate for the diagnosis of cancer.

Patient information

Gynaecological patients require considerable support and assistance when dealing with decisions about treatment particularly surgery. The most important factor is the manner in which the patient understands the impact of the operation upon herself, particularly her sexuality. The surgeon must be prepared to spend a considerable amount of time discussing and explaining the content of any surgical procedure. This important process is frequently aided by the use of literature and drawings, copies of which should be included in the medical record. The patient should also be supplied with copies to take home, and encouragement should be given to invite further questioning by direct contact with the clinician or through the clinical staff or the internet. Departmental websites and contact numbers are of great assistance.

It is at this point that the clinician may feel the need to involve other expertise including nurse specialists, psychologists, stoma therapists and psychiatrists. It is often of enormous reassurance to the patient to meet other patients who have been treated for a similar problem and who have experienced similar procedures.

Clearly such a detailed approach is not practical for all procedures especially minor ones; however, it is important not to trivialize minor procedures especially those involving anaesthesia as complications can and will occur, and warning of the possibility and appropriate consenting is vital for all operations even those of a diagnostic nature carried out in the outpatients under local anaesthetic. It is also important in the editor's opinion not to 'talk down' to patients, always to use accurate terminology with appropriate explanation and to resist the temptation to use gross inaccuracies, which become perpetuated in the mythology of the subject such as the vaginal hysterectomy being described as a 'suction' hysterectomy.

In an increasingly litigious world, the careful but not necessarily cautious doctor who keeps good records and takes the time to communicate and document all meetings will to a significant extent protect himself from the very distressing circumstances of litigation.

History taking and documentation

As the clinician progresses through training every effort should be made to concentrate on developing a style of clear and concise history taking. Initially, this process of meticulous systematic questioning may seem cumbersome. However, with constant practice an abbreviated technique will develop which concentrates on the major fields of interest but also allows for peripheral areas of relevance to be included.

Documentation of the history is vital for medicolegal purposes, for transmission of information to colleagues and for analysis in clinical research and audit. The editor's department has over many years organized complete standardized questionnaires for all patients, the details of which have build up a complete picture of each patient, their cancer and their progress through therapy. This huge database allows rapid access for office administration, audit, research and analysis.

Ward procedure book

Just as it is vital that the patient should be fully informed of her management, the editor feels that the ward staff, be they medical, nursing or from professions allied to medicine, should all be fully aware of these details. It has been found to be very valuable to have a ward procedure book which details the scope of the various surgical procedures, the patient preparation required, the postoperative management and the follow-up protocols. This type of document is doubly valuable because of the frequent rotation of ward staff. It is important not to presume that these ward practices are common knowledge.

General advice

Smoking continues to be generally very prevalent in society, especially among women where a large increase in smoking in younger women has been observed with a consequent increase in smoking-related diseases including lung cancer. The visit to hospital is a good opportunity to impress on the patient the importance of stopping smoking. However, it must be remembered that if a heavy smoker stops smoking shortly before receiving a general anaesthetic, there is a possibility of reducing the cough reflex, resulting in stasis of secretions in the postoperative period. With this single caveat, smoking should be discouraged and the patient persuaded that the proposed operation is an excellent time to break this damaging habit.

Oral contraceptive pills are widely used. When the thrombosis risks of using the oral contraceptive pill were first demonstrated it was advised that the pill should be stopped for at least 1 month before surgery. This is now felt to be impractical and unnecessary because of the widespread use of low-dose pills. The risk of thromboembolism appears to rise with the oestrogen content. Thus, it is felt to be unnecessary to stop the pill before minor surgery and for major surgery; only those patients at high risk should have their pill stopped and careful prophylaxis introduced.

Prophylaxis

Since the 1970s, there has been general agreement that efforts to reduce the incidence of thromboembolism must be made for virtually all patients undergoing major surgery. There has been a considerable debate as to the relative efficacy of either calf compression techniques both intra- and postoperatively versus the use of heparin prophylaxis, 5000 IU subcutaneously twice daily, beginning at or about the start of surgery and continuing into the postoperative period until the patient is fully mobilized. Currently the choice is based on a variety of reasons including usage, availability of nursing staff and patient compliance.

For the patient with a very high risk of thromboembolic disease a fractionated heparin is advocated. For patients at low risk the use of thromboembolism stockings is common, to be worn until normal mobilization is achieved.

Prophylaxis for thromboembolic disease must be considered for all major procedures. Patients should be screened for high risk factors including:
1 Previous thromboembolic phenomena.
2 Radiotherapy prior to surgery.
3 Obesity.

4 Stasis generated by prolonged bed rest or immobility. This is particularly common in older patients.
5 Smoking.
6 Pregnancy.
7 A haematocrit below 30%. The risk is increased in blood group A and reduced in blood group O.
8 An intravenous long line in place.

Obesity

Obesity has become a scourge of modern society with up to 10% of patients being obese and a smaller percentage morbidly obese. Obese patients have a poor exercise habit and tolerate the stress of surgery badly. The problems generated include difficulties of access, difficulties with anaesthetics, stasis of fluid in the limbs and secretions in the lungs, problems of movement and mobilization in the peri- and postoperative period. Thromboembolic prophylaxis is made difficult due to problems of fitting compression equipment and the difficulty of estimating appropriate dosages of heparin.

Unfortunately, the practice of sending the patient away for some time to 'lose weight' is often counterproductive as the gynaecological problem of the patient may be a factor in their eating and exercise problems. It is the editor's policy to simply work out ways of performing the operation in the obese patient so that there is no delaying of treatment. It is helpful to utilize epidural or spinal anaesthesia in order to reduce intraoperative bleeding and postoperative ooze. The siting of the wound is also very important. In very obese women, the thinnest part of the abdominal wall is often a transverse line running roughly across the line of the pubic hair in the equivalent position to a high Pfannenstiel incision. If the panniculus of fat is elevated and tied to the bed head of the operating table, the abdomen can be entered relatively easily through little fat. This incision can be used for radical surgery if the rectus muscles are cut or dislocated from their inferior insertion on the pubis.

Preoperative investigations

The majority of investigations can be organized prior to admission for surgery on an outpatient basis, or programmed to be performed on the day before surgery so that all results are available for the surgeon and the anaesthetist at the time of consent. In many modern centres, preassessment clinics have been set up, run by nursing staff, where all preoperative investigations and admission procedures can be performed. This is excellent where the patients live close to the hospital; however, making an extra journey to the hospital is either inconvenient or impossible for patients who have to travel any distance, as is found in association with centralized services such as oncology. It is vital to avoid the older method of admitting patients some days before surgery for a leisurely performance of preoperative test. This practice is not only wasteful of valuable inpatient resources, it has the major disadvantage of causing patients to become static, increasing the risk of development of thrombosis, and also exposes the patient to hospital infections which can be extraordinarily difficult to eradicate, particularly MRSA bacterial infection.

Early admission may be necessary on occasions for patients who have specific problems which may need to be corrected prior to surgery.

1 Infections of the operative field should be cleared if possible; this particularly applies to the vagina, e.g. the infected and oedematous skin associated with the long-term use of a vaginal pessary. Large infected tumours of the vulva can be improved by intensive cleansing for 48 hours prior to surgery using simple skin cleansing agents.

2 Control of diabetes may require hospitalization but normally it is better to have the patient balanced and settled on her regimen whilst ambulant, the possible exception being where oral hypoglycaemics are being changed to insulin before the procedure. Any signs of infection in the diabetic patient should be rigorously dealt with, usually with the consequence that the diabetes is easier to control.

3 Nutritional improvements are often advantageous especially in the patient suffering from cancer of the ovary or chronic fistulae. The advice of nutritionists and the use of parenteral or intravenous nutrition is often necessary to achieve a positive nitrogen balance and to give the patient sufficient calories to cope with the rigours of the surgical procedure. In debilitated patients it is advantageous to continue the parenteral nutrition well into the catabolic postoperative period.

4 The anaesthetist may request preoperative physiotherapy and bronchial decongestion prior to anaesthesia. Most patients are now 'scored' by the anaesthetists, using the ASA physical status score:

I Healthy patient
II Mild systemic disease—no functional limitations
III Severe systemic disease*—definite functional limitations
IV Severe systemic disease* that is a constant threat to life
V Moribund patient not expected to survive 24 h with or without operation.

In the editor's own practice of gynaecological oncology in 2000, 75% of patients were ASA II or greater, reflecting the ageing population which now commonly presents to surgeons.

Specific preoperative investigations

It is not the place of a surgical text to detail exhaustively all preoperative investigations. The specific test will be outlined in relevant chapters; only a general outline will be provided here.

1 *Haematological investigations.* Every patient should have a full blood screen performed to include haemoglobin, haematocrit, white count and differential, platelets and a blood film where indicated.

For all procedures where there is a significant risk of blood transfusion, typing and retention of serum should be performed so that blood and blood products can be obtained at short notice. In recent times acceptance of lower haemoglobin levels, especially postoperatively, coupled with a lay nervousness about blood and blood products have led to a marked reduction in the use of transfusion. A postoperative haemoglobin level of 9 or even 8 g/dl is often treated with oral iron.

2 *Biochemical investigations.* In most centres it is customary to use computerized assessment of blood which allows a large range of investigations to be performed rapidly on a small volume of blood. For the majority of procedures the assessment of the blood electrolytes and liver function test are appropriate.

3 *Urinalysis.* Using simple 'stick' tests a range of analyses can be performed accurately and rapidly on the urine obtained on admission. These are usually screening tests leading the clinician to more detailed tests where necessary.

4 *Radiological investigations.* Chest X-ray, pelvic, abdominal and vaginal ultrasound, CT scan, MRI and other contrast radiology may all be helpful in making a

*Whether or not the systemic disease for which the patient is undergoing surgery.

preoperative diagnosis. Their specific indications and value will be discussed in the individual chapters.

5 *Assessment of other medical conditions.* Cardiovascular disease, hypertension, diabetes, pulmonary disease and mental state may all require an input from an expert in the field. It is important to allow adequate time for appropriate consultation and correction of problems prior to surgery. Often the expert anaesthetist will be able to give a clear opinion on the physical state of the patient. It is the editor's opinion that the decision to anaesthetize is taken by the anaesthetist and the decision to operate by the surgeon following on.

Obtaining consent for operation

In recent years, considerable effort has been expended in trying to improve the whole process of consent. The main reason for this is the extensive publicity given when operations are allegedly performed without 'proper' consent.

Patients must give consent for operation in the light of full knowledge of the procedure. For the under age patient and in circumstances of extreme emergency or non-competence where the patient is not fit in the medical or legal sense, arrangements must be made for a competent person to give consent. Such a person must also be given the same information so as to be fully cognisant of the content and consequences of the operation.

The consent of the husband is not required for procedures to be performed upon the wife/partner and vice versa. However, it is considered prudent that, if possible, the husband/partner should be involved in any decision making and fully understand the procedures. These discussions are particularly important when sterilization or termination procedures are concerned. If the woman does not wish her husband to be involved, this fact must be recorded in the notes. The potential impact upon future life must be clearly and accurately described so that both partners understand the implications. This approach will save considerable heartache and friction in the future. Even in those circumstances where there is not complete accord between husband and wife it is in their best interests to be present when procedures are being explained.

Conversely, if the wife clearly expresses a wish that the husband is not informed of the procedure, the surgeon must respect her wishes after impressing on her the advantages of a frank discussion with both partners.

If there have been difficulties in the discussion, the surgeon should accurately record such facts in the clinical notes, confirming that the partners have had the facts and implications of the procedure explained, and that they have understood and accepted them.

Information notes and drawings

Clinical information
If at all possible, information in written form should be sent to patients prior to the first visit. This should not only include details of appointments, parking facilities, transport access, etc., but also as many broad details as can be envisaged. This should include warnings about examination, time involved and the advisability of having a partner or companion present. For many specialist clinics, such as colposcopy, specific details of procedures can be outlined.

Drawings
Drawings of procedures indicating tissues to be removed with small annotations alluding to potential complications and future difficulties are of enormous value. Such drawings, however crude and simplistic, are often critical when complaints or legal proceedings occur. The drawings should be made in the clinical record and preserved.

Information sheets
At the end of the clinic visit it is of inestimable value to be able to give the patient and her companion a sheet of information with an outline summary of what has been said and discussed in the clinic. The type of document will usually have space for drawings and hand-written notes. If the sheet can be of a 'carbon copy' type the patient will be able to take home an exact copy of the sheet which is stored within the clinical record.

Contact telephone numbers
A preprinted list of contact telephone numbers for the patient to take home is valuable. This list should contain internet websites as well as fax and telephone numbers.

The timing of consent

There has been considerable discussion but no firm conclusions about the best time for consent for an operation to be carried.

The taking of consent as part of the clinic visit has been viewed by supporters of such a step as enabling the patient to take this important step away from the stress of admission to hospital and an imminent operation. The contrary view is that at the time of the clinic visit there is far too much information to be taken in and that the patient is suffering from information 'overload' and will have problems in making a sensible balanced decision.

The taking of consent at the time of admission for surgery has been viewed as incorrect because of the stresses already mentioned. This problem may be exacerbated as we move more and more to admission times very close to the moment of surgery. The positive side of this approach is that the patient has had time to weigh the points of management which have been put to her at the original clinic visit. Contact may have been made in the interim and further concerns dealt with.

Waiting times for surgery

Many governments and their chosen deliverers of care, including insurance companies, now set time constraints for the delivery of a package of care. This has particularly occurred in cancer care where arbitrary time limits of 2 weeks have been set for the inception of management from the point of first complaint of symptomatology suggestive of cancer.

There is thus a pressure on clinicians to deliver information rapidly, to begin complex care pathways and most importantly for the patient to become a willing partner in this process. For some patients the process is 'too fast'—they have difficulties in understanding the concepts involved and in taking in the plethora of information which is presented to them. The explanation of every small potential complication, although encouraged, can result in a mind-numbing terror in the patient. Although doctors are criticized for being patronizing and God-like to their patients, the complete transference of all decision making to patients is equally flawed. Many patients do not have the mental capacity to cope with concepts of 'risk', they certainly do not have the training, and they are not in any posi-

tion to dispassionately weigh options for care which affect themselves so critically.

The team approach to gynaecological surgical care

It is unreasonable and unrealistic for one individual to be capable of dealing with all the multifaceted problems associated with surgical care. The pelvic surgeon will be pivotal in the system of multidisciplinary care which will involve the following:
1 *The primary care physician.*
2 *The pelvic surgeon.*
3 *The nurse specialist.*
4 *Professions allied to medicine.*

Type of consent form

There are many and various patterns of consent form available, though within the National Health Service there is a move to a single standard form. The most important element in any form is that it should be acceptable to the clinicians and legal experts of the hospital. Specific segments dealing with high risk areas of practice including minimal access surgery are acceptable.

The form should also contain a clause which allows the surgeon to exercise judgment intraoperatively in the event of untoward events or findings which may warrant different management.

Preoperative preparation

Preoperative discussion of the scope of surgery

This discussion should be a continuation of the information given at the first clinic visit. Many of the details outlined at the first visit may have been forgotten or misunderstood; therefore, it is recommended that the clinician repeats the whole explanation of the need for the operation, the expected findings and outcome. In particular this should include all that the patient may expect to happen in the postoperative period. The presence of drips, suction drains, catheters and patient-controlled analgesia devices must be described. The likely timing of their removal is often reassuring, especially if the proposed timetable is adhered to.

This treatment plan allows the patient to see ahead

and to be uplifted as the targets are met and recovery proceeds.

Complex postoperative needs such as the possibility of stomas or prolonged application of devices is often best described by experts such as the stoma therapist.

Preoperative visits by the anaesthetist

It is the editor's practice to give to each patient a 'pre-anaesthetic assessment form' which contains a series of questions about the patient's personal health and is then sent directly to the anaesthetist in charge. This simple form provides a large amount of information prior to surgery and allows the anaesthetist to have a preview so that any special test or investigation can be organized well in advance of hospital admission.

For most patients the major fear associated with surgery is related to the anaesthetic. Consequently, a sympathetic, reassuring and confident anaesthetist will help to allay most phobias; some patients have fears about needles, some about masks. The skilled anaesthetist will be able to promise that a particular technique will or will not be used. Clearly it is important that the person visiting the patient is the clinician who will be present at the anaesthetic.

Preoperative medication may be prescribed at this visit and its timing carefully organized to fit in with the timing of surgery. The advantages of the surgeon and anaesthetist working together as a team can clearly be seen. The drugs to be prescribed are recorded on the anaesthetic record so that the actual time of administration can be checked by the anaesthetist in theatre.

Preoperative preparation

Skin

The most important part of skin preparation for the gynaecologist is for the patient to be shaved. Traditionally, all patients were shaved, but it is now felt that unless an incision is made in the skin a full shave of the abdomen and pudenda is not necessary. For operations such as laparoscopy patients should not be shaved.

All patients should be encouraged to bathe on admission, in the evening prior to operation and on the morning of operation if possible. It is counterproductive to use strong antiseptics in a misguided attempt to 'sterilize' the abdominal skin; the end result is to remove the patient's natural protective bacteria, allowing colonization by more sinister hospital-based organisms.

Similarly, no disinfectant or sterilant should be put in the water used for bathing.

Bowel

Minor procedures do not require significant bowel preparation; usually, two suppositories on the morning of surgery will suffice. If the patient is habitually constipated, then it will be necessary to extend the period of bowel preparation to the previous day, giving the patient oral laxatives with the addition of suppositories or an enema prior to the procedure.

Major procedures where it is envisaged that bowel will not be resected should receive more extensive preparation in the form of an oral aperient on the day of admission and an enema on the evening prior to operation. This enema may be repeated on the morning of operation if there has not been a good result.

Major procedures where bowel is to be resected will require that the bowel content be reduced to a minimum and sterilized. This is best achieved by putting the patient on a low residue diet for 2 days prior to operation and giving strong aperients. A non-absorbable antibiotic such as neomycin should be given for 48 hours prior to surgery.

Augmentation of this preparation with enemas may be necessary; however, purgation should be not so fierce as to render the patient debilitated from this exercise.

Vagina

Preparation of the vagina should be considered as part of the general skin preparation. For the post-menopausal patient exhibiting atrophic changes, there is a place for the use of vaginal oestrogens to improve the quality of the epithelium; rendering it more resistant to infection and improving healing.

Further reading

Textbooks

For most gynaecologists who have carried out higher training in general surgery, the text *General Pathology* by Walter and Israels will bring back many happy memories. It is a marvellous book for giving the trainee a sound guidance in all the problems that should be looked for in the surgical patient. It also clearly identifies those areas of difficulty which may jeopardize the patient's progress intra- and postoperatively.

References

Clarke-Pearson DL, Olt G. Thromboembolism in patients with gynaecologic tumours: risk factors, natural history and prophylaxis. *Oncology* 1989;3:39–45.

www.doh.gov.uk/consent A government website covering consent. This document covers the importance of uniformity of consent and information required for patients.

www.nice.org.uk The National Institute of Clinical Excellence (NICE)—recommendations covering pre-operative assessment.

4

Operations on the cervix

Dilatation of the cervix

This is the most frequently performed surgical procedure in gynaecology. Consequently, it should be carefully learned and practised, with close attention being paid to the potential pitfalls and complications.

Indications

Dilatation of the cervix is an important preliminary to many gynaecological procedures, including uterine curettage, early termination of pregnancy, cervical cautery and intracavitary radiotherapeutic procedures. It is also associated with Manchester repair and conization of the cervix, and will sometimes be necessary prior to hysteroscopic examination of the uterine cavity. There are now few circumstances when dilatation is used alone except for post-traumatic or atrophic stenosis of the cervix and for the relief of postradiotherapy pyometra and post-surgical haematometra. Dilatation of the cervix is no longer indicated for the treatment of dysmenorrhoea.

Instruments

A prepacked dilatation and curettage set is well worth developing for all gynaecological theatres (gynaecological minor set; see Chapter 2). It should include a vaginal speculum (either an Auvard's or a Sims'), a uterine sound, a toothed vulsellum and a single-toothed tenaculum, graduated uterine dilators, a pair of narrow ovum forceps, and small, medium and large uterine curettes.

Preparation of the patient

There is no necessity to shave the patient preoperatively. She should be asked to empty the bladder immediately before going to theatre, as a full bladder may distort the pelvic anatomy and makes examination more difficult and inaccurate. If there is doubt about the emptiness of the bladder it should be catheterized prior to the procedure.

A general anaesthetic is usually required even though dilatation is part of a minor procedure, and as most modern hospitals are well organized to perform day case surgery of this type, the editor does not advocate the use of local cervical analgesia.

The operation

Initial examination and assessment of the pelvis
The patient is placed in lithotomy position with the buttocks projecting slightly over the end of the operating table (Fig. 4.1). The vulva and vagina are swabbed using Savlon or aqueous Hibitane (chlorhexidine gluconate) solution, and draped. A bimanual examination is now performed. This is the most important part of the procedure as it allows the surgeon to examine fully the pelvis with the patient totally relaxed. Often, features which were not elicited in the consultation room are found and slightly worrying findings put into perspective. As with examination of the whole abdomen at laparotomy, the junior surgeon should develop a habit of careful preoperative pelvic examination prior to even the most minor of procedures. The vulva is also inspected, the labia are gently drawn apart and the introitus viewed; the editor has seen early carcinomas of the

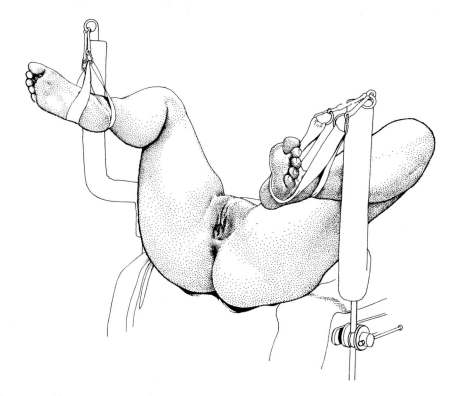

Fig. 4.1 Lithotomy position.

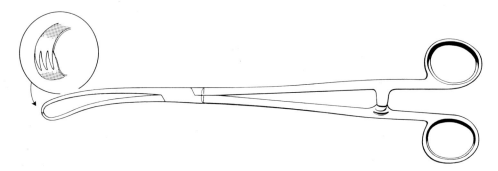

Fig. 4.2 Cervical volsellum.

vulva missed because the surgeon did not carry out this simple process meticulously. Two fingers of the right hand are now inserted into the vagina, and with the left hand on the lower abdomen the entire pelvic contents can be assessed.

Sounding of the uterus
The vaginal speculum is now inserted into the vagina allowing access to the cervix. From the pelvic examination the surgeon will have determined the size of the vagina and an appropriately sized speculum should be chosen. The anterior lip of the cervix is grasped with the vulsellum (Fig. 4.2) and, holding this in the left hand, the cervix is drawn down towards the introitus. This has the effect of straightening the endocervical canal and easing the passage of the instruments.

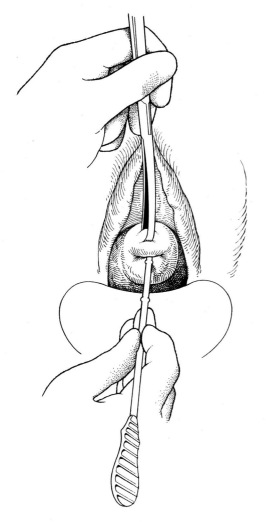

Fig. 4.3 Passage of uterine sound.

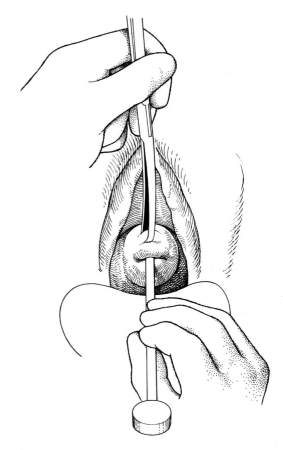

Fig. 4.4 Dilatation of the cervix.

With a pregnant or recently pregnant uterus the volsellum may easily cut out from the tissue of the cervix and should be replaced by either multiple instruments or a sponge holder. The position of the uterus has already been noted at pelvic examination and is confirmed by the gentle passage of a uterine sound (Fig. 4.3). This allows measurement of the uterocervical canal (UCC) length, which should be recorded.

Cervical dilatation
Dilatation of the cervix is now carried out using the graduated dilators in order, beginning with a size close to that of the sound, unless there is evidence of a patulous or partially dilated cervix. Remember the larger dilators are potentially less likely to perforate the uterus than the smaller. The surgeon should be able to feel the dilator gently touch the fundus of the uterus as each one is inserted. He must remember never to pass the dilator for a greater distance than the sounded length of the uterus. The amount of pressure on the dilator calls for considerable judgement which can only be built up by extensive practice. The pressure can be more easily controlled if the surgeon rests the heel of the left hand and lower forearm against the patient's right thigh and the heel of the right hand against the patient's left buttock (Fig. 4.4). The right and left hand are thus providing traction and countertraction, both of which are totally controlled. The dilator should be held in the right hand with the thumb posteriorly counterbalanced by the first

three fingers along the length of the instrument. If this technique is adopted, considerable 'feel' can be achieved and any significant obstruction will cause the dilators to slide between the thumb and the fingers. The surgeon should be building up in his mind a three-dimensional picture of the inside of the uterus, noting and mentally recording any obstructions or irregularities.

Extent of dilatation

The degree of dilatation will depend on the procedure to be performed. For most simple curettage procedures the cervix will not need to be dilated to more than 7 mm, whereas for suction termination of pregnancy the optimum is 10 mm.

Similarly, for adequate assessment of large possibly carcinomatous uteri more rather than less dilatation is an advantage. In virginal patients the surgeon should consider using the smallest possible instrument (such as a Novak curette or a Vabra aspirator) through a smaller cervical os to cut down the risk of trauma and long-term incompetence of the cervix.

For all patients, excessive force or roughness must be avoided.

Difficulties in performing the dilatation

Inability to pass a sound or dilator

If the patient has a menstrual history, the os must be patent; patience and careful technique will always be successful. The position of the uterus must be carefully reassessed — extreme retroversion or retroflexion may be corrected manually. Traction on the vulsellum straightening the endocervical canal will also assist. A gentle touch with the sound will define the nooks and crannies of the endocervical canal. Finally and surprisingly, a slightly larger dilator will often pass into the uterus as it rides over the small cul-de-sacs in the canal.

Cervical rigidity or spasm

This problem manifests itself as an inability to proceed with the dilatation beyond a small dilator. The cure is to leave the maximum sized dilator in the canal for a short while to allow the spasm to relax. If this is unsuccessful the problem may be due to old scarring from previous surgery or childbirth, and the surgeon may then have to accept limited dilatation and modify his technique by using smaller instruments. Otherwise the risk of a cervical tear will be significant.

Difficulty with dilatation

As dilatation proceeds it may be noted that the dilators do not pass in as far as the earlier ones. This is because the operator is not passing the dilators the full length of the UCC and the internal os is not being dilated. The solution is to begin again and feel the uterine fundus as each dilator is passed.

Dilatation of a false passage or diverticulum

If this is not noticed, the end result may be rupture of the cervix or uterus. This problem is obviated if the surgeon meticulously follows the axis of the uterus as defined at bimanual examination.

Complications of dilatation

Tearing and laceration of the cervix

The pregnant cervix is at very great risk of laceration, particularly by the traction on the vulsella. However, it is at relatively less risk of laceration from the process of dilatation than the non-pregnant cervix unless dilatation is performed to excessive levels, i.e. greater than 12 mm. Laceration is most likely to happen if excessive force is used, the cervix is dilated too widely or if spasm of the cervix is not allowed to relax before proceeding.

A sudden 'give' as dilatation is being carried out is very suspicious of a tear. Usually these tears are small and out of sight in the endocervical canal; rarely, they extend rapidly through the full thickness of the cervix into the vaginal fornices, or from the internal os into the body of the uterus, rupturing through into the broad ligament. If the surgeon suspects that a tear may have occurred, he must cease dilatation immediately. If the laceration is visible and bleeding, suture of the damage is mandatory. Even when there is no bleeding, suturing will restore the anatomy and obviate bleeding developing later, but will probably not restore the functional integrity of the cervix if the internal os is damaged. Late complications of laceration are bleeding, infection and cervical incompetence.

Early bleeding

This may be of varying amounts; usually, it is slight if the tear is small and ceases as the cervix resumes its normal shape after dilatation has stopped. Occasionally, significant haemorrhage may occur from a ruptured branch of the cervical arteries. This may be dealt with by either direct suturing if the offending vessel is visible or a pressure pack if it is not. The second course has a number of significant pitfalls: it is possible that the haemorrhage will continue, dilating the uterus or even extending into the broad ligament if the uterine lower segment has been damaged. It is therefore vital that the patient is carefully monitored in the postoperative period, elevations of pulse, lowering of the blood pressure and untoward pain being reported immediately. If a laceration has been suspected, the recovery room staff must be made aware of the possible consequences.

If the bleeding is considerable and coming from an invisible site in the upper cervix, packing should not be considered. The cervix should either be split to demonstrate the bleeding point, or, if the site cannot be identified, the uterine artery on that side should be exposed as in a vaginal hysterectomy and separately ligated. Usually the treatment of the descending branch alone will allow the surgeon to deal effectively with bleeding on one side of the cervix. Very rarely, it may be necessary to open the abdomen and deal with the artery directly. However, the surgeon should remember the enormous collateral circulation, especially of the pregnant uterus, and realize that he may have to tie off both internal iliac arteries or carry out a hysterectomy if the haemorrhage fails to settle. Haematomas of the broad ligament will distort the anatomy, and the close relationship of the ureter must be remembered; failure to pay adequate attention may well turn a disaster into a tragedy.

Late bleeding

Rarely, profuse secondary haemorrhage will occur, usually the consequence of an unnoticed laceration or haematoma becoming infected and rupturing a significant cervical or lower uterine blood vessel. Packing and transfusion are the mainstay of management as it is wise to avoid surgical procedures in this infected area. Broad-spectrum antibiotics, together with one specific for anaerobes, should be given immediately following the taking of specimens for bacteriology. If the bleeding persists, the abdomen should be opened. Occasionally, ligation of the internal iliac arteries will suffice, but the surgeon should not expect this procedure to always produce the desired effect. Hysterectomy may be the final solution.

Perforation of the uterus

Perforation may occur into the peritoneal cavity, the broad ligament, the bladder or, more rarely, into an adherent viscus. The accident is frequently blamed on the inexperience of the surgeon, but it is more closely related to dilatation of the pregnant or recently pregnant uterus and of the uterus affected by carcinoma. A prior knowledge of the position and attitude of the uterus cannot be stressed enough in the prevention of this complication. Figure 4.5 shows the ease with which a perforation can be performed in the retroverted gravid uterus. The dilators should be extensions of the surgeon's hands and should follow the contours of the uterine cavity. A sudden release of pressure suggests a perforation; the position of the dilator or sound should be noted and the procedure terminated. The exception to this will be when evacuation of the uterus is imperative, such as in termination of a pregnancy, in which circumstances the remainder of the procedure should be performed with extreme gentleness and care. When the suspected perforation has occurred during a clean procedure, such as a curettage for menorrhagia or for endometrial sampling, observation of the patient by half hourly pulse and blood pressure is all that is necessary. If there is suspected infection, the same observation should be accompanied by antibiotic cover for at least 7 days. If malignancy is demonstrated, treatment at the earliest possible moment is essential.

Peritonitis due to perforation Most perforations produce no major or long-term sequelae. However, when associated with infection, perforation may progress to peritonitis (see below). This is due to direct transfer of pathogens either to the peritoneal cavity or to the opening of the infected area allowing access. Symptoms may not develop for 12–24 h, appearing as abdominal pain and discomfort with muscle rigidity and pyrexia. The classical signs of gas under the diaphragm may not be present and laparoscopy is of enormous value in order to determine the diagnosis accurately.

Peritonism Douching and washing of the uterine cavity with saline or antiseptics are now rarely performed, so the risk of escape of the irritant douche into the peritoneal cavity is small. The most common cause of peritonism is irritation by escaped blood, the patient complaining of extreme and persistent lower abdominal pain in the postoperative period. If the patient has been lying in a slight Trendelenburg position, shoulder tip pain may also be a feature and is almost diagnostic. If the bleeding persists, features of a pelvic haematocele supervene with tenesmus, frequency and a bearing down sensation accompanied by backache. Treatment may initially be conservative with antibiotics if there is

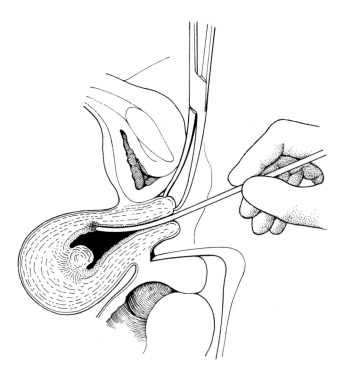

Fig. 4.5 Damage to the anterior wall of a retroverted gravid uterus.

any evidence of infection. However, if the patient shows evidence of progression, more active management, including laparoscopy and laparotomy, must not be delayed. The laparotomy must include a full inspection of the bowel, particularly the small bowel which may have been lying close to the uterus as well as the genital organs.

Bowel damage Reports of bowel damage following perforation still occur and should serve to warn the operator of the consequences of a careless approach to the seemingly simple process of cervical dilatation. If the operator suspects that the bowel has been damaged, an immediate laparotomy should be performed, the entire bowel inspected and any trauma dealt with (see Chapter 26). The bowel must never be returned to the abdomen and ignored—to do so is reprehensible and may cost the woman her life.

Perforation into the broad ligament This complication is usually secondary to laceration of the cervix at or close to the internal os. Progressive dilatation then causes the laceration to deepen as the dilators are thrust

deeper into the tear, culminating in lateral rupture of the uterus into the broad ligament. If the tear has not involved large vessels or has not occurred in the presence of infection or carcinoma, the problem often resolves with conservative treatment. However, all too often the uterine arteries or their major branches are damaged, resulting in significant haemorrhage into the broad ligament. Pain is the commonest initial symptom accompanied by the usual signs of acute blood loss; examination reveals a growing doughy mass in the broad ligament. If the haemorrhage is torrential, the patient will become rapidly shocked with signs of retroperitoneal haemorrhage, including gross intestinal dilatation due to disruption of the splanchnic nerves. Rapid emergency management, including fluid and blood replacement and laparotomy is essential.

Trauma to preceding pelvic disease
It is possible during the examination phase of the dilatation procedure that preceding disease present in the pelvis may be disturbed. This will include rupture of the pyosalpinx, stimulation of salpingitis, and rupture of adhesions and cysts of the ovary and tube. Each of these

complications may be treated conservatively with the addition of antibiotics where appropriate, unless there is evidence of haemorrhage or progressive pelvic irritation. Extreme peritonism may be seen after rupture of a pyosalpinx or of an endometriotic cyst. The laparoscope is a useful tool in these circumstances and may produce a firm diagnosis without the patient having to undergo a formal laparotomy.

Peritonitis due to infection

As well as peritonitis following perforation, rupture of a pyosalpinx or tubo-ovarian abscess, or simply following dilatation, the problem may be consequent upon infection in a wound in the endometrium. The peritonitis is usually localized to the pelvis and may appear as a minor lower abdominal upset or may be of rapid onset and life threatening. When the infection is of lesser degree, the tubes and ovaries rapidly become matted together and are palpable as a mass behind the uterus and broad ligament. In more severe disease, the patient rapidly develops toxaemia with collapse and signs of bacteraemia and septic/endotoxic shock.

Pelvic cellulitis and parametritis

It is not uncommon following minor procedures on the cervix to see evidence of inflammation and minor infection of the tissues alongside the cervix and uterus (parametritis). This is manifested as pain in the lower abdomen and back with associated dyspareunia and pain on pelvic examination and movement of the cervix. Occasionally a thickening of the parametrium may result. The treatment is conservative with antibiotics and local heat. If a mass is palpable, fine-needle aspiration will confirm the presence of pus, which should be drained.

Cauterization of the cervix

In the past an enormous number of unnecessary cauterizations were performed on the cervix. Many patients seen at postnatal clinics with a normal postpartum ectropion were subjected to this operation. It is not necessary to carry out this procedure for cervical ectropion following pregnancy, nor for ectopic columnar epithelium on the ectocervix unless the patient has significant symptoms. Even those patients who have discharge from a cervix which becomes infected are probably better served by cryosurgery without the need for a general anaesthetic. Rarely, chronic cervicitis and infected Naboth's follicles warrant the use of cautery or electrodiathermy. Currently, the most important use of electrodiathermy is in the treatment of cervical intraepithelial neoplasia (CIN), diagnosed following colposcopic assessment. In Britain this technique is now relatively rarely used, having been superseded first of all by CO_2 laser ablation and more recently, in the last decade, by the use of excisional techniques such as loop diathermy excision.

Instruments

The gynaecological minor set, as described in Chapter 2, and an electrodiathermy machine are required.

Patient preparation

No special preparation is required as most procedures will be performed on a day case basis.

Anaesthesia

For most cauterizations a light general anaesthetic is required because heat transfer from the cervix to the uterus can result in severe pain. Very short procedures can be carried out without anaesthesia since the cervix itself is relatively insensitive to heating. Electrodiathermy of CIN should always be carried out under either general anaesthetic or a wide local anaesthetic.

The operation

Do not use any antiseptic containing alcohol in the preparation of the patient. Every year reports describe accidental burns to patients because of this error, which is now quite indefensible. The cervix is exposed by inserting a Sims' or Auvard's speculum into the vagina and then drawing down the cervix using a toothed vulsellum. For superficial cauterization the ball electrode is moved over the area of ectopic columnar epithelium, taking care not to touch the vagina and clearing the char from the electrode during the procedure. Modern Teflon-coated electrodes reduce the build-up of char.

If radical electrodiathermy is performed in the treatment of CIN it is important to use a slightly different technique. The cervix is first incised in a radial fashion using the needle electrode to a depth of approximately

3–5 mm. The area to be incised has been defined using the colposcope and outlining the abnormal tissue with iodine. Again, this iodine must be an aqueous solution and not in alcohol. The ridges of tissue lying between these radial cuts are now removed using the ball electrolode. At the end of the procedure the cervix should look as though a shallow cone of tissue has been removed which, when radical electrodiathermy is being used to treat CIN, the cone should reach a depth of 7 mm.

Following electrodiathermy, healing is generally excellent with very occasional reports of infection occurring during the healing phase. Secondary haemorrhage does occur and is comparable to that following cone biopsy or other local ablative techniques. This secondary haemorrhage is most frequently associated with secondary infection.

Cervical scarring and stenosis is more common than following cryosurgery or laser ablative therapy, and may give problems during subsequent pregnancies. This complication, however, is rare and generally does not cause difficulties. Haematometra and pyometra have been reported but are easily treated by dilatation of the cervix and drainage of the fluid from within the uterine cavity.

Cryosurgery

Cryosurgery has largely superseded elecrocautery as the optimal treatment for benign epithelial abnormalities of the cervix.

The principle

Cryosurgery depends on the cooling effects of a rapidly expanding gas. This is achieved by venting the gas (usually nitrous oxide) through a narrow jet into a space behind a probe tip and then exhausting the gas via a large diameter port (similar to the Venturi effect). The subsequent cooling is transferred to the cervix through the metal cryoprobe. The resultant cooling and indeed freezing of the cervical epithelium extends inwards for a depth of between 4 and 7 mm and is adequate for killing cells to that depth.

Instruments

There are many cryosurgical sets available, all with similar characteristics. A variety of probe heads are available which are interchangeable and can be sterilized, and an appropriate one should be chosen prior to engaging in treatment. A large Cusco's or Sims' speculum is necessary so that the entire cervix can be exposed with an adequate clearance around the cervix so that the vagina is not involved in the treatment.

Anaesthesia

Cryosurgery has a very high patient acceptability; only rarely will patients feel any discomfort, which is usually described as like a period cramp. Therefore, neither anaesthesia nor analgesia is usually necessary. Almost all procedures are performed on an outpatient basis.

The operation

Exposing the cervix
The patient is placed in lithotomy position and partially draped for her own modesty. No preparation of the vulva or vagina is necessary. The Cusco's speculum is inserted following lubrication of the outer part of the blades. The largest comfortable speculum should be used so that the entire cervix can be visualized, and the vagina held away from the edges of the cervix.

Defining the lesion
If the patient has a precancerous lesion on the cervix, colposcopy must be performed in order to outline the lesion. Treatment should not be performed unless the entire limits of the lesion are visible and accessible, the histology and cytology reports taken at a previous examination are available, and there is no gynaecological indication for surgical excisional treatment. Schiller's or Lugol's iodine may be used to outline the area requiring treatment, but is not as accurate as colposcopy using acetic acid. Its use is not generally recommended by the editor.

Cryosurgery
A cryoprobe head is chosen which will cover the entire lesion. If this is not possible the lesion should be divided into segments and treated piecemeal. The cryoprobe head is gently pressed against the cervix and freezing begins. Within a few seconds the probe will be felt to 'stick' to the cervix as the ice crystals form on the back of the probe. The probe should be kept clear of the vagina to avoid unnecessary damage.

Timing of the freeze
For a benign lesion a single freeze of 60 s will suffice, whereas for treating precancerous conditions a freeze/or refreeze technique of 120 s on, 120 s off and 120 s on has proved to be most effective. The timing should begin from the moment the operator can see a clear rim of approximately 4 mm of frozen tissue around the cryoprobe head.

Postoperative care
No special precautions are necessary; the patient should be given a sheet of instructions informing them of the following:
1 They should not have intercourse for 4 weeks.
2 They should not use tampons for 4 weeks.
3 They should not use intravaginal creams.
4 Any untoward pain or bleeding must be reported to their doctor.
5 The patient should expect to have a profuse watery vaginal discharge which will last for 2–3 weeks and then cease.

Factors which influence the success of cryosurgery

The most important factors to determine successful treatment of precancerous lesions are:
1 Size of lesion.
2 Irregularity of the cervical surface.
3 Cryoprobe tip selection.
4 Nitrous oxide bottle pressure.
5 Depth of gland crypt involvement.

There does not appear to be any increased failure rate associated with more severe grades of CIN. In general, cryosurgery is recommended for the treatment of all benign epithelial conditions of the cervix, but does not produce the high clearance rates which published series have demonstrated to be achieved with either laser ablation, cold coagulation or electrodiathermy.

Cold coagulation

The SEMM cold coagulator was introduced into gynaecological practice in 1966. Initially it was used for the local destruction of benign cervical lesions, but many authors have confirmed its wide applicability to the treatment of precancerous conditions of the cervix. The equipment works by raising the temperature of the surface epithelium of the cervix to approximately 110°C.

Instruments

The SEMM cold coagulator is required together with a large Cusco's or Sims' speculum as for cryosurgery.

Anaesthesia

Although this procedure has been extensively used without anaesthetic it is probably necessary for the cervix to be infiltrated with local anaesthetic in order to reduce discomfort to a minimum.

The thermoprobe is applied to the lesion and using two to five overlapping applications the entire abnormality is covered. The thermoprobe heats the tissues to between 110 and 120°C and thereby literally boiling the tissues. Cell death is virtually instantaneous and the results of treatment are comparable with those following a radical electrodiathermy and laser ablation.

Complications are as for cryosurgery or laser ablation or electrodiathermy.

Laser ablation

The CO_2 laser is an accurate surgical tool allowing the surgeon to remove a measurable block of tissue from the cervix. The instrument became widely used during the early 1980s, mainly for the local treatment of pre-cancers or cancers of the cervix, vulva and vagina. Its use in the abdomen and other sites has enjoyed rather less popularity. The CO_2 laser is a powerful device and complications and dangers may occur if a simple safety code is not adhered to:
1 The clinical area where the laser is to be used must be clearly marked by warning signs, ideally of the type which illuminate when the laser is in use.
2 The area must have access doors which are not in the line of use of the laser.
3 A minimum of personnel should be present when the laser is in use.
4 The laser must only be used by trained medical staff and those in training must be supervised at all times.
5 All individuals in the laser area should wear safety glasses, especially when 'freehand' lasering treatment is being performed. The use of safety glasses is not neces-

sary for the operator using a laser via an operating microscope.

6 The CO_2 laser must not be used when the helium-neon (HeNe) laser beam is not functioning.

Non-reflective equipment has been sold by a number of manufacturers for use with the laser. This is not of proven value as the reflection of laser light is almost as high from a matt surface as it is from a polished one, and the reflected light may not be of the same wavelength as that absorbed.

Instruments

The laser

The most important requirement for a CO_2 laser is that it has adequate power. Initially this was between 20 and 35 W, but more modern lasers are much more powerful with considerable flexibility. Most lasers have a device which allows the spot size to be altered so that different power densities can be applied to the tissue to be treated. The beam of the CO_2 laser is in the infrared part of the spectrum and is therefore invisible to the human eye. The energy produced is at a wavelength of $10.6\,\mu\mathrm{u}$ and is normally allied with a second laser of a HeNe variety which is visible to the human eye and allows the invisible CO_2 laser to be guided by this red spot.

The two beams of the HeNe and the CO_2 laser are guided by being reflected from a surface reflective mirror which is rotated by a micromanipulator stick guided by the operator.

The smoke extractor

The CO_2 laser functions by vaporizing tissue. Its power is entirely absorbed by the first water-bearing surface that it meets, the resultant steam with carbon particles admixed is generated as 'smoke'. It is therefore essential if the operator is to be able to see the operative field that this smoke is removed. This is best achieved using a sucker attached to the upper part of the speculum which can run continuously during the procedure.

Anaesthesia

For many patients, possibly up to 50%, there is either no pain or only minimal discomfort. For the remainder, local analgesia or, occasionally, full general anaesthetic is required. Larger lesions, particularly those extending on to the vagina or vulva, and where the patient is nervous, should be selected for full anaesthesia. For the remainder laser ablation can be performed as an outpatient procedure.

The operation

Exposure of the cervix

This is as described for performing cryosurgery, except that the Cusco's speculum should have a suction tube attached to the smoke extractor.

Defining the lesion

Colposcopy is performed and the lesion identified. The same criteria as defined under cryosurgery must be met.

Ablating the lesion

The laser is switched on and the lesion is outlined with the laser, leaving a margin of 3 mm clear around the lesion. The operator then begins at the bottom of the lesion and steadily vaporizes tissue down to a depth of approximately 7 mm. Small blood vessels will be easily dealt with by the laser; so long as the vessel is completely transected it will retract and stop bleeding. If only part of the vessel is cut it will continue to bleed because the side of the vessel is held open by the cervical stroma. A rapid circling movement with the laser will complete the transection and stop the haemorrhage. If bleeding does continue the vessel should be occluded by applying a swab stick or cue tip for a short time; in the meantime the operator should proceed with lasering other parts of the cervix. He can then return to the swab stick and vaporize it and the vessel.

Attempts to laser through bleeding vessels can produce a considerable build-up of carbon which has to be vaporized; as the laser burns this away the increased heat produced is transferred to the uterus, with a consequent increase in pain and blood supply.

In order to reduce pain and bleeding to a minimum, the lasering time must be short. This is achieved by using a high power density (greater than $1000\,\mathrm{w/cm^2}$ per second) with a spot size of approximately 1.6 mm.

Completing removal of the cylinder of tissue

As the lasering proceeds, the surgeon should attempt to vaporize a cylindrical block of tissue with vertical side walls and a slightly domed base, similar to that removed at the laser cone biopsy (see Figs 4.10 and 4.11).

This will remove any precancerous lesion which may have entered the cervical glands. At the end of the procedure, the cervix is dry and the patient is given an instruction sheet as described for cryosurgery.

Complications common to all local ablative treatment methods

Pain

Pain appreciation varies considerably from one patient to another and it does not appear to be possible to forecast which patients will or will not feel pain. In general, the higher the temperature of the treatment and the longer the application, the greater the pain. Thus, electrodiathermy, which utilizes extremely high temperatures, produces intolerable pain and must be used under general or wide local anaesthesia. General anaesthetic is not usually necessary for the other treatment modalities, and any pain appreciated always disappears at the end of the treatment. When patients are informed of this and are then supported by a 'chatty' nurse, most can be treated without analgesia. A confident team of doctors and nurses produces the best results.

Pain occurring after treatment in the healing phase is usually due to infection of the cervix or the pelvic organs and should be investigated by pelvic examination, inspection of the cervix, and culture of a high vaginal swab and midstream specimen of urine. It is important to differentiate the pain due to local infection from other causes such as ectopic pregnancy or appendicitis. Laparoscopy or laparotomy may be indicated. Chronic pelvic inflammatory disease may flare up after laser treatment and must be actively managed with antibiotics and surgery if necessary.

Cryosurgery appears to be the best tolerated technique and for most patients is pain free. Occasionally a period-like cramp is experienced, and may be associated with vasovagal attacks shortly after the procedure. Normally neither local nor general anaesthetic is required.

In laser treatment pain is felt by 50% of patients, 10% having severe pain. The pain is appreciated as either a sharp 'multiple pin prick' sensation and/or a dull, cramping period-like pain. The former is felt when the laser is actually working and the latter is a function of the heating effect on the cervix. If, during treatment, pain becomes intolerable, 2–4 ml of 2% lidocaine should be directly injected into the cervix using a fine needle attached to a dental syringe.

Discharge

Discharge occurs after any operative manipulation of the cervix but is most commonly seen after cryosurgery.

Almost all patients have a profuse watery discharge lasting for 2–4 weeks after cryosurgical treatment. The discharge is clear and rarely becomes infected, but may be so profuse as to require sanitary protection. All patients must be forewarned of this complication.

After electrodiathermy, the mucus produced becomes mixed with the charred material remaining on the cervix producing a discoloured discharge which responds to local cleansing, and only rarely needs treatment with antibiotics if pelvic infection supervenes.

Following laser treatment, discharge occurs relatively rarely but when profuse it is associated with cervicitis or pelvic infection and should be actively treated with antibiotics.

Bleeding

This problem is never seen during cryosurgery but can appear when slough separates from the cervix during healing, or when infection occurs.

Using a laser, bleeding can be a significant problem during and after treatment. Patients who have evidence of cervical infection, especially *Trichomonas vaginalis*, *Neisseria gonorrhoea* and *Gardnerella* infestations, should have treatment prior to lasering, otherwise very troublesome bleeding will occur.

After electrodiathermy, bleeding varies from none to severe and may on occasion require admission to hospital, packing the vagina, suturing and/or blood transfusion. Most patients experience no unusual bleeding or, at worst, a blood-stained discharge.

Complications of healing

After cryosurgery, healing occurs rapidly and is associated with slight shrinkage of the stroma of the cervix, resulting in radial ridging. The squamocolumnar junction is frequently resited in the lower part of the endocervical canal; therefore, follow-up of precancerous conditions must rely on cytology, since colposcopy is frequently unsatisfactory. It will be necessary to utilize an endocervical brush technique as a method of surveillance in these patients.

Stenosis of the cervical os and bridging of the epithelium have been reported but these rarely give problems during menstruation or pregnancy. Intravaginal creams are not of proven protective value and do not affect the rate of healing or the subsequent position of the squamocolumnar junction. Following treatment using electrodiathermy healing is usually excellent, comparable with that following laser treatment, although in some patients the squamocolumnar junction may be resited in the endocervical canal. Stenosis of the cervix can occur and may require dilatation under general anaesthesia and haematometra and dysmenorrhoea have been reported. The possibility that more scarring will occur after electrodiathermy than with other techniques has not been borne out in published series, and the subsequent obstetric performance of these patients is comparable to that of patients after other ablative techniques.

In the healing phase after laser treatment the edges have a tendency to roll in producing a narrow sulcus around the rim. The base of the cylinder covers over with columnar epithelium which over a period of time (up to 6 months) is replaced with squamous epithelium by a process of squamous metaplasia. Until this occurs the columnar epithelium is very vulnerable and may easily be traumatized, producing bleeding which may worry the patient. The area may be re-lasered but if this fails the application of cryosurgery usually promotes rapid cover with squamous epithelium. Occasionally, a rim of vascular 'lakes' appear around the edge of the lasered area but unless they bleed, no further attention is required.

Menstrual alteration

The menstrual period following local ablative treatment may be delayed or the flow greater than usual. Attempts to avert this problem by synchronizing treatment to the first half of the menstrual cycle are rarely successful and quite impractical in a busy clinic. Intermenstrual and postcoital bleeding associated with the healing process can occur but other gynaecological causes must first be eliminated.

No particular ablative technique is more prone to this complication than any other and patients should be advised to consult their own doctor or to return to the clinic if they are concerned about significant alterations in menstrual pattern.

Subsequent obstetric performance

Patients who have had local ablative therapy are no more likely to develop obstetric complications than the normal population.

Patient information

Complications can be markedly reduced if patients are kept fully informed about likely problems associated with the procedure. This should be complemented by the use of closed circuit television during diagnosis, and information sheets explaining potential complications following treatment. The information sheet must warn the patient of any discharge, pain or abnormal bleeding which may occur and, where appropriate, advise against intercourse or the use of intravaginal tampons and creams for a short period after therapy.

Excisional techniques

The use of excisional techniques has been for many years the mainstay of the management of CIN. In the past the predominant technique was the cold knife cone biopsy, but to this has been added the laser cone biopsy and large loop excision of the transformation zone (LLETZ). For the occasional patient with persistent problems or with associated gynaecological problems, hysterectomy—whether abdominal or vaginal—has been the final excisional treatment of choice.

Cold knife cone biopsy

Instruments
The instruments required for this procedure are those described in the gynaecological minor set (see Chapter 2). The knife itself may have a pointed blade thus facilitating the formation of the conical excision.

Anaesthesia
This procedure should be performed under general anaesthetic, although rarely it is possible, though not in the authors' view desirable, to use a paracervical or wide local infiltration.

Patient preparation

The patient should be prepared as for any vaginal procedure. Shaving is not necessary. All cone biopsies should be carried out under colposcopic control to be certain of identifying the ectocervical limits of the colposcopic abnormality. Schiller's or Lugol's iodine may be used as an alternative, but is not essential. Usually the cone biopsy is being performed because the endocervical limits of the lesion cannot be seen at colposcopy, or where there is a suspicion of invasive carcinoma. The use of techniques to assess the depth of involvement by CIN of the endocervical canal have been many and various. Contact hysteroscopy and colpohysteroscopy have been used but are not generally employed.

The operation

Lateral haemostats The patient is draped in the lithotomy position and an Auvard's or Sims' speculum inserted into the vagina. The cervix is visualized and colposcopy performed. Iodine may be applied as described previously. The cervix is then grasped above the anterior limit of the ectocervical lesion using a toothed vulsellum. By drawing the cervix to one side and then to the other access is gained to place a deep lateral haemostatic stitch on either side of the cervix (Fig. 4.6). The stitch is inserted to ligate the descending branch of the uterine artery which passes along the lateral side of the cervix deep to the epithelium. The stitches, usually of Dexon or Vicryl, may be left long and attached to artery clips in order to manoeuvre the cervix later in the procedure.

Incising the cone The cervix is now drawn down using the volsellum and, taking a pointed bladed scalpel, the cone is cut beginning at the posterior part and cutting around the anterior area (Fig. 4.7). As soon as the initial encircling incision has been made it is a great advantage to grasp the specimen with a Littlewood's tissue forceps to infold the ectocervical epithelium upon itself (Fig. 4.8). The deeper part of the cone can then be cut under direct vision. Holding the specimen in the tissue forceps also protects the ectocervical epithelium and produces an intact specimen for the pathologist. This is of particular importance when dealing with high-grade CIN as there appears to be reduced tissue adhesion between the dermis and the subdermal layers in this condition.

Repairing the cervix For many years the standard re-

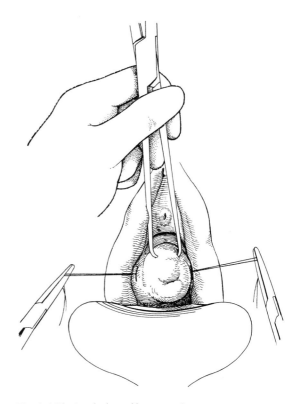

Fig. 4.6 Placing the lateral haemostatic sutures.

pair after cone biopsy was to insert Sturmdorf sutures, producing a very ugly cervix often with ectocervical epithelium infolded and hidden or epithelial cells drawn down stitch tracks, producing a potential danger of hidden precancerous change. The editor has for many years used a simple and effective technique of inserting a cryoprobe head into the cone base and then freezing the area to stop bleeding. The vagina is then packed, the bladder catheterized and the patient returned to the ward. Occasionally it is necessary to augment this technique by using either isolated sutures to the edge of the cone or an encircling continuous suture around the edge, or by tying across the front of the cone the lateral haemostats (Fig. 4.9). The great advantage of these simple methods is that the squamocolumnar junction is still accessible for future assessment for both cytology and colposcopy.

Dilatation and curettage Many surgeons routinely perform this procedure with a cone biopsy. Unless there

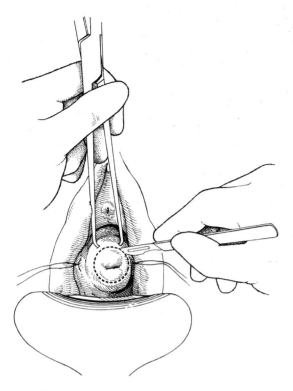

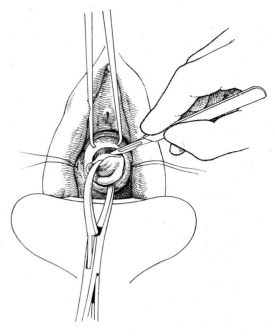

Fig. 4.8 Grasping the cone biopsy.

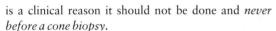

Fig. 4.7 Cutting of the cone biopsy.

is a clinical reason it should not be done and *never before a cone biopsy*.

This latter practice usually results in there being no epithelium left on the cone specimen and leaves the poor pathologist unable to make any realistic report. There is also no advantage in attempting to dilate the cervix to reduce the risk of stenosis. Scarring and stenosis are more likely to occur after the enthusiastic insertion of Sturmdorf sutures.

Laser cone biopsy

The CO_2 laser is an excellent instrument, not only as a vaporizing instrument, but also when the spot size is reduced to 1 mm or less as a slow cutting device. This facility to reduce the spot size and thus increase the power density of the beam gives the surgeon a very accurate instrument with which to remove lesions from the cervix, vulva, etc. In many centres laser cone biopsy has effectively replaced the cold knife conization procedure because of its accuracy, relatively small blood loss,

low complicational rate and the potential to remodel the cervix. Although the procedure is bloodless, the major drawback is the extreme slowness of the procedure and, in inexperienced hands, the tendency to produce significant heat trauma to the specimen.

Patient preparation
The patient is prepared as for a cold knife cone biopsy.

Instruments
Apart from the minor gynaecological set the laser device fitted with a micromanipulator is necessary.

The operation
Outlining the limit of the lesion The patient is colposcoped and the ectocervical limits of the lesion are outlined using the laser at its smallest spot size. If the cone is to be very small, it is important to leave at least 3–4 mm between the outline and the lesion so as not to jeopardize the specimen by thermal damage. This initial outlining (Fig. 4.10) is now deepened, particularly anteriorly and posteriorly, to at least 4–5 mm (Fig. 4.11).

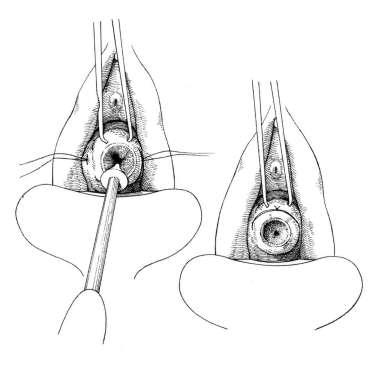

Fig. 4.9 Freezing of the cone base and tying the lateral haemostatic sutures anteriorly.

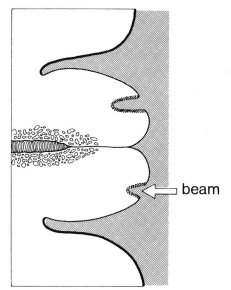

Fig. 4.10 Outlining the laser cylinder.

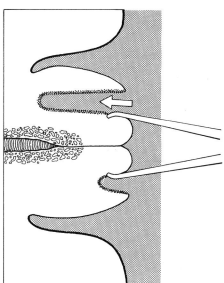

Fig. 4.11 Deepening the cut for a laser cylinder/cone.

Developing the cylinder A long straight Allis tissue forceps is inserted into the anterior and posterior 'slots' cut in the cervix (Fig. 4.11). The laser beam can now be used down the narrow sulcus without further charring of the central cylinder. The block of tissue is manoeuvred with one hand while the beam is guarded with the other. This calls for considerable dexterity and all too frequently the surgeon may find that he has lasered his

41

own fingers. As the circular sulcus develops, the central cylinder of tissue is drawn out of the cervix. Although some surgeons have advocated using a knife for the final cut at the bottom of the cylinder, the editor performs the complete procedure with the laser, usually without any blood loss or excessive thermal damage.

Postoperative care It is not usually necessary to pack the vagina and the patient goes home either the same day or the following morning.

Large loop excision of the transformation zone

Wire diathermy loops have been used for many years to remove both large and small lesions from the cervix. They have all the advantages of other minimally invasive conservative therapies and the added bonus that a large block of material can be obtained for pathological assessment. The technique when used in conjunction with the well-developed colposcopic assessment has proved to be extremely popular for the majority of patients and is now in most Western countries the most popular technique for treatment of CIN.

Patient preparation

The preparation of the patient is as for local ablative techniques. Most large loop excisional procedures are carried out in outpatients under local anaesthetic. The patient is colposcoped in the usual manner and in those circumstances where a high-grade cytology has brought the patient to the clinic, the technique of loop diathermy is used in a 'see and treat' policy, as in these circumstances it is possible to confirm the existence of a significant lesion on the cervix consistent with the high-grade cytological abnormality, and to diagnose and treat it effectively with the one procedure.

The equipment

The systems that are currently available consist of combined cutting and coagulating facilities. These can be blended and used with a single device. Although a wide variety of shapes and sizes of loops are available, in broad terms these consist of an insulated barrel inserted into a standard diathermy hand piece with buttons for cut and coagulation available to the operator. A stainless steel wire is either made in a thin flexible form or a thicker more rigid form. The rigid form is easier to use but does produce more thermal damage to the specimen. The fine flexible wire requires a delicate touch and an understanding of the memory facility of the wire so that a satisfactory loop specimen can be generated.

The operation

As with other conservative techniques the patient is advised of the procedure, both verbally and in writing. The patient is put in lithotomy position with a Cusco's speculum with a smoke extraction facility attached. The cervix is exposed and colposcopy performed in the standard manner. The limits of the lesion are identified. It is not usually necessary to outline the lesion with iodine and at this point local anaesthetic is injected directly into the cervix. The preferred agent is Citanest 3%, with Octapressin which is prilocaine, hydrochloride 30 mg/ml and felypressin 0.03 IU/ml. This combination of local anaesthetic agent and vasopressor gives adequate analgesia and reduces blood loss. The agent is delivered with a fine dental syringe. The injection is given into both anterior and posterior lips of the cervix and sometimes also at 3 and 9 o'clock in larger cervices. It is important to inject superficially so that blanching of the epithelium occurs. If the injection is put in too deeply the agent is rapidly absorbed with minimal effect on the cervix.

An appropriately sized loop is chosen to encompass the entire lesion so that the specimen can be removed in one block. In the editor's experience it is rarely necessary to use more than one sweep, and in his series over a 10-year period where a total of 4944 loops were performed, 80% were made with a single sweep, 15% required two sweeps and the remaining 5% required more than two sweeps.

The loop is laid over the transformation zone so as to encompass the lesion comfortably. If the fine wire loop is used slight pressure is put on the loop so that it adopts a curved attitude to the cervix. The 'cut' button on the hand piece is pressed, and after a few seconds the wire begins to enter the cervix (Fig. 4.12). The surgeon should then follow the wire very gently as it cuts through the cervix taking out a scoop of tissue to the required depth. It is also possible to cut deeply into the cervix by inserting the wire in the long axis of the cervix so as to cut directly in, and then it is gently drawn backwards so that a much deeper scoop is performed.

At the end of the cut the block of tissue which usually sits in the cervix can be removed (Fig. 4.13). Minimal bleeding is experienced and the base of the loop can

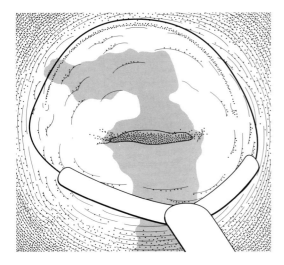

Fig. 4.12 The loop is laid over the transformation zone to encompass the lesion comfortably.

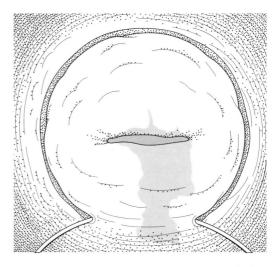

Fig. 4.13 The wire is then 'followed', rather than pushed, through the cervix so that it exists below the lesion on the posterior lip.

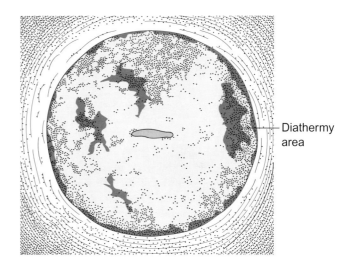

Diathermy area

Fig. 4.14 The completed treatment leaves a shallow scoop defect in the cervix with a completely sealed surface.

then be diathermied using a ball electrode (Fig. 4.14). At the end of the procedure the patient can be allowed home.

Complications
These tend to be minimal but are very similar to other local ablative techniques. Most commonly that of bleeding, discharge and occasionally infection.

The major advantages of the loop excision is that it can be used in the outpatient department under local anaesthetic, and also that it generates a block of tissue which can be easily orientated by the pathologist, and in general terms has minimal heat artefact associated with it.

Hysterectomy is described in Chapter 7.

Complications of cervical conization

Haemorrhage is the most important and common problem encountered. The bleeding may be primary or secondary, usually associated with the former occurring in the first 24 h, and associated with reactive bleeding, the latter some 10 days postoperatively and often associated with infection. Vaginal packing is often all that is required, but the cervix should be inspected and any local bleeding points dealt with individually. Of the techniques for conization mentioned in this chapter, no single one has an advantage. Therefore, the method which produces the least trauma to the cervix should be chosen. Infection will occur from time to time producing haemorrhage, discharge and occasionally progressing to pelvic infection. It should be actively treated by a combination of local vaginal cleansing and systemic antibiotics, especially the antibacteroides.

Cervical stenosis may occur and should be treated by simple dilatation; rarely does it cause a problem in labour.

Mid-trimester spontaneous abortions have been said to be increased following cone biopsy, but there is a considerable amount of conflicting evidence. In the editor's department a case-matched study showed no difference in the abortion rates following cone biopsy when compared with the normal population.

Trachelorrhaphy

The description of this procedure is taken from previous editions of the text. It has been included once more as there may be occasional indications for its use. Usually this is treatment of tears of the cervix following delivery or enthusiastic dilatation. However, if the cervix is hypertrophied it is probably better to perform an amputation and then remodel it.

Instruments
The gynaecological minor set will be required.

The operation
Defining the laceration The cervix is exposed using a Sims' or Auvard speculum. The cervix is then drawn down with the vulsellum and the endocervical canal dilated to 8 mm. The laceration is exposed and, if necessary, a second vulsellum is attached to the opposite side of the cervix (Fig. 4.15).

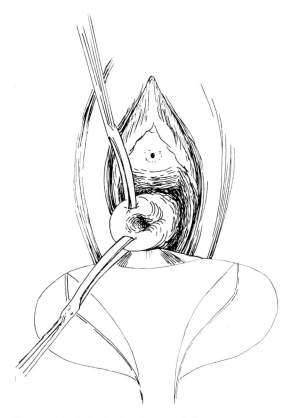

Fig. 4.15 Trachelorrhaphy: exposing the laceration.

Excision of the scar The entire scar is now excised by removing a wedge of tissue and exposing the canal (Figs 4.16 and 4.17).

Suture of the laceration Now the wedge-shaped incisions can be apposed. This is best done using a series of interrupted sutures ensuring that the stitches reach the endocervical canal surface in order to achieve complete apposition and haemostasis (Fig. 4.18).

Cervical incompetence

The signs and symptoms of cervical incompetence include:
1 One or more mid-trimester spontaneous abortions, often preceded by painless rupture of the membranes.
2 An unusually patulous cervical os easily admitting the index finger.

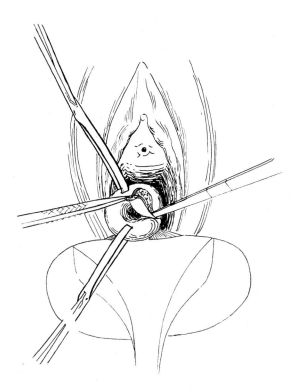

Fig. 4.16 Trachelorrhaphy: excision of the cervical scar.

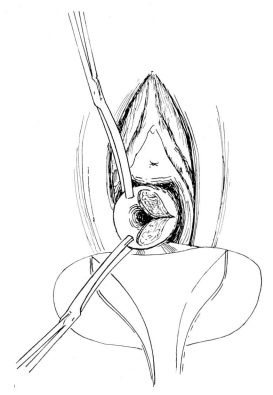

Fig. 4.17 Trachelorrhaphy: raw areas left after excision of the cervical scar.

3 A history of previous cervical surgery or a previous rapid delivery with cervical trauma.

4 If the patient is examined during the pregnancy the membranes may be seen to protrude from the cervical os; occasionally, even at this stage, the pregnancy may be saved by judicious insertion of a suture to support the integrity of the os.

There is no doubt that the name of Shirodkar will always be associated with this operation. His pioneering work and the widespread use of his procedure have saved countless pregnancies over the years. However, in Western practice the classical Shirodkar operation has been overtaken in popularity by the simpler McDonald operation, which is described here.

Indications

If the patient gives a history of previous mid-trimester loss or even of recurrent premature delivery she should be considered for the procedure. In modern-day practice a type of McDonald suture may be placed in the cervix following the procedure of trachelectomy used for the management of early invasive cancer where the cervix and uterus have to be preserved.

The operation is best planned when the patient is booked for delivery. It is usual to carry out the operation between 12 and 14 weeks gestation, although with patients who consistently miscarry at an earlier time the suture may be put in prior to 12 weeks or even before conception. It is important to perform an ultrasound scan in order to exclude fetal abnormality before embarking on the procedure. The McDonald suture consists of a length of Mersilene (Terylene) tape swaged directly onto a large needle to cope with the width of the tape.

Instruments

The instruments required are found in the gynaecological minor set described in Chapter 2.

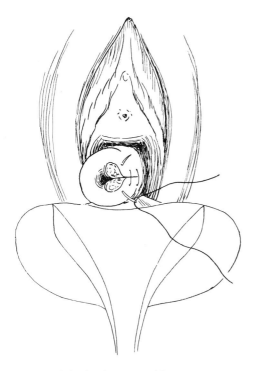

Fig. 4.18 Trachelorrhaphy: suture of the raw areas to reconstruct the cervical canal.

Patient preparation

It is of value for the patient to be put on prophylactic antibiotics and β-sympathomimetics prior to surgery.

Anaesthesia

Either a light general anaesthesia or an epidural is ideal for carrying out this procedure.

The operation

Exposing and grasping of the cervix

The patient is placed in the lithotomy position and the cervix exposed by placing an Auvard's or Sims' specu-lum in the vagina. The cervix is grasped using two or more sponge holders, one on the anterior and one on the posterior lip of the cervix. The cervix is gently drawn down, exposing the length of the cervix. By drawing the sponge holders first to one side and then the other the lateral parts of the cervix can be easily reached with the needle.

Insertion of the suture

The large needle with the Mersilene tape threaded onto it is now passed through the substance of the cervix in three places, beginning at 12 o'clock to 10 o'clock, then 8 o'clock to 6 o'clock and completing the encircling from 4 o'clock to 2 o'clock. The suture is then tied between 2 o'clock and 12 o'clock. Practice will determine the correct tension, which should be tight enough to just close the os but not so tight as to produce a pallor of the cervix.

Removal of the suture

An anaesthetic is not required. Removal must be performed before labour becomes established and is easily accomplished by exposing the cervix and cutting the suture at any of the points where it is visible on the exterior of the cervix, and then by simply pulling the knot.

The patient must be informed of the importance of early attendance at the hospital if there is a suggestion of labour beginning. Management is particularly difficult when the patient goes into premature labour and the decision to cut the suture or to leave it and possibly conserve the pregnancy has to be made.

Further reading

Singer AS, Monaghan JM. *Lower Genital Tract Precancer*, 2nd edn. Oxford: Blackwell Science, 2000.

5 Operations on the uterine cavity

Assessment of the uterine cavity remains a significant part of the work of the gynaecologist. Alterations in menstrual pattern require assessment and evaluation. Often these changes, which include menorrhagia, polymenorrhoea, intermenstrual and postcoital bleeding, and postmenopausal bleeding, have increasingly become the area of activity preferentially seen in rapid access clinics.

All such patients should be assessed with a comprehensive personal, menstrual and hormonal history. The patient's cervical cytology record must be reviewed.

A full pelvic examination should be performed including visualization of the cervix and palpation of the pelvic organs. All findings should be recorded. Although in many countries colposcopy forms part of this process, it is not necessary in a patient who has a normal smear history (see Chapter 4). For many patients, particularly the young, bleeding problems are often associated with hormonal ingestion as part of a contraceptive programme.

Rapid access clinics

It is now commonplace for hospitals and surgeries to run rapid access clinics for special problems which are amenable to ambulant or outpatient care. The rapid access bleeding clinic (RABC) is appropriate as modern pelvic/vaginal ultrasound and endoscopic uterine sampling lends itself to this approach.

Patients can access the clinic via a phone, fax or email appointment via their own general practitioner or primary care physician. In many cancer networks standard proforma faxes have been developed which cover all documentation required for rapid processing. The clinics must be available on a frequent basis throughout the working week. Many clinics are run almost entirely by nursing and ultrasound staff who have been trained in history taking, endometrial sampling techniques, and abdominal and vaginal ultrasound.

Ideally, all results of investigations should be available on the same day. For histopathology this can be achieved using microwave processing systems which produce a high-quality histopathological specimen for the pathologist to report within 2–3 h of sampling.

Such a complex system of care requires considerable organization and commitment of skilled individuals. There has to be a critical mass of patients with a special facility on one site. Equipment has to be of a high order with rapidly available and appropriate skills on tap. Cover for holidays and other absences dictates that the whole process is expensive to run but does provide an immediate high-quality service.

In many hospitals, the RABC concept is fragmented because of variable availability of skills and equipment. Many centres can provide elements of care, such as outpatient endometrial sampling with Pipelle or other systems linked to an ultrasound assessment of endometrial cavity structure and endometrial thickness measurement. However, drawing all these skills and facilities together may be difficult.

Following history taking, visualization of the cervix and pelvic examination, an assessment of the endometrium can be performed using an outpatient technique such as endometrial cytology, or more satisfactorily by techniques which obtain a quantity of endometrium suitable for histopathological assessment, such as the Vabra aspirator or the Pipelle sampler.

Pipelle sampling of the endometrium

The Pipelle endometrial sampler is currently one of the most commonly used techniques of obtaining a sample of endometrium in the outpatient setting without need for anaesthetic or admission.

The device consists of an outer tube measuring 3 mm in diameter within which is a closely fitting rod, which when withdrawn creates a vacuum which sucks in a section of endometrium sufficient to give a histological report on. The diameter of the whole instrument is such that for many patients it is easily introduced into the uterine cavity and a satisfactory sample obtained. Unfortunately, the technique has a tendency to fail because there can be difficulties in introducing the sampler particularly in the postmenopausal patient or that the specimen generated is inadequate for pathological reporting.

Where outpatient sampling fails or the specimen is unsatisfactory, the gold standard assessment technique is hysteroscopy and curettage.

Outpatient hysteroscopy

Some centres have developed outpatient hysteroscopy using either a low-viscosity liquid or a gas (CO_2) expansion technique. It is important to understand that this process is entirely diagnostic. This technique, which relies on either a rigid (4–4.6 mm) or a flexible (3.6 mm) hysteroscope is frequently successful in expert hands. If the cervical os is tight the use of a local anaesthetic may be helpful. It is important to realize, however, that a separate sampling method has to be used and that the limitations of the Pipelle are even more pronounced with the larger diameter instruments.

Vasovagal attacks can be pre-empted to some extent by giving the patient intramuscular atropine 0.5 mg 15 min prior to the procedure. Similarly, cramping of the uterine muscle can be reduced by asking the patient to take a prostaglandin synthetase inhibitor some 2 h before the procedure.

Day case or ambulant hysteroscopy

Although many patients have hysteroscopy performed under local anaesthetic, the author utilizes a brief general anaesthetic particularly where significant operative manoeuvres are involved. Recovery from modern anaesthesia is so rapid that the use of local anaesthetic techniques is unnecessary.

The instruments

The hysteroscope should comprise a 3 mm 30° scope in a 4.6 mm sheath linked to a continuous flow pressure system. The procedure should be performed in a fully equipped day case operating theatre with full recovery facilities available.

When an intervention is required such as sampling of the endometrium the gynaecological minor set is necessary. Excision of lesions identified can be performed either with a simple curettage or with endoscopic electrodiathermy resection equipment (resectoscopes).

The cavity of the uterus requires distension for the various procedures. CO_2 gas has already been described for outpatient hysteroscopies, but for most diagnostic and minor procedure hysteroscopies dextrose/saline 5% is cheap and safe.

However, whenever electrical energy is used within the uterus a non-conducting medium is essential, as is a high flow rate of clean new fluid in and contaminated fluid out. The two most commonly used are 1.5% v glycine and sorbitol. Both these agents can cause hyponatraemia if excessive absorption occurs. Haemolysis is also possible. A meticulous account of fluid in and out of the systems is essential during any operative procedure.

The operation

The procedure should ideally be performed in the first half of the patient's menstrual cycle. The technique should be 'no touch' where possible.

The patient should be asked to empty her bladder immediately prior to going to theatre.

A rapid acting anaesthetic used with a laryngeal mask is given and the patient brought into the theatre and put into lithotomy position. The vulva and vagina is swabbed down with a non-alcoholic skin preparation. The legs and lower abdomen are draped.

The patient is examined using a bimanual technique to ascertain the shape, size, consistency and position of the cervix, uterus and adnexae.

A Sims' speculum is inserted into the posterior vagina and an Auvard's speculum may be used for improved access. The cervix is grasped on its anterior lip using a multitoothed volsellum forceps. The cervix and uterus is then gently drawn down and forwards to place the uterus on slight tension. This effectively straightens the endocervical canal and provides countertraction when dilatation of the cervix is necessary. The cervical canal and uterus is gently sounded to determine the length of the cavity, the attitude of the uterus having already been determined. This length will be recorded in the notes. Some experts do not recommend sounding; however, the author feels that the information gained is not disadvantaged by any potential risks of trauma.

For most parous patients it will be unnecessary to dilate the cervix prior to inserting the hysteroscope. If the scope does not pass easily, gentle dilatation of the endocervical canal can be performed up to 6 mm. It is important not to over dilate the cervix as the uterine cavity will not be expanded due to escape of the expansion medium.

The scope should be inserted gently along the anticipated line of the endocervical canal and the uterine cavity determined by the prior examination and sounding. The continuous flow of fluid should begin as the scope is inserted, aiding the opening of the canal. Visualization of this process is best achieved if a video camera is attached to the scope. Pressure to achieve expansion of the uterine cavity is produced either passively by elevating the bag of fluid at least 1 m above the level of the uterus or by applying a pressure bag to the fluid maintaining a pressure of 150 mmHg.

Once the hysteroscope is within the cavity of the uterus after a short time any debris will clear giving a superb view of the entire field.

The findings should be described systematically beginning with the endocervical canal, continuing into the cavity and ending with the tubal ostia. Positive and negative findings should be recorded. A full description with a drawing or ideally a photograph of the interior of the cavity is essential for adequate documentation.

Once the hysteroscopy is completed it is common for a sampling of the endometrium to be performed. This is best achieved using a curettage system.

Curettage
A small sharp curette is all that is required for the procedure. The small curette can be inserted without the need for further dilatation after the hysteroscopy. A systematic approach to sampling is required remembering that the uterine cavity consists of essentially an anterior and a posterior surface plus two cornu and a

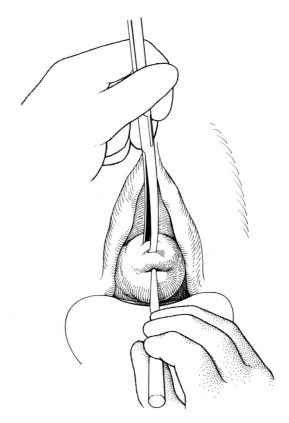

Fig. 5.1 Curettage of the uterine cavity.

fundus. If the curette is gently but firmly scraped first length wise down the posterior surface using three separate strokes followed by the same down the anterior surface and finally scraping right to left and then left to right across the fundus, the whole surface will be effectively sampled. The action of curettage is a gentle one with the curette lightly held in the first three fingers and the thumb of the right hand (Fig. 5.1). As the surgeon's experience grows a considerable amount of 'feel' will develop distinguishing irregularities, soft areas, septae and synaechiae seen on hysteroscopy. The specimens produced should be drawn out of the cervix and delivered onto a swab which has been placed just under the posterior lip of the cervix, in the posterior fornix. The swab is then taken, excess blood or mucous is removed and the curettings are immediately fixed in preservative.

At the end of the procedure the vagina is swabbed clean and a formal count of all swabs and instruments made and recorded.

Variations in technique
Fractional curettage This technique has been largely superseded by the use of hysteroscopy. However, it may have a value in separately curetting the endocervical canal when localized cancer is suspected. Material generated from each separate area of curettage is placed in clearly marked pots for histopathological assessment.

Removal of retained products of conception The most important aspect of this procedure is to remember the softness of the cervix and the body of the uterus and to use the utmost gentleness in all movements. The cervix should be grasped with sponge holders rather than a volsellum, and curettage performed with a large blunt curette. The author does not recommend digital exploration or the use of a flushing curette, although the latter is used by some surgeons as a large curette, without the flushing mechanism.

If there is any evidence of infection, bacterial swabs should be taken, antibiotics given before and during the procedure and all material send for pathological examination, otherwise a molar pregnancy may be missed.

All pregnancy-related curettage should be performed using prophylactic antibiotic cover.

Complications and dangers Trauma to the cervix and uterine wall are the commonest dangers and can be avoided with meticulous, gentle technique.

Infection is a significant risk with pregnancy-related procedures.

There is a small risk of adhesions in premenopausal patients which rises in the postmenopausal group.

Removal of endocervical mucous polyps and endometrial myomatous polyps
Endocervical polyps Most endocervical polyps are symptomless and are found at routine gynaecological examination such as the performance of a cervical smear. Less commonly they produce symptoms such as intermenstrual and postcoital bleeding.

When the polyps are small (<1 cm), they can usually be easily avulsed in the clinic by grasping them with small polyp forceps and rotating the forceps until the polyp falls off (Fig. 5.2). The specimen should be sent for pathological examination. Where polyps are large or have broad sessile bases, the procedure may require to be carried out under general anaesthesia. The polyp should be grasped and the base sutured in a purse string

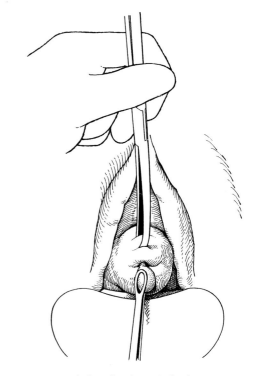

Fig. 5.2 Removal of small endocervical polyps.

pattern, or a small forceps placed across the base. The polyp is then removed with a knife taking care not to cut the suture, and the suture tied firmly. The placing of the suture prior to removal of the polyp is obvious as it is not uncommon for the base to retract into the endocervical canal making haemostasis difficult.

Fibroid polyps Occasionally, the uterus extrudes small submucous fibroids outside the cervix. The technique described by Bonney and shown in Figs 5.3–5.6 remains the ideal to this day. If the polyp is large and distends the cervix, it is best to try and identify the base and then to gently incise around the base, clamping bleeding points as necessary. Sometimes it is easier, as Bonney described, to enucleate the fibroid to render access easier and then deal with the pedicle (Fig. 5.6).

Endometrial polyps These are often identified at hysteroscopy and can be removed simply by inserting a small polyp forceps into the uterine cavity, grasping the polyp and avulsing it/them.

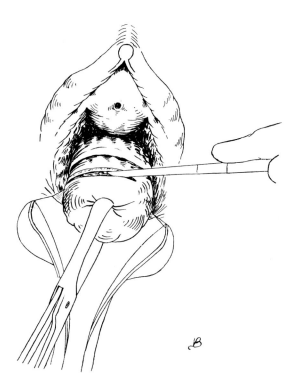

Fig. 5.3 Removal of a large myomatous polyp: incising the capsule.

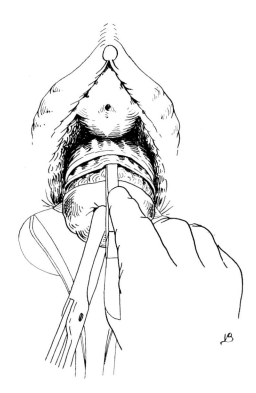

Fig. 5.4 Reflecting the capsule.

Resectoscopes Where the polyp is large or sessile the use of a resectoscope or laser may be necessary. The resectoscope used is virtually identical to the systems used in urology and have developed as part of the endometrial resection techniques used for persistent menorrhagia. The technique performed under continuous measured flow of distension media allows direct resection of the lesions identified. The specimens generated can be sent for pathological examination albeit in fragments. However, as has been noted above, the polyp can be released from its base and then left for the uterus to extrude naturally.

Lasers The lasers used are either YAG or Nd:YAG which can be transmitted down flexible fibre optic cable into the uterine cavity. Then, by direct contact or non-contact application to the area to be treated, the laser will cut or coagulate the tissue to a controlled depth of approximately 7 mm. It is important to use hysteroscopes with quite separate media in flow and out flow channels. This technology is particularly valuable in the treatment of submucous fibroids.

Fluid media measurement It is vitally important when using any operative hysteroscopic technique to have a meticulous technique of fluid inflow and outflow measurement. The risks and problems associated with fluid overload are well known and can be avoided by careful, well-monitored technique.

Surgical technique Preoperative reduction of the endometrium with either danazol (400–600 mg for 3 weeks) or gonadotropin-releasing hormone (GnRH) agonist (3 months of treatment) is usually used.

Uterine fibroids have been arbitrarily classified into four groups to facilitate indications for treatment and analysis of results:

Type I   Pedunculated fibroids.
Type II   Submucous fibroids.
Type III Small intramural fibroids.
Type IV   Large intramural fibroids.

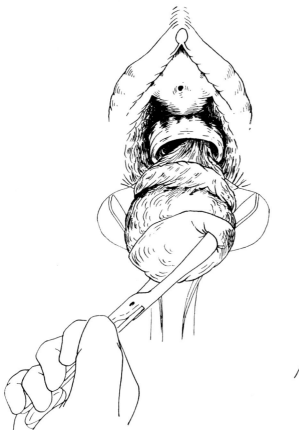

Fig. 5.5 Enucleation of the tumour.

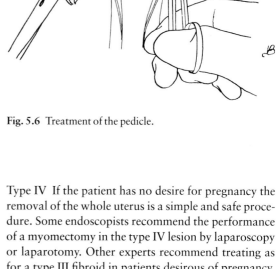

Fig. 5.6 Treatment of the pedicle.

Type I The Nd:YAG laser is used in the non-contact mode to coagulate the base of insertion of the fibroid, then in the contact mode the pedicle is cut and the fibroid is left in the cavity of the uterus unless it is small enough to be extracted at the end of the procedure.

Type II Ablation is achieved by passing the laser tip through the base of the fibroid to release the fibroid progressively. The fibroid is then left in the cavity as before to be naturally expelled.

Type III The dome of the fibroid is incised and resected and the centre of the fibroid is myolized using a non-contact technique to a depth of 5–7 mm. This results in significant volume reduction allowing removal in a second procedure some 12 weeks later.

Type IV If the patient has no desire for pregnancy the removal of the whole uterus is a simple and safe procedure. Some endoscopists recommend the performance of a myomectomy in the type IV lesion by laparoscopy or laparotomy. Other experts recommend treating as for a type III fibroid in patients desirous of pregnancy, or laparoscopic resection.

Endometrial ablation There has developed an increasing demand from patients for less invasive ways of dealing with dysfunctional uterine bleeding.

Numerous techniques have developed effectively to reduce or remove endometrium. The resectoscope, the Nd:YAG laser thermal balloons and the Mirena IUCD have produced acceptable effective long-term results.

Further reading

It is superfluous to produce a further reading list for procedures on the cavity of the uterus except to say that the tyro should carefully read as many standard texts as possible in order to reinforce the simple rules of care and safety for this, the most basic of gynaecological procedures. No amount of further reading will replace careful and meticulous practice of these commonly used techniques.

6

Opening and closing the abdominal cavity

Opening and closing the abdomen should be one continuous movement.

JM Monaghan

The length and position of the abdominal incision will depend on the purpose of the operation and on the physical state of the patient. Complicated and time-consuming incisions are inappropriate for emergency surgery, and small, cosmetic incisions are of little use for the removal of large masses: conversely, it is wrong to produce large unsightly scars after performing simple pelvic procedures. Just as the operation is planned the incision must allow the surgeon to carry out the procedure with ease and full access to the operative field. The incision must allow an adequate exploration of the abdomen, especially if there is any possibility of pathology other than that expected.

The patient should be left with a scar that is neat and, like the memory of the surgical intervention, fades with time. An unsightly scar will continuously remind the patient of the procedure, bringing back memories of the worst aspects of the operation. Most gynaecological procedures are best performed through one of two incisions—the subumbilical mid-line incision or the low transverse incision (Pfannenstiel).

Paramedian and high transverse (Maylard) incisions have their limited place and will be mentioned in the appropriate chapters.

Instruments

The instruments required are those described in Chapter 2 in the general gynaecological set.

Subumbilical mid-line incision

This is adequate for most gynaecological operations; it should extend from the skin fold below the umbilicus down as far as the hair line or one finger's breadth above the symphysis pubis. The incision can be easily extended for removal of very large intra-abdominal masses or for better operative access. This extension should be carried out upwards either through or around the umbilicus. There is little to be gained by cutting into the hair-bearing area; in fact it could lead to more bleeding and an unsightly scar.

Operative stance

The surgeon must be comfortable when he is operating; the young surgeon will realize very quickly that he has a preferred side to stand. The editor stands on the patient's right, as did Bonney; this allows the dominant right hand to perform all the dissecting, cutting and suturing procedures while the left hand is used for tying, putting tissues on tension and displaying the operative field. The tyro can frequently be seen leaning and contorting as though glued to the spot. He should remember that the feet can be moved to obtain a more comfortable operating position and, if a part of the procedure is more easily performed from the opposite side of the table, he and his assistance should not hesitate in changing places.

The table should be adjusted for the surgeon's requirements to give him a comfortable operating position and the very best access to the operative field. The editor uses varying degrees of head down tilt for most abdominal procedures; this allows the bowel to be easily packed out of the pelvic field and ensures minimal blood pooling in the lower limbs. However, it does make for poor visibility for the scrub nurse and second assistant, and means that special care has to be taken to ensure that the patient does not slide off the operating table. The editor remembers well performing a radical operation on a large patient under epidural analgesia, with the table steeply tilted; all went well except that the patient continuously assisted the surgeon by wriggling back up the table!

When laparoscopic surgery is being performed only a minor degree of head down tilt is required as it is usually very simple to move the bowel contents from the pelvis and to obtain a clear operative field during any minimal access surgery. Relatively rarely special positions of the patient may be required to obtain access to specific areas of the pelvis and external structures.

Draping the patient

Drapes should be applied to the abdomen so that the bony landmarks are visible and accessible. At the mid-line and Pfannenstiel incisions these are the anterior superior iliac spines and the symphysis pubis. The umbilicus should also be visible for the mid-line incision. Some surgeons use plastic adhesive drapes for skin cover and cut through the surface; the editor feels that these are unnecessary for most procedures and reserves their use for covering over and sequestering potential sources of wound infection, such as stomas and sinuses.

The drapes must be placed accurately, as they offer lines which the surgeon will use to orientate himself. An untidily draped abdomen will all too frequently result in a squint ugly scar. It is of paramount importance that the drape clips should not be put into the patient's skin; these small wounds will often cause more discomfort than the incision itself. The incision should also lie within the drapes; the cut must not reach into the towels and if extension is necessary and there is not enough room available, the patient should be redraped. Consequently a very wide area of the abdomen must be prepared for this eventuality.

In modern practice the use of self-adhesive paper drapes is becoming increasingly common. These drapes are of high quality. The adhesion to the skin is firm and complete and does not allow soiling beyond the adhesive area. They can be placed very accurately assisting the surgeon's orientation prior to the incision.

Very few surgeons use skin towels as a separate part of the draping procedure and they will not be described at this stage.

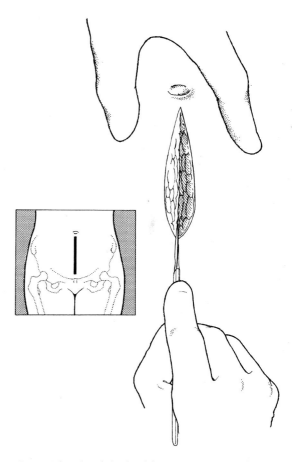

Fig. 6.1 The subumbilical mid-line incision, incising the skin.

The incision

Once the patient has been draped, and the scrub nurse and the anaesthetist are ready, the incision can be performed. The surgeon places his left hand across the upper part of the incision site with the fingers and thumb outstretched; the knife is grasped firmly in the palm of the right hand with the index finger along the length of the handle. A bold stroke is now made accurately down the mid-line the full length of the required incision (Fig. 6.1). The first cut should extend well down into the fatty layers; these are then separated with the knife down to the rectus sheath, which is incised for a short distance in the same line. Small vessels in the fatty layer bleed and may be clipped and tied or diathermied. In the interests of speed some surgeons ignore these small bleeding vessels and simply pick them up at

55

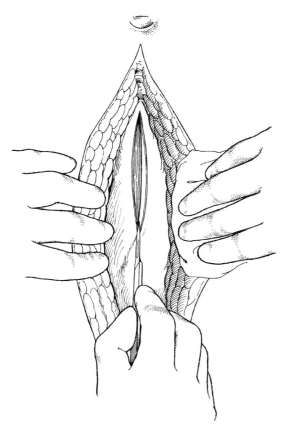

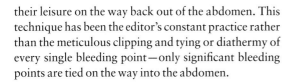

Fig. 6.2 Incising the rectus sheath.

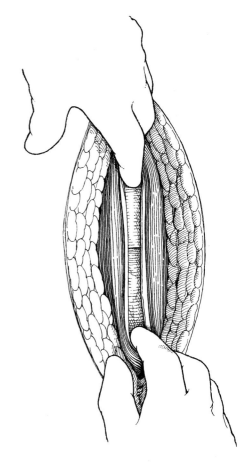

Fig. 6.3 Separating the rectus muscles.

their leisure on the way back out of the abdomen. This technique has been the editor's constant practice rather than the meticulous clipping and tying or diathermy of every single bleeding point—only significant bleeding points are tied on the way into the abdomen.

Extending the rectus incision
The small incision in the rectus sheath has now extended the full length of the skin incision using either the scalpel (Fig. 6.2) or the dissecting scissors. The editor uses the scissors as they allow easy and bloodless separation of the rectus sheath prior to cutting by the simple expedient of running the scissors under the sheath in the fascial plane and opening the blades. The scissors that the authors uses are either Mayo's angled or flat (Bonney's) or lighter scissors of his own design (Monaghan's).

Separation of the recti
The mid-line is identified and the recti separated by using either a knife or the scissors to cut down through the fascia to the posterior layer of the rectus sheath. The incision is now extended the full length of the wound by inserting the index finger of each hand and drawing the hands apart (Fig. 6.3). The fingers run easily along the plane completely separating the muscle and bringing the posterior rectus sheath and the peritoneum into view.

It is important not to deviate from the mid-line as it is easy to traumatize vessels which run along the posterior surface of the rectus sheath, causing troublesome bleeding and haematoma formation. Similarly division of the muscle longitudinally should be avoided.

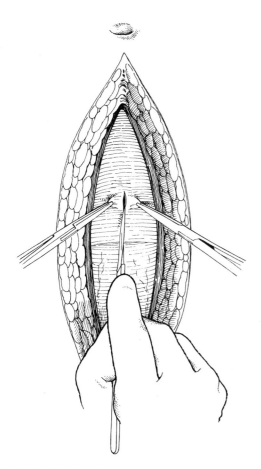

Fig. 6.4 Incising the peritoneum.

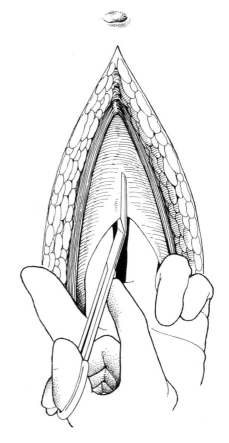

Fig. 6.5 Cutting the peritoneum along the full length of the wound.

Peritoneal incision

The peritoneum is now in full view except in the obese patient where a layer of fat of variable thickness may be present. This fat should be separated gently with the fingers or the dissecting scissors. The peritoneum is now picked up at the junction of the mid and upper third of the wound using two small artery forceps. The mid-line can often be easily identified by the presence of the urachus and the obliterated umbilical arteries shining through the peritoneum. If the urachus is grasped the abdomen can be entered confidently without fear of damage to underlying bowel or bladder.

The surgeon and first assistant now slightly elevate the forceps, the surgeon palpates the fold of peritoneum between finger and thumb to make sure there is no bowel included and then makes a short incision in the

peritoneum (Fig. 6.4). As air enters the cavity of the abdomen the bowel falls away from the abdominal wall and the surgeon can now lengthen the incision under direct vision. If it is clear that there are extensive adhesions beneath the peritoneum then it is prudent to move to another part of the incision and enter the abdominal cavity away from the adhesions.

The edges of the incision are now picked up either by the surgeon and assistant hooking their index fingers under the peritoneum, or by the surgeon elevating the peritoneum with two fingers of the left hand (Fig. 6.5). The opening is extended longitudinally using the scissors for the full length of the wound. Care is taken at the lower end of the wound to be sure that the bladder is not damaged; occasionally, small vessels are cut in this area and require special attention and ligation.

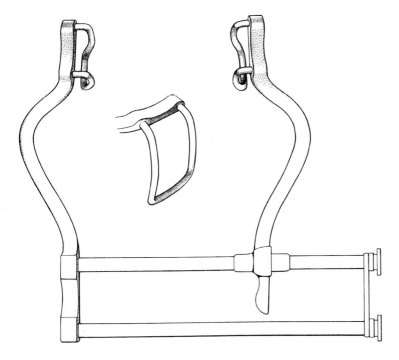

Fig. 6.6 The Balfour self-retaining retractor.

Exploration of the abdomen and retraction

The authors would advocate a combination of manual and authors exploration carried out before and after introducing the self-retaining retractor. The habit of routinely exploring the entire abdomen is one that should be adopted early in the surgeon's career; the process takes a very brief time and can be extremely rewarding. It is of particular importance in cancer surgery where for many tumours the process is part of the surgical staging. If there is any suggestion of malignancy, biopsies and peritoneal washings should also be taken at this time. The development of this habit will allow the surgeon to build up a comprehensive knowledge of normal abdominal organs so that any minor variations will register as his experience increases.

The choice of retractor is very much a personal decision, the editor preferring a Balfour self-retaining retractor (Fig. 6.6) for most routine gynaecological procedures, dispensing with the lower blade and replacing it with a Morris retractor held by the second assistant for all cancer or complicated surgery (Fig. 6.7). This second option allows the bladder to be moved and protected, producing the tissue tension in the parametrial and paravesical areas which is so valuable during dissection of the ureters. Great care should

be taken if the self-retaining retractor is kept in position for an extended period of time, as bruising and even necrosis of the rectus muscles may occur (this is reduced if the patient is fully relaxed). It is interesting that Bonney and Wertheim both preferred manual retraction of the abdominal incision edges by the surgical assistant. This dynamic manual retraction is said to be less traumatic than the use of self-retaining retractors. The choice of retraction technique will clearly depend upon the surgeon's own personal choice and his training.

Packing away the intestines

In order to facilitate access to the pelvis, all small bowel, omentum and redundant loops of the sigmoid colon must be removed from the pelvis. This is achieved by a combination of Trendelenburg or head down positioning and packing away of the intestines. The bowel is removed from the pelvis by the left hand with the fingers spread; a large pack is then spread over the fingers and, by sliding out the left hand, the right hand can then gently lift the bowel above the pelvic brim. Packing is best performed using one very large pack rather than a number of small ones. The pack must have a Raytec radio-opaque marker sewn into it and a long tape attached which is brought out of the abdomen and

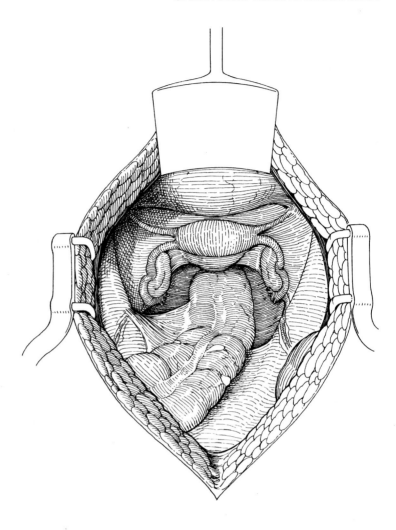

Fig. 6.7 The incision retracted using the
Balfour and Morris retractors.

marked with a clip. It is very important to use wet packs dampened by saline or water; the packs must not be hot, blood heat is all that is required. This wetting and normal temperature is important in order to reduce damage to the bowel and the subsequent increased risk of adhesions.

The authors routinely use very steep Trendelenburg for most procedures; with modern operating tables it is now not necessary to use shoulder rests with all their attendant dangers of nerve compression, but it does help if the table is broken at the knee level so that the Mayo table, if used, can be placed at the lower end of the operating table. All patients should have prophylactic calf compression systems attached prior to their placing on the operating table.

Special circumstances

Previous scar

The surgeon should not feel constrained to utilize a previous scar if that route is inappropriate for the planned procedure. For example, it is folly to attempt to remove a large tumour or cyst through a low transverse incision simply for cosmetic effect. However, if it is necessary to make a different incision it is frequently found that healing may be impaired at the junction of the two scars.

If it is decided to enter the abdomen through the previous scar, the surgeon must decide whether to remove it or to simply incise through it. As a general rule, if the scar is thin it is easier and quicker to simply cut through it; if it is broad or there has been keloid formation, the old scar should be excised. Excision is most easily performed by picking up the ends of the scar using tissue forceps such as Littlewood's forceps. With the assistant holding the scar up the surgeon can cut accurately down either side of it.

Adhesions to the old scar

Previous surgery markedly increases the risk of the development of adhesions, particularly to the back of the scar. Entry into the abdomen must therefore be carried out in a circumspect way. If bowel is adherent to the anterior abdominal wall it should not be separated by pulling or rubbing with a swab. If there is no obvious plane of separation, the 'postage stamp' technique should be used. This involves removal of a 'stamp' of peritoneum with the bowel so that there is no danger of damage to the bowel wall.

Extension of the wound

This only applies to the mid-line and paramedian incisions. For the mid-line incision a lot has been written about how to handle the umbilicus, varying from cutting straight through to circumnavigation and even a curious oblique incision. Extension can be easily and accurately performed if the surgeon and his assistant elevate the upper part of the wound using the index fingers, and the surgeon cuts through all layers with a knife, keeping the abdominal contents in full view. The umbilicus is therefore easily circumnavigated using this technique.

Closure of the abdomen

At the end of the surgical procedure, having made certain that there is no untoward bleeding, the abdominal pack is removed; the swab, instrument and needle count is carried out and reported and confirmed to be satisfactory. There is no great advantage in bringing down the omentum to lie in the pelvis unless there is a wide defect in the peritoneum (see Chapter 12). The abdominal wall can now be closed, maintaining the patient in Trendelenburg whilst the various layers are sutured.

Closing the peritoneum

There is considerable discussion as to whether the abdominal peritoneum should be closed. There is no absolute certainty as to the correct procedure in these

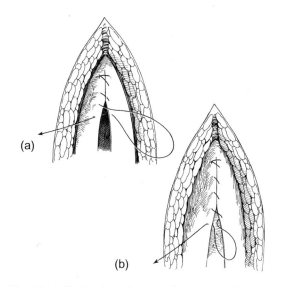

Fig. 6.8 (a) Closing the peritoneum; (b) rectus sheath.

circumstances and therefore we will describe its closure. The peritoneum should be identified and raised by straight tissue forceps attached to the mid points of the wound on either side and at the lowest point. The surgeon then begins to appose the peritoneum from the uppermost part, using an absorbable suture of the modern type such as Dexon or Vicryl. The suture is inserted in a continuous manner, the assistant keeping an even tension on the stitch so that the peritoneum is neither bunched nor so slack that windows appear. The editor often advises assistants that this should be a case of appose and not necrose (Fig. 6.8a).

Closing the rectus sheath

The sheath is closed in the same line as the peritoneum using a similar continuous absorbable suture (Fig. 6.8b).

Fat stitch

In very thin patients it is unnecessary to suture the fat. However, in the majority of patients, fat stitches should be used as a series of interrupted sutures to obliterate any potential space (Fig. 6.9a). Critics state that it is impossible to stitch fat. This may be so, but in women Scarpa's fascia is often well developed and is well worthwhile suturing.

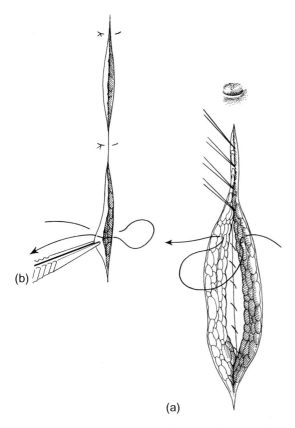

(a)

Fig. 6.9 (a) The fat stitch and skin closure; (b) the fat stitch with interrupted stitches.

Wound drains
Unless there has been exceptional oozing from a very deep abdominal wound, there is no necessity for drains. Infection of the pelvis should always be drained through a separate abdominal stab wound.

Skin closure
There are many techniques of skin closure varying from metal clips through silk to stainless steel. In the editor's experience closure should be by interrupted and not by a continuous method (Fig. 6.9b). This allows any serous or bloody ooze to drain from the wound. The materials which produce least skin reaction and scarring are monofilament materials such as nylon or, more ideally, stainless steel staples in a preloaded stapling device (Fig. 6.10). It is the editor's experience that subcuticular techniques, using absorbable sutures, produce a

thick tender scar. This may be reduced by using a nylon subcuticular stitch, which is removed after a few days.

Variations in technique
Deep tension sutures. If there is a significant risk of wound infection and/or breakdown, e.g. if there has been wound soiling or there is extensive intraperitoneal carcinoma, then it is prudent to support the wound as much as possible. This is best done by using deep tension sutures. The sutures should be of a monofilament material to reduce the introduction of further infection. It is best to use a large curved atraumatic needle. The suture should pass through all layers, being placed wide of the wound edges, so that when it is tied, following the normal layered closure, the plastic tube spacers lie across the wound edges (Fig. 6.11). Usually between four and six deep tension sutures are required.

Mass closure. This technique, which uses a 'far and near' continuous suture technique (Fig. 6.12), has gained in popularity as it provides a simple strong closure with a very low dehiscence rate. Although not so aesthetically satisfying, it is a sound closure system, especially for patients at high risk of wound breakdown.

Transverse or Pfannenstiel incision

The single most important value of this incision is cosmetic. It is important for many women that their abdomens should remain apparently untouched by the surgeon's knife, and using this technique the illusion can be maintained. The incision follows Langer's lines, a short distance above the symphysis pubis, usually just within the pubic hair line. Most minor pelvic surgery can be easily performed through this incision and as the surgeon develops his skills he will find that most hysterectomies, minor tubal and ovarian surgery, and lower segment caesarean sections come within the compass of this route of access. In the author's view, the use of this incision for more radical surgery and particularly Wertheim's hysterectomy should be eschewed, although some clinicians do utilize it in these circumstances.

This incision is also of particular value when operating on the *extremely* obese patient, for the area a short distance above the symphysis pubis is often the thinnest part of the abdominal wall, and if the massive abdominal pannus is lifted up and held out of the way

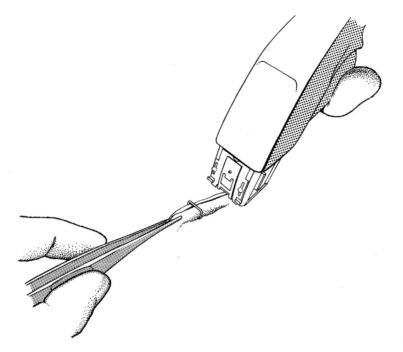

Fig. 6.10 Stapling the abdominal skin.

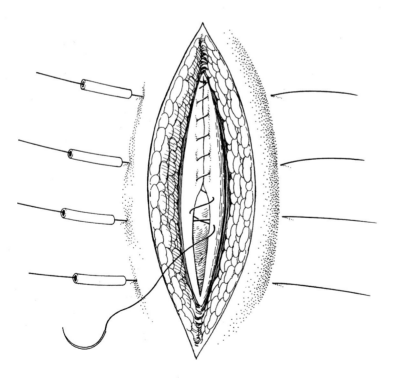

Fig. 6.11 Deep tension sutures.

by large Lane's forceps, access to the abdomen is often amazingly easy.

The incision is not advocated for extreme emergency situations as it takes significantly longer to enter the abdomen using this technique. The incision is also more vascular than the mid-line alternative.

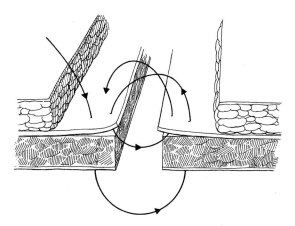

Fig. 6.12 The mass closure technique.

The incision

It is extremely important that the initial skin incision is level and symmetrical. A skewed scar after this incision is less acceptable than after any other. The landmarks of the symphysis and the anterior superior iliac spines must be accessible and not covered by drapes. The drapes must be accurately and evenly placed so as not to mislead the surgeon. The incision should be approximately 12 cm long for a hysterectomy, shorter for more minor procedures. The initial cut is made cleanly through the skin, slightly convex towards the pubis (Fig. 6.13). The fat is incised down to the rectus sheath and the aponeurosis of the external oblique muscle. As the incision is completed, the surgeon should make short cuts into the sheath on either side of the mid-line. Small vessels in the fat are more numerous than in the mid-line incision and must be clipped and tied or diathermied. In particular, a large vein at each lateral edges of the incision are often seen and should be incised and tied unless they can be gently pushed on one side. The techniques of tearing the fatty layers have been advocated and although functionally satisfactory, they are not aesthetically so.

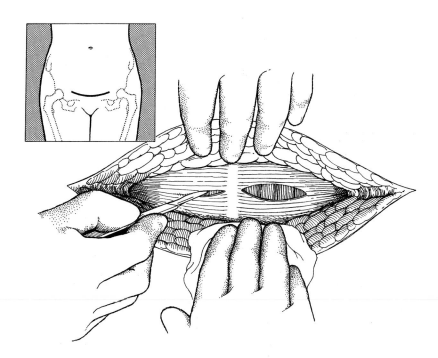

Fig. 6.13 The Pfannenstiel incision.

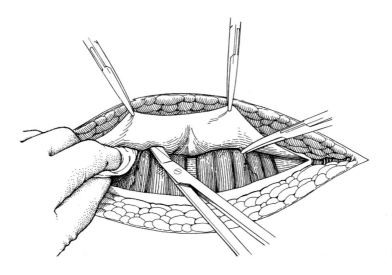

Fig. 6.14 Dissecting the rectus sheath.

Incision of the aponeurosis

The short incisions in the rectus sheath are now extended for the full length of the skin incision using either a scalpel or the Bonney's dissecting scissors. The upper and then the lower edges of the incision are now grasped in turn by small artery forceps, elevated and the underlying muscle separated from the sheath by a combination of blunt (swab) and sharp (scissors) dissection (Fig. 6.14). Small vessels running parallel to the midline are clipped and tied. The rectus muscles are now separated vertically and the peritoneum visualized.

Opening the peritoneum

This is performed in the same manner as for the midline incision, keeping a watchful eye on the upper limits of the bladder. It is usually easy to see the upper limit of the bladder by identifying urachus as it appears as a narrow fibrous band in the mid-line. Grasping the urachus and incising it is a simple way of entering the peritoneal cavity.

Closure of the abdomen

Closing the abdomen

This is carried out as in the mid-line incision, using a continuous absorbable suture material for the peritoneum and sheath. It is superfluous to suture the rectus muscles together as the design of the wound gives adequate strength.

Fat stitch

This is particularly useful in this incision as Scarpa's fascia is well developed and easily defined. All subcuticular space should be obliterated if possible since this vascular incision has a significant risk of haematoma formation.

Wound drains

It is the editor's impression that the transverse incision requires drainage more frequently than the mid-line. However, this is not a significant disadvantage and the use of wound drains should not be regarded as a mark of failure. If there is evidence of more oozing than usual, and this may occur particularly after multiple entries in the same site, the surgeon is well advised to utilize the drainage procedure. As soon as drainage has ceased, often within 24 h, the drain can be removed without great discomfort to the patient, and without any residual scarring.

Further reading

Te Linde RW, Mattingly RF. *Operative Gynaecology*, 4th edn. Philadelphia: Lippincot, 1970. This is one of the great standard textbooks of gynaecological surgery with excellent descriptions of the methods of entering and closing the abdomen.

Joel-Cohen S. *Abdominal and Vaginal Hysterectomy*, 2nd edn. London: William Heinemann, 1977. This covers the various techniques in full and is a mine of useful information.

For the student who feels that a study of potential problems is essential, the editor would recommend the early sections in the text *Complications of Surgery in General* by J.A.R. Smith (1984), published by Baillière Tindall, London. The author extensively discusses the various techniques of opening and closing the abdomen, listing all the advantages and disadvantages of each approach.

In the text *Wound Healing for Surgeons* (1984) by Bucknall and Ellis, published by Baillière Tindall, London, Professor Harold Ellis reviews the many factors which a surgeon must take into account when making and closing an abdominal wound (pp. 124–42).

We also recommend the readers to review chapter 9 in the *Atlas of Pelvic Surgery* by C.R. Wheeless, published by Williams & Wilkins, 3rd edition, 1997.

7

Total abdominal hysterectomy

It is interesting that Bonney used the more correct title for this chapter of 'Abdominal total hysterectomy'; the current editor has changed to the present form so that the accepted abbreviation of TAH is consistent. This operation remains the accepted basic procedure for removing the uterus in the management of benign disease; it is also used in oncological care for the management of cervical intraepithelial neoplasia (CIN), cancer of the corpus uteri and ovary.

Once a decision to perform a hysterectomy has been made, the surgeon must decide and recommend to the patient the most appropriate route. The choices available currently include abdominal, vaginal, laparoscopically assisted vaginal and subtotal. Various forms of total laparoscopic hysterectomy are rarely indicated or performed. The factors determining the choice are discussed in Chapter 8.

The technique described here is inevitably a melange of many influences upon the author, not least previous editions of this book.

Instruments

The gynaecological general set described in Chapter 2 is used.

Patient preparation

The patient is usually admitted as close to surgery as possible; when the operation is planned for the morning, the day before is the usual admission time. If an afternoon list is planned, the morning of operation is most appropriate. Increasingly patients are reviewed and preplanned in preadmission clinics, which reduce the preoperative admission times significantly.

It is essential that the patient fully understands the scope of the surgery intended, particularly in relationship to the removal or preservation of the ovaries. Occasionally, fashions concerning preservation or removal of the cervix will appear. The patient must be quite clear as to the extent of any surgery.

Preadmission clinics and early admission will be an opportunity to go through the procedure with the patient. The blood should be taken for a full blood count, grouping of the blood type and the preservation of the sample in case a transfusion is required. Transfusion for most hysterectomies is rarely required. Patients will be reviewed and consented by the anaesthetist and any extra investigations organized.

It remains traditional to shave the abdomen for an abdominal procedure; in the author's view this is only necessary for the visible part of the pubic hair. The traditional 'through and through' technique is unnecessary. Conversely, for a vaginal hysterectomy, only the pubic area needs shaving. It is important to perform any shaving as close to surgery as practicable. It is also unnecessary and potentially dangerous to over clean the abdominal wall with antiseptics as recolonization with more malign bacteria may occur prior to surgery.

The balance between late admission and reducing preoperative tension is a fine one. A good night of sleep before operation is advantageous and this may best be achieved in the patient's own bed. Some patients may require sedation prior to surgery others will not.

The operation

Following general anaesthesia, the vulva and vagina are cleaned and the bladder catheterized and emptied. Usually if the hysterectomy is being performed as the only procedure, and the patient is fit, an indwelling catheter is not necessary. If the procedure is part of the management of, for example, ovarian cancer an indwelling catheter will greatly assist fluid assessment both intraoperatively and postoperatively.

The use of intravaginal dyes or packs is superfluous. Suturing and occlusion of the cervix when dealing with corpus cancer is also quite unnecessary.

The incision
The choice of incision is dealt with in Chapter 6.

Exploration of the abdomen and pelvis
This important preamble is dealt with in Chapter 6.

Clamping and dividing the round and infundibulopelvic ligaments
The uterus is elevated by placing the surgeon's left hand into the pouch of Douglas and lifting the body of the uterus to put the uterosacral ligaments on the stretch. A medium-sized straight pressure forcep is placed on either side of the cornu to include the origins of the tubes and the round ligament approximately 1 cm from the uterine wall (Fig. 7.1). When the handles of the two clamps are placed together and held in the left hand, the whole uterus can be manoeuvred. When the uterus is elevated, the round ligaments become prominent bands passing anterolaterally behind the peritoneum towards the inguinal ligament. The round ligaments are picked up at roughly their mid points with a medium-sized pressure clamp and then incised on their medial side (Fig. 7.1). This clamp is handed to the assistant thus opening the anterior part of the broad ligament. The soft areolar tissue within the leaves of the broad ligament is now revealed.

The author recommends that at this point the simple manoeuvre of opening up the retroperitoneal space down the point at which the ureter is visible is an important practice which once learned can be applied to virtually all pelvic procedures. This technique allows the ureter to be visualized in the upper pelvic part of its course where it lies close to the infundibulopelvic ligament, a site of all too frequent clamping of the ureter.

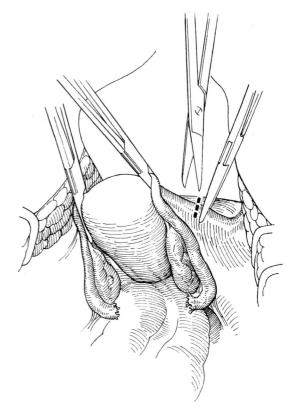

Fig. 7.1 Cutting the round ligaments.

Once the course of the ureter has been identified, the index finger of the left hand can be used to elevate the infundibulopelvic ligament allowing a clamp to be placed either on the medial or the lateral side of the ovary dependent on whether these structures are to be preserved or removed (Fig. 7.2). If the ovaries are to be removed they can be moved medially on the index finger and a clamp applied directly to the vessels within the infundibulopelvic ligament. If the ovaries are to be preserved, the clamp is simply placed on the medial side of the ovary and the tube and ovarian ligament are cut.

Ligation of the round and infundibulopelvic ligaments
It is useful to ligate these ligaments at an early stage in the procedure to leave the operative field as clear as possible. The pedicles may be stitch ligatured or simply tied, as is authors' practice. The round ligament tie can be 'left long' and attached to a small Spencer Wells clip, thus maintaining tension on the peritoneum

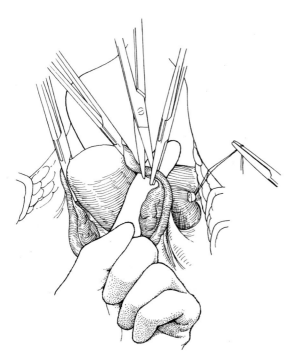

Fig. 7.2 Cutting the infundibulopelvic ligament.

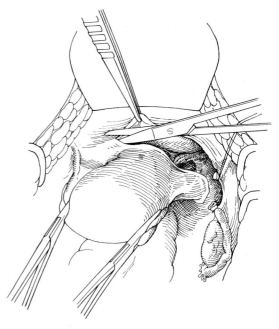

Fig. 7.3 Incising the uterovesical fold.

laterally and assisting in 'opening up' the lateral broad ligament space, providing improved access to the parametrial tissues. *NB*: a clip should never be left on a pedicle containing a blood vessel such as the infundibulopelvic ligaments.

Reflecting the bladder

It is logical to incise the peritoneum overlying the bladder along the line of the uterovesical fold at the same time as the round ligaments are divided. With the scissors in the surgeon's right hand and the assistant elevating the peritoneum over the bladder with Mayo toothed forceps, it is very simple to run the scissors under the tented peritoneum separating the bladder and then to incise the peritoneum in a curved line across the front of the uterus to meet up with the round ligament on the opposite side (Fig. 7.3). If the level of incision is too high the peritoneum will not separate from the front of the uterus and if too low bleeding will occur from the small vessels on the surface of the bladder.

Once this incision is complete, the bladder can be gently separated from the anterior surface of the uterus and then the cervix. The technique to achieve this ma-

noeuvre will vary; the authors' preferred choice is to use the relatively blunt closed tips of the Monaghan scissors to gently push and occasionally incise the tissues attaching the bladder to the uterus. If the surgeon begins close to the mid-line and gently separates, staying close to the uterus and the cervix, a clean plane will be identified. A thin gauze swab over the finger may be used to push the angles of the bladder away from the cervix if preferred (Fig. 7.4). This entire process is assisted by the surgeon maintaining tension of the uterus by gently drawing it upwards using the clamps originally placed close to the cornu.

The lower limit of the cervix can be readily identified by observing the indentation as the cervix ends and the anterior fornix begins. It is important to be sure that the lateral parts of the bladder are adequately reflected as the ureters are very close to the upper vagina at this point. If the patient has had a previous lower segment caesarean section, the dissection may be more difficult and will require significantly more sharp dissection in order to release the scar tissue; this sharp dissection is in fact less traumatic and fundamentally safer than blunt pushing of the tissues. Close attention should be paid to the tissue plane on the surface of the lower uterus and cervix, as this is the optimal and safest position for any sharp dissection.

Where the uterus is a little immobile it often helps if the surgeon puts the left hand into the pouch of Douglas, bringing the thumb around the uterus to the anterior part at the level of the junction between the corpus and the cervix; the fingers of the left hand pressing into the posterior fornix will cause the cervix to protrude forwards and the position of the anterior fornix becomes more obvious. The effect of this step is to make the application of clamps to the parametrium and the paracervical tissue easier as well as causing the bladder to drop 'below' the level of the cervix.

Clamping the uterine vessels and the vaginal angles
The uterine arteries arise from the anterior division of the internal iliac arteries deep in the lateral pelvis at the level of the obturator fossa. They then pass medially, overlying the ureter as it approaches the lateral part of the cervix. The artery divides close to the uterus at the level of the internal os into a descending and an ascending branch. The ascending branch, which is larger, runs close to the lateral sides of the uterus and can be seen as it passes in a tortuous fashion from below upwards feeding small branches into the substance of the uterine corpus. This vessel is clamped by placing a pressure forcep with the tip abutting onto the myometrium at right angles to the long axis and at roughly the mid point of the length of the uterus (Fig. 7.5). The pedicle is divided as close to the forcep as possible. The same procedure is performed on the opposite side. A further forcep, ideally one with longitudinal ridges such as a Zeppelin,

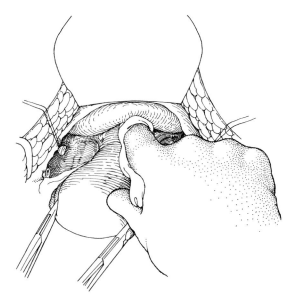

Fig. 7.4 Separating the bladder.

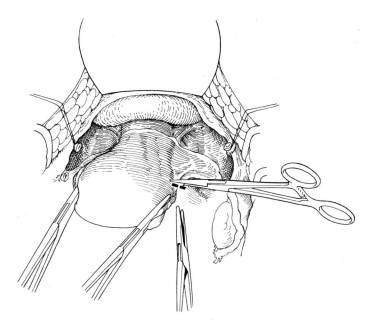

Fig. 7.5 Clamping the uterine artery.

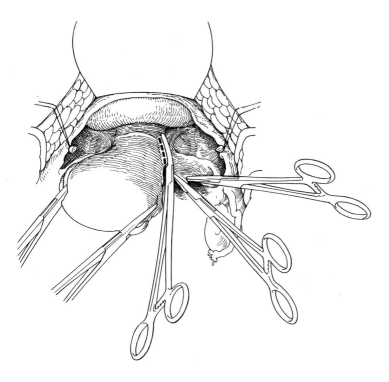

Fig. 7.6 Clamping the parametrium.

is now placed parallel to the cervix, squeezing the paracervical tissue off the side of the cervix. It is advantageous to incise on the medial side of the forcep before placing the one on the opposite side as this step reduces tension on the tissues, allows the forcep to be placed very close to the cervix and reduces the risk of the tissue sliding out of the forcep. This is particularly important if the cervix is bulky and access is limited. These forceps may be curved or angled (the author prefers a slight curve as the forcep can be used to 'fit' the shape of the cervix to a very high degree). Each forcep should be placed so as to reach the vaginal angles but should not include the tissue of the vaginal epithelium (Fig. 7.6). The tissue on the medial side of these forceps is now incised either with powerful scissors such as the Bonney or with a knife for greater accuracy.

Clamping the uterosacral ligaments
It is not the authors' constant practice to clamp and divide the uterosacral ligaments. However, if the uterus is not mobile and is clearly bound down by contracture of these ligaments due to scarring from previous endometriosis or infection, then mobility can be advantageously achieved by clamping and cutting the ligaments used a curved Zeppelin or similar forcep.

Opening the vagina and removing the uterus
The surgeon should now draw up the uterus with the left hand and clearly identify the vagina using the techniques described above (see Ligation of the round and infundibulopelvic ligaments, p. 67), making sure that the bladder is safely reflected. A knife is now plunged into the anterior fornix (Fig. 7.7), often accompanied by a hiss of air entering the vagina; the knife blade is then run to the right and to the left using the tips of the lowest forcep as the lateral landmark. The editor would now recommend the clamping of the uterosacral ligaments at this point. This is done by passing the curved Zeppelin clamps backwards so that each blade comes to lie on either side of the vagina in the lateral part of the posterior fornix. This has the effect of clamping the uterosacral ligaments close to their attachments to the posterior part of the cervix. The tissue in these last two clamps is now incised and the uterus removed from the pelvis. The entire circumference of the vagina is now visible.

Ligating the lateral uterine and cervical pedicles
The two or perhaps three pedicles on either side are now stitch ligatured using a 0 or 1 Vicryl or Dexon suture; with these materials there is no need for double suturing of the pedicles.

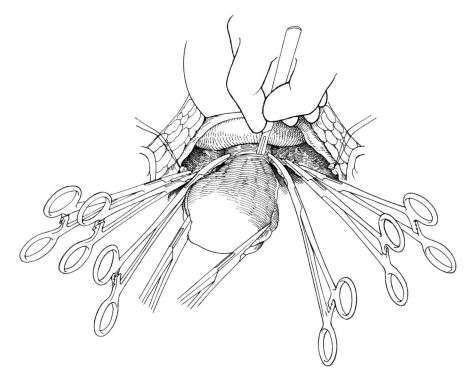

Fig. 7.7 Incising the vagina (showing all clamps in place).

It is important to obliterate any 'dead space' between pedicles as these may be or become the site of troublesome bleeding in the intra- or postoperative period. Accurate placing of the sutures allows an overlapping technique to be used, obliterating any spaces.

Dealing with the vaginal edge

It is frequently recommended that the vaginal edge be grasped with a tissue forcep for identification and manoeuvring purposes. The editor would recommend abandonment of this technique and its replacement by simply picking up the posterior edge of the vagina with the stitch that is to be used to suture the vaginal edge. The long free end of the stitch can be grasped with a clip which is placed over the edge of the wound (Fig. 7.8), and used to place light tension on the vaginal edge, allowing the needle to be accurately placed as the edge is sutured circumferentially. Whether the vagina is left open or closed, this technique is simple and allows maximum access with minimal equipment in the wound. The excellent visibility can be further improved by adopting the following suture technique.

The posterior vaginal suture should be placed at approximately 5 mm intervals and the suture locked in a form of 'blanket' stitch. This has the effect of rolling the vaginal edge inwards. Once the corners of the vagina have been reached, carefully identified and sutured, the stitch should change to a 'rolling' pattern causing the anterior edge to evert, thus making the inner edge of the vagina totally visible and accessible.

This part of the procedure can be performed without any active participation of the assistant. It has been the editor's practice to leave the vault of the vagina 'open' although there does not appear to be a great deal of evidence of the value of either 'open or closed'.

Closing of the abdominal peritoneum

The pelvis is finally checked for haemostasis and the pedicle stitches on the round ligaments are cut. Since the eighth edition of this book it has become clear that there is no need to close pelvic peritoneum and indeed there may be significant disadvantages. If the pelvic peritoneum is observed as the tension on the abdominal wall retractor is relaxed, it will be seen that

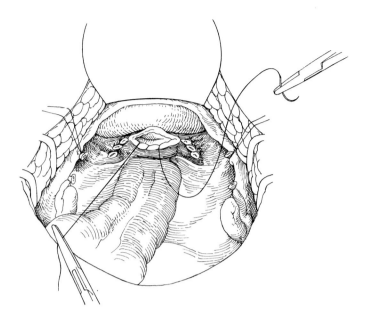

Fig. 7.8 Suturing the vaginal edge.

the peritoneal edges lie close together transversely across the pelvis. All that is required is that the abdominal pack be removed and the sigmoid colon lain down into the pelvic cavity. It is superfluous to draw down the omentum as so many surgeons ritualistically do.

Drains should only be very rarely required following a hysterectomy.

Closing the abdominal cavity
This is described in Chapter 6.

Prophylactic antibiotics
The majority of surgeons would now regard the use of intraoperative antibiotics as the norm. It is important to be cognisant of any allergies and to make sure that the manufacturer's time cover is observed; it may be necessary to repeat the antibiotics if the surgery is unduly prolonged. The reduction in postoperative febrile morbidity is well proven, especially when antibiotics efficacious against *Bacteroides* are used.

Variations in technique

There are many modifications to this technique. This one described is an evolution of constant analysis over 30 years. Each surgeon should first learn a standard procedure from their chiefs and then by dint of careful analysis and modification develop their own 'style'. This analysis should take the form of constantly questioning the value of every move, determining whether the step can be eliminated or improved and made more efficient. Always, the aim must be to reduce tissue handling and improve patient recovery times.

Subtotal hysterectomy

The editor has to declare that to date he has never performed such an operation and to this day does not see any indication or value in such a procedure. He also acknowledges that we are once more passing through a fashion for the occasional performance of this operation. This fashion is driven by a misguided belief that the procedure reduces the risk of post-hysterectomy prolapse and facilitates the orgasm. We know of no such evidence.

Further reading

There are many textbooks of gynaecological surgical technique, each confidently extolling its own perfect method of performing this standard procedure. As stated in the first chapter in this text, the trainee should avidly read every available book on each operation, carefully studying every variation and nuance, and then develop his own style.

If there was one name which the editor would recommend to every trainee and gynaecological surgeon it would be that of Joel-Cohen. His writings always stimulate; one can feel the enthusiasm exuding from the page. The editor does not agree with all that he says and writes but always finds conversations and correspondence with him thought-provoking, and they frequently make him seriously review his practice. One such chapter is Chapter 2 in *Clinics in Obstetrics and Gynaecology* vol. 5, no. 3, December 1978, 'Gynaecological Surgery' David Lees and Albert Singer (eds), published by W. B. Saunders, London. The chapter is a wealth of argument and idiosyncracy; it is written from the heart of one of the finest thinking gynaecologists of the present day. The chapter also demonstrates Joel-Cohen's technique for opening the abdomen, which has aroused so much controversy world wide.

The editor finds it interesting that Joel-Cohen also roundly condemns the subtotal hysterectomy.

8 Total hysterectomy for cervical and broad ligament fibroids

Victor Bonney developed, in the course of his surgical career, a particular skill in dealing with fibroids/leiomyomas in almost every site within the pelvis. As with the previous edition, therefore, it would be insulting to the memory of the master surgeon to attempt to rewrite this chapter. Very few minor modifications have been made to the text in an attempt to place the techniques previously described in context with contemporary gynaecological surgical practice, which hopefully add to the exemplary account of these procedures that has gone before.

A large cervical fibroid growing from the supravaginal cervix is not usually suitable for treatment by standard hysterectomy techniques. This is because the tumour may be impacted in the pelvis and overhang the vaginal vault so much that this cannot be reached until the myoma is dislocated upwards or removed by myomectomy. In order to understand the technique of the removal of these tumours an appreciation of their anatomical relationships is necessary.

Cervical fibroids may be classified as:

1 *Anterior*, where a tumour arising from the superficial muscle of the anterior lip of the cervix bulges forwards and undermines the bladder.

2 *Posterior*, where a tumour of the posterior part of the cervix either flattens the pouch of Douglas backwards, compressing the rectum against the sacrum or, in the rarer form, undermines the peritoneum in the bottom of the pouch of Douglas and obliterates the cul-de-sac, lifts the serous membrane off the anterior surface of the rectum and sacrum, and pushes down between the vagina and rectum, separating Waldeyer's fascia.

3 *Lateral*, where the myoma, starting on the side of the cervix burrows out into the broad ligament and ex-

pands it. These tumours in their growth outwards may fill the whole broad ligament and sometimes find their way between layers of the mesocolon and the bowel lying upon them.

Their relation to the ureter is most important. Most commonly, this structure is underneath the fibroid and to the lateral side. Very rarely, when the fibroid begins to develop under the ureter, it may be lifted onto the upper surface of the tumour. However, wherever the ureter and uterine artery may be in relation to the fibroid, they will always be extracapsular. A knowledge and appreciation of the importance of this fact will turn a potentially dangerous procedure into a relatively safe and easy operation.

4 *Central*, where the tumour, either of interstitial or of submucous origin, expands the cervix equally in all directions. This variety of tumour may present all the anatomical vagaries mentioned in connection with the other three varieties. Upon opening the abdominal cavity, a central cervical myoma can be recognized at once because the cavity of the pelvis is more or less filled by a tumour, elevated on top of which is the uterus like 'the lantern on the top of St Paul's'. This characteristic appearance does not occur when there are two or more fibroids in the body of the uterus. Occasionally, a submucous fibroid arising in the fundus of the uterus may burrow downwards to lie in the position of the cervix and may form a pseudocervical fibroid, but these are exceedingly rare.

5 Lastly, cervical fibroids may be *multiple*, so that a lateral myoma may be present on both sides, or an anterior myoma may be coexistent with a posterior tumour, or a lateral myoma may complicate either an anterior or a posterior one.

The operation for the removal of a cervical myoma can be difficult, and may at times be an extremely formidable undertaking. We have knowledge of patients with this condition whose abdomens have been closed as inoperable even by senior surgeons who were obviously unaware of the steps described below to make the operation relatively simple and safe. Surgical difficulties associated with this operation are, however, greatly enhanced by a lack of knowledge of the technique most suitable to the particular occasion and ignorance on the operator's part of the altered anatomical relations of the surrounding structures. It is for this reason that we have laid such stress upon the disturbance of the normal anatomy by cervical myomas.

Instruments

The gynaecological general set described in Chapter 2 is used.

Patient preparation

It is not the authors' practice to pretreat these women with gonadotropin-releasing hormone (GnRH) analogues in an attempt to shrink the fibroids and reduce their vascularity. A major concern with the use of these agents is that they can destroy the fine plane of cleavage between the capsule of the tumour and the surrounding structures, thus eliminating one of the very few 'godsends' that are available when attempting to deal with these conditions surgically.

The preamble described in Chapter 7 is followed, although an indwelling catheter may be advisable as these complex operations can be prolonged, and with an over-zealous anaesthetist, an enlarging bladder during the course of the operation can become an unnecessary cause for frustration.

The incision

The discussions previously given in Chapter 6 are particularly apt when dealing with these conditions.

Hysterectomy for a central cervical myoma by transverse incision

The operation

Opening of the abdominal cavity
As cervical myomas usually raise the bladder much above its normal level, special care must be taken not to injure it.

Examining the abdomen and packing off the intestines
See Chapter 6.

Clamping and dividing the ovarian vessels and round ligaments
The upper part of the broad ligament, containing the ovarian artery and ligament, is clamped and divided in the usual way on each side (Chapter 7, see Figs 7.1 and 7.2). In many of these cases, however, the uterine vessels are so elevated on the surface of the tumour that they run almost parallel with the ovarian vessels, the result being a formidable vascular leash converging towards the cornu on each side. In such circumstances, the separate clamping of the ovarian contingent is almost impossible, and the whole mass must be seized and divided. From the many vessels thus opened up, very brisk haemorrhage may occur, which must be immediately controlled by the application of several pressure forceps. It is most important to make sure that the ureter has not been displaced upwards so that it is lying in association with these vessels. Many ureters have been severed or damaged during the surgical treatment of cervical myomas.

The clamping of the uterine vessels is merely temporary, as these vessels will presently be divided again lower down.

In some cases, the ovarian vessels can be isolated by first dividing the round ligament and then inserting the finger through the hole in the peritoneum, thus undermining them and lifting them up, so they can be easily secured.

Dissecting down the anterior flap of peritoneum
An incision is made between the points where the round ligaments have been divided, through the upper limit of the loose peritoneum in front of the uterus and well above the level of the bladder reflection (Fig. 8.1). The bladder is then separated, together with the anterior flap of peritoneum, from the surface of the expanded

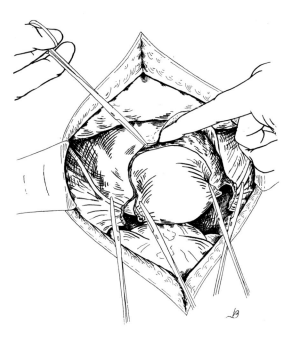

Fig. 8.1 Reflecting the anterior peritoneal flap.

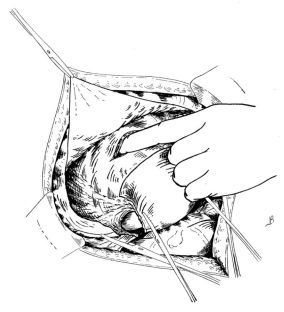

Fig. 8.2 Opening the capsule of the tumour.

supravaginal cervix and continued down until the vagina is reached. Due to stretching and displacement of the bladder, many of the fine adhesions between the anterior aspects of the uterus/cervix and the bladder are often eliminated thus allowing this step to be completed with surprising ease. Steps described in the technique of total hysterectomy (see Chapter 7) to safeguard the uterovesical angle should be followed in detail. Special care must be taken to see that the bladder is not injured, as it will probably be considerably displaced upwards. If there is difficulty in identifying the superior aspect of the bladder, after incising the uterovesical peritoneal fold between the two round ligaments, pick up the superior flap of peritoneum with a pair of dissecting forceps and strip the peritoneum off the underlying structures using the Monaghan scissors, taking care to remain superficial. This dissection is continued until the dense attachment between the peritoneum and the upper aspect of the uterus is reached. By de-peritonealizing the anterior area of the uterus, the superior aspects of the distorted bladder are more easily identified.

Ascertaining the plane of cleavage
The capsule of the tumour formed by the tissues of the expanded supravaginal cervix is incised with a scalpel

for about 5 cm. The index finger of the left hand is inserted through the incision and the exact plane of separation between the tumour and its capsule is defined (Fig. 8.2). The capsular incision may be either transverse or vertical. The advantage of the former is that it can be placed well above the level of bladder reflection and so reduce the risk of vesical damage. The disadvantage is that it cuts across vessels, which results in increased haemorrhage. The vertical incision, on the other hand, can be placed over the most avascular area, usually the mid-line, and can extend up into the body of the uterus if necessary so as to expose the upper limits of the tumour. The transverse incision was used extensively by Bonney, and is preferred by the authors.

Enlarging the incision in the capsule
The incision is now extended across the supravaginal cervix (Fig. 8.3).

It is at this point, when incising the capsule of the tumour that the bladder is most at risk of being injured.

Enucleation of the tumour
A volsellum is fixed on to the anterior surface of the tumour, now exposed through the incision in its capsule. The tumour is then pulled upwards as much as

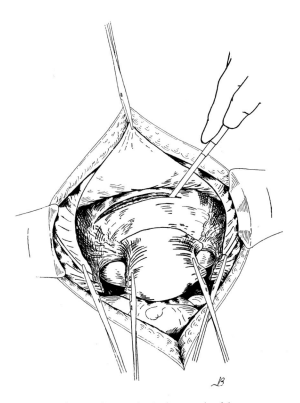

Fig. 8.3 Enlarging the opening in the capsule of the tumour.

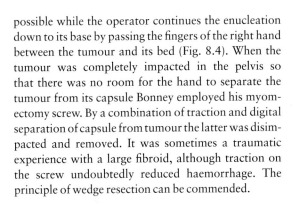

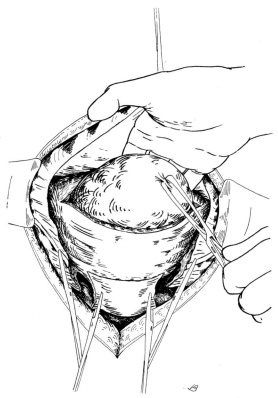

Fig. 8.4 Enucleating the tumour.

possible while the operator continues the enucleation down to its base by passing the fingers of the right hand between the tumour and its bed (Fig. 8.4). When the tumour was completely impacted in the pelvis so that there was no room for the hand to separate the tumour from its capsule Bonney employed his myomectomy screw. By a combination of traction and digital separation of capsule from tumour the latter was disimpacted and removed. It was sometimes a traumatic experience with a large fibroid, although traction on the screw undoubtedly reduced haemorrhage. The principle of wedge resection can be commended.

Removal of the uterus
After the removal of the tumour, the uterine vessels can be clamped under direct vision. The anatomy of the parametrium will be disturbed by the expanded cervix and one or more clamps may be needed on each side to secure the enlarged vessels of the descending branch of the uterine artery (Fig. 8.5). These clamps should be

placed close and parallel to the lateral border of the cervix. The limit of the cervix can now be felt by finger and thumb and the vagina transected at the correct level (Fig. 8.6). Apart from these minor modifications, the operation proceeds as already described under total hysterectomy (see Chapter 7).

Ligation of the ovarian and uterine vessels
See Chapter 7.

Suturing the broad ligaments and peritoneal flaps
See Chapter 7.

Closing the abdominal cavity
See Chapter 6.

Difficulties and dangers

The surgeon may find some difficulty in enucleating the tumour; this is nearly always due to the fact that his

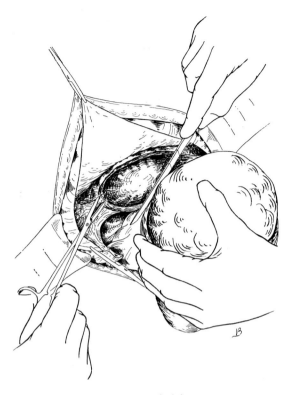

Fig. 8.5 Hysterectomy: securing the left uterine artery.

fingers are not within the true capsule. The commonest error is to attempt to peel off the peritoneum only; or, again, there may be one or two layers of connective tissue under the peritoneum which, partly separating, are mistaken for the capsule. Lastly, the incision to open up the capsule may be too deep, and the operator, unknowingly, may be trying to separate the outer layer of the tumour from its deeper parts. If the right plane between the capsule and the tumour is identified, the latter can generally be freed quite easily.

If the tumour has been or is inflamed, the capsule may be adherent to it, and the adhesions may have to be cut through.

Advantages of the method

This special method is applicable to all cases of central cervical myomas, whatever their size, except in those unusual cases in which the bladder is so raised on the front of the uterus that it is impossible to get at the vaginal vault. The enucleation being accomplished within the capsule, all danger of wounding such important structures as the ureter, rectum and bladder is avoided, whereas an attempt to perform total hysterectomy by

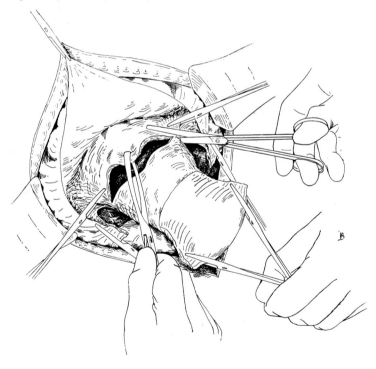

Fig. 8.6 Removing the uterus.

the usual method will be fraught with a risk to those structures that increases with the size and fixity of the tumour.

Hysterectomy for an anterior cervical myoma

An anterior cervical myoma takes up one of two positions: either it undermines the bladder and elevates it on its upper surface or it forces its way up between the peritoneum covering the posterior wall of the bladder and the musculature of the viscus. In the first case, unless the displacement of the bladder is appreciated, it will stand a good chance of being wounded when the parietal incision is made. It should also be borne in mind that the round ligaments may be so elevated that they form the highest ridge in the broad ligament, and that, because the tumour bulges into the wound and retroverts the body of uterus, the landmarks of the ovary and the fallopian tubes are hidden from the operator. In these circumstances, we have seen the round ligaments mistaken for the fold containing the ovarian vessels, and clamped and divided as such, with the result that this division, being extended too far forwards, has opened the elevated bladder. Because of this elevation of the bladder, it is more than ever necessary to exercise care in opening the abdomen; the peritoneal cavity should be opened at the top of the incision, which should be extended upwards when this is necessary for safe entry.

The operation

Opening of the abdominal cavity
Comments previously made should be considered.

Examining the abdominal cavity and packing off the intestines
See Chapter 6.

Clamping the round ligaments
The round ligaments, having been very carefully identified and their relation to the bladder defined, are clamped and divided close to their attachment to the uterus. If there is difficulty in identifying the round ligaments at the onset of the operation as a result of anatomical distortion, a loose flap of peritoneum on the lateral pelvic side wall should be incised allowing entry

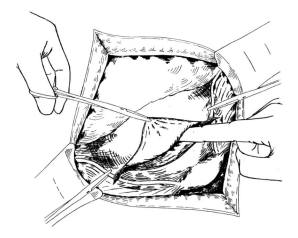

Fig. 8.7 Hysterectomy for anterior cervical myoma; separating the anterior peritoneum.

into the retroperitoneal space. The incision is then extended caudally and medially until the thick band of the round ligament is identified, at which point it can be clamped and divided safely under direct vision.

Incising the peritoneum and capsule over the tumour
The peritoneum covering the expanded supravaginal cervix, together with the round ligaments, is now divided at the upper limit of the loose attachment of the peritoneum to the uterus, this point being, if necessary, defined beforehand by undermining the peritoneum with the finger, or the assistant elevating the tissue with a pair of toothed dissectors. The incision commences on the left-hand side just external to the point where the round ligaments are clamped and extends to a similar point on the opposite side (Fig. 8.7). The anterior peritoneal flap is now pushed off the surface of the expanded supravaginal cervix until the reflection of the bladder is reached and the capsule of tumour is then divided just above the level of bladder attachment. It must be remembered that no myoma, however superficially placed, is truly subperitoneal; there is always a thin layer of expanded uterine muscle covering it.

Enucleation of the base of the tumour
The peritoneum and capsule are now together carefully pushed off the face of the tumour, which is gradually enucleated with the first and second fingers of the right hand as far as its base, care being taken not to injure the bladder. This enucleation is assisted by fixing the

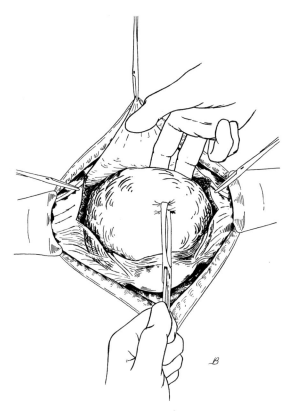

Fig. 8.8 Enucleating the tumour.

volsellum to the tumour and pulling on this with the left hand (Fig. 8.8).

Securing the ovarian vessel
Directly the tumour has been raised from its bed, the upper parts of the broad ligaments containing the ovarian vessels are brought into view. These are divided on each side between two pairs of forceps in the usual way (Fig. 8.9).

Clamping of the uterine vessels and removal of the uterus
The tumour, together with the uterus, is drawn out of the wound. The uterine vessels are then clamped on each side and total hysterectomy performed by first opening the anterior vaginal wall as described in Chapter 7.

Ligating the vessels
See Chapter 7.

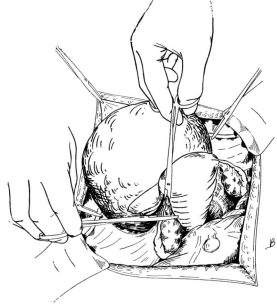

Fig. 8.9 Clamping the ovarian vessels.

Treatment of the vaginal vault
See Chapter 7.

Suturing the peritoneal flaps
See Chapter 7.

Closing the abdominal cavity
See Chapter 6.

Hysterectomy for a central cervical myoma by hemisection of the uterus

Central cervical myomas are frequently best removed by hemisection of the uterus followed by hysterectomy, a technique originally introduced by Rutherford Morrison. This method is particularly indicated when the tumour, either central or posterior, so raises the bladder that, on the abdomen being opened, the uterovesical pouch is found obliterated and the uterus is so covered by the bladder that only its fundus presents. In such cases it is impossible to adopt the method of transverse section of the capsule described before in this chapter, as the intervening bladder cannot be sufficiently pushed down.

The operation

Abdominal incision

The abdominal cavity is opened by the method described above, taking the same care to avoid the bladder.

Examining the abdomen and packing off the intestines

See Chapter 6.

Clamping and dividing the ovarian vessels and round ligaments

See Chapter 7.

Separation of the anterior peritoneum and bladder

An incision is made from one round ligament to the other at the level of the upper limit of the loose attachment of the peritoneum where it is stretched over the tumour and the anterior surface of the uterus. The peritoneum, together with the bladder, is now pushed downwards with a swab as far as possible off the face of the expanded supravaginal cervix as in Fig. 8.1.

Hemisection of the uterus

The operator then seizes the fundus on each side with volsellum forceps; he hands the left pair of forceps to his assistant and, grasping the right pair in his left hand, steadies the uterus and divides its body in half with a scalpel in the relatively avascular mid-line. The incision is carried downwards well into the tumour so that the plane of its capsule is easily distinguished (Fig. 8.10).

Enucleating the tumour

The capsule having been defined, the tumour is seized with a volsellum and enucleated whole by means of the fingers (Fig. 8.11).

Securing the uterine vessels and removing the uterus

The bisected uterine body and the collapsed cervix are now easily pulled up, the uterine arteries secured in the usual way, and total hysterectomy performed as described in Chapter 7.

Closing the abdominal cavity

See Chapter 6.

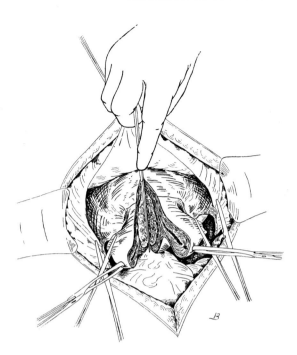

Fig. 8.10 Hysterectomy for a central cervical myoma by hemisection of the uterus.

Hysterectomy for a posterior cervical myoma

There are two methods of dealing with a posterior cervical myoma, depending on its variety. If the rarer form is present where the tumour, undermining the peritoneum at the bottom of the pouch of Douglas, strips the serous membrane off the anterior face of the sacrum and rectum, and pushes down between the vagina and rectum, or by the side of the latter, the uterus will be found to have been bodily elevated on the myoma in a position of retroversion. In this case the bladder will be found to overlie the front of the mass entirely, and the best technique to adopt will be to bisect the uterus in the manner previously described. The bisection will be principally carried out on the posterior wall of the uterus, as the presence of the bladder in front generally prevents the incision being carried very far down on the anterior wall.

If the tumour is of the commoner variety, namely that which projects into the pouch of Douglas, the method to be described should be followed.

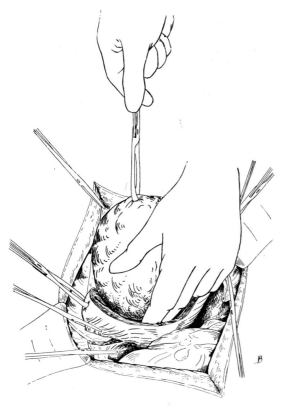

Fig. 8.11 Enucleating the tumour.

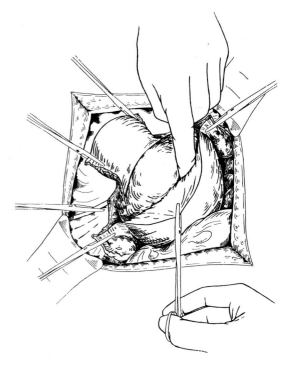

Fig. 8.12 Hysterectomy for a posterior cervical myoma: reflecting the posterior peritoneum.

The operation

Opening the abdominal cavity
Comments previously made should be considered.

Examining the abdomen and packing off the intestines
See Chapter 6.

Clamping and dividing the ovarian vessels and round ligaments
These are clamped, divided and tied as described in Chapter 7.

Incising the peritoneum and capsule
The peritoneum and capsule at the junction of the uterus are incised and reflected (Fig. 8.12).

Enucleation of the base of the tumour
The tumour having been pulled forward by the volsellum, the fingers are now forced between the capsule and the tumour, and the latter is enucleated down to its lower pole. To effect this in difficult cases, the fingers may have to be inserted a distance equal to almost the whole length of the vagina. With large tumours the removal of a central wedge, as previously described, will facilitate their removal. In fact, a large mass of tumour can be removed safely in this way to give the surgeon far better access to the vessels.

Reflecting the anterior flap of peritoneum towards the bladder
Next, the peritoneum over the anterior surface of the supravaginal cervix is reflected as far as the attachment of the bladder.

Clamping the uterine vessels and removing the uterus
Strong traction is now made on the tumour, which, together with the freed uterus, can be easily pulled up with a volsellum so that the uterine vessels on each side are brought into view and then clamped (Fig. 8.13). After this the uterus is removed by total hysterectomy, first opening the anterior vaginal vault.

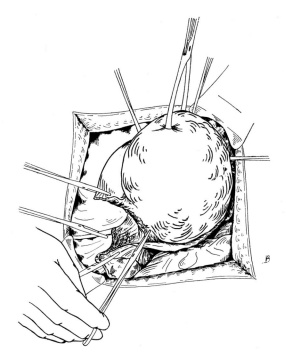

Fig. 8.13 Clamping the uterine artery.

Ligating the ovarian and uterine vessels
See Chapter 7.

Suturing the peritoneal flaps
See Chapter 7.

Difficulties and dangers

It is most important to get into the plane of cleavage between the tumour and its capsule of expanded cervical muscle; otherwise, troublesome bleeding and risk to the organs around will occur.

Hysterectomy for broad ligament myomas

Broad ligament myomas are divisible into two classes. The first variety is the true broad ligament myoma, and springs from the muscle fibres normally found in the mesometrium. Such tumours may, therefore, be found in at least three situations:

1 In the round ligament.
2 In the ovariouterine ligament.

3 In the connective tissue surrounding the ovarian or uterine vessels.

As a rule, tumours growing in the first two situations are of small size, and can be enucleated as described in Chapter 9. Tumours growing in the third situation frequently attain a large size; they distend the broad ligament so that the fallopian tube is stretched and lies sessile on their upper surface as in a broad ligament cyst. Having exhausted the capacity of the broad ligament, the tumour pushes its way upwards, stripping the peritoneum off the lateral wall of the pelvis and iliac fossa, and on the left side it often burrows between the layers of the pelvic mesocolon, the bowel itself then lying upon the tumour. If the operator is not familiar with the anatomy of these tumours he may believe that this condition of the bowel is due to adhesions, and may abandon the attempt to remove the tumour, when, as a matter of fact, a plane of easy cleavage lies between the muscularis of the intestine and the surface of the tumour. The ureter and vessels supplying the intestine can be in danger and great care is necessary not to damage either structure.

True tumours of the broad ligament can be distinguished by the fact that they are entirely separate from the uterus, which they displace but do not deform. Their relation to the uterine artery should be remembered; it lies beneath and on the inner side of the tumour, while the ureter is displaced inwards, and will be found running in the posterior peritoneal layer of the broad ligament, after which it courses under the tumour to reach the bladder.

There are two methods of dealing with true broad ligament myomas. The tumour may be enucleated in the manner described in Chapter 9. If the tumour is very large, vascular or adherent, it may be necessary also to remove the uterus, principally as a means of controlling the haemorrhage easily. This method will be described in the operation for the second variety of broad ligament myoma.

The second variety may be termed the 'false' broad ligament myoma. In this case the tumour springs from the lateral wall of the uterine body or of the cervix, and bulges outwards between the layers of the broad ligament. The uterus is, therefore, an integral part of the tumour. These tumours distend the broad ligament, and at times raise the lateral pelvic peritoneum and invade the mesocolon.

Besides its relation to the uterus, the second variety differs from the first variety in that it displaces the uterine artery outwards and upwards, so that in extreme cases the uterine and ovarian vessels are approximated and run parallel on the top of the tumour. The ureter is displaced outwards to the pelvic wall and, as a rule, lies under the tumour, except in the rare lateral cervical myomas already referred to, when, together with the lateral angle of the bladder, it may be undermined by the tumour and elevated on its upper surface. These tumours can be enucleated, but when large or associated with other fibroids in the uterus it is often best to deal with them by hysterectomy.

It is better, if possible, to begin the removal of the tumour by attacking the healthy side of the uterus. The reasons for this are first, that haemorrhage can be better controlled and secondly, that the uterus itself constitutes the firmest attachment of the tumour which is elsewhere surrounded by cellular tissue and peritoneum. The greatest difficulty in these cases is the control of the uterine vessels on the side of the tumour, and it is often impossible to secure them until the tumour is removed from the field of view. The concluding stage of its removal has, therefore, often to be effected as quickly as possible, and this is materially aided by the previous removal of the uterus and clamping of the uterine vessels on the healthy side.

The operation

Opening the abdominal cavity
Comments previously made should be considered. With a large tumour, the bladder may be elevated towards the umbilicus and to avoid damaging it care must be taken to open the peritoneal cavity at the top of the incision. This must be extended upwards where necessary.

Clamping and dividing the upper parts of the broad ligament on the healthy side
This is carried out as though performing a standard hysterectomy (see Chapter 7).

Stripping the anterior peritoneal flap
The peritoneum is incised across the uterus and tumour; the incision, commencing at the healthy side and passing across the tumour, divides the round ligament and is extended upwards to just short of the ovarian vessels. The peritoneum is now stripped from the upper surface of the tumour as far as possible, and the bladder is pushed down (Fig. 8.14).

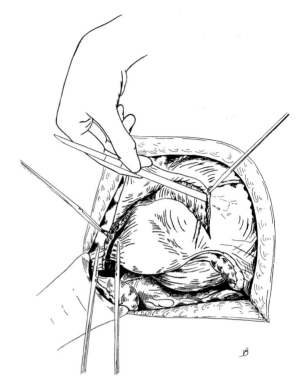

Fig. 8.14 Hysterectomy for a broad ligament myoma: separating the peritoneum off the upper pole.

Clamping the ovarian vessels on the diseased side
The index finger of the operator's left hand is then inserted between the cut edges of the peritoneum and forced under the fallopian tube and ovarian vessels, which are thus separated from the tumour. The upper parts of the broad ligament and the round ligament are then divided between forceps (Fig. 8.15).

Freeing the upper part of the tumour
The upper part of the tumour is now freed from its attachments, leaving only its base.

Clamping the uterine vessels on the healthy side
The uterus and tumour are now strongly pulled over to the side of the tumour and the uterine vessels on the healthy side are clamped and divided, as in a standard hysterectomy.

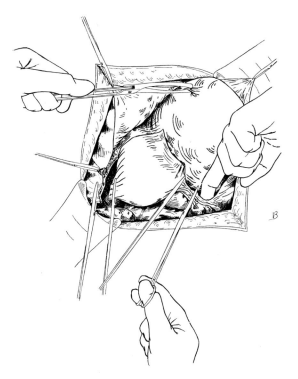

Fig. 8.15 Separating the fallopian tube and ovarian vessels from the tumour.

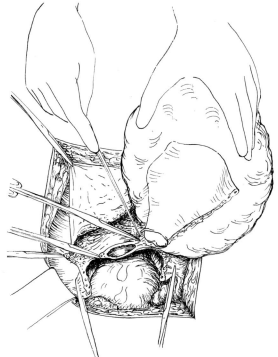

Fig. 8.16 Securing the uterine artery on the side of the myoma.

Removing the uterus

The fundus of the uterus is drawn over towards the side on which the tumour lies, and total hysterectomy is performed.

Dividing and clamping the uterine vessels on the diseased side

Just before the hysterectomy is completed, the uterine vessels on the same side as the tumour come into view. Remembering the proximity of the ureter, these vessels should be defined clearly and clamped before they are cut. If this is not done, an inexperienced operator troubled by the extent of the haemorrhage may inadvertently damage the ureter when endeavouring to control the bleeding (Fig. 8.16).

Removal of the uterus and tumour

The assistant pulls the uterus strongly towards the side of the tumour, and the operator, passing the fingers of his left hand between the tumour and the base of the broad ligament, frees its lower surface and thus enucleates it.

Ligating the uterine and ovarian vessels and round ligaments

This is easily performed and completes the removal phase.

Closing the abdominal cavity (See Chapter 6)

Occasionally, a fibroid, lateral to the uterus, so displaces this organ downwards and to the opposite side that the vessels on the healthy side cannot be reached in the manner described. In such circumstances the tumour must first be enucleated or partly enucleated after the ovarian vessels spread out on its upper surface have been clamped and divided. During enucleation the fingers must be kept close to the tumour. The enucleation effected, the uterus rides up, and the vessels on the healthy side become accessible. Because of probable displacement of the ureter, it is necessary to define its exact position in relation to the vessels before they are clamped. This can be done, preferably by exposing it to view as it runs on the posterior layer of the broad

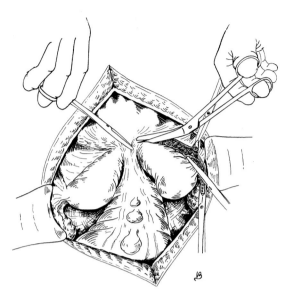

Fig. 8.17 Hysterectomy for a double uterus: dividing the vesicorectal fold or median raphe.

ligament or by careful palpation. If in doubt, the ureter at the brim of the pelvis should be identified and followed down from a position of anatomical certainty and safety.

Difficulties and dangers

The operator must remember the various displacements to which the ureter is liable, and if he cannot be sure of its exact position, must minimize the danger of wounding it by keeping as close to the tumour as possible during enucleation. It is very important to ligate all bleeding points left in the cavity after the removal of the tumour, otherwise a large haematoma may form. If suction drainage is not instigated and haemorrhage does occur, vaginal examination 10 days or more after the operation will usually reveal a mass in the area of the broad ligament. It should be left alone and will slowly absorb over a period of weeks.

Hysterectomy for a double uterus

The technique of hysterectomy for a double uterus does not differ materially from that for the single organ except in certain particulars. When two complete organs are present (uterus duplex), a pronounced fold of peritoneum exists (median raphe) which joins the bladder to the rectum in the middle line, separates the two corpora and divides the uterorectal pouch into two lateral compartments. This fold should be divided by the same incision through the peritoneum that demarcates the anterior peritoneal flap, and the operator must make sure that the bladder is pushed well forward and the rectum well backward before he proceeds with hysterectomy (Fig. 8.17).

With a double corpus and a single cervix (uterus bicornis unicollis) the fold may not be present.

In uterus duplex, the two cervices, though complete in themselves, are joined together by a block of tissue, which is continued downwards as a median vaginal septum. There is only one uterine artery to each half of a double uterus.

Further reading

The editor would refer the student to the end of Chapter 9 for further reading.

We would also recommend the readers to look into *An Atlas of Gynaecologic Oncology, Investigation and Surgery* by Smith, Del Priore, Curtin and Monaghan. Published by Martin Dunitz (2000).

Myomectomy and management of fibroids in pregnancy

Myomectomy

The name of Victor Bonney will always be associated with the development of myomectomy so as to preserve uterine function. At the time he was working, a subtotal hysterectomy was considered to be the treatment of choice for fibroids. He demonstrated that fibroids could be removed, the uterus preserved and successful pregnancies achieved.

Fibroids or leiomyomas occur in approximately 20% of women; there is a clear relationship with infertility and in those patients who have a myomectomy performed there is a marked improvement in subsequent fertility. Fibroids are also frequently seen in association with endometriosis; in neither of these conditions is the causal relationship to infertility clear.

The fibroid, a benign overgrowth of the muscular elements of the uterine wall, may develop in any part of the genital tract but almost always within the myometrium. Any effects of the fibroid will depend on the position and size of the tumour. Fibroids which impinge on the cavity of the uterus are most commonly associated with infertility and, in later life, with alterations of menstrual pattern produced by a combination of expansion of the endometrial surface and irregularities of that surface.

Those tumours within the myometrium may grow to a very large size and be entirely symptomless, growing steadily and forming a false capsule by compressing surrounding tissues. This false capsule allows the surgeon to enucleate the fibroid with ease using the tissue planes so formed as a simple line of cleavage. The fibroid picks up its blood supply from adjacent arteries, but as it grows develops anoxic areas in the centre of the tumour which not infrequently undergo degeneration.

Fibroids lying more superficially may become pedunculated and may at times undergo torsion. They are frequently mistaken for ovarian tumours.

In pregnancy, fibroids may undergo 'red degeneration', which manifests itself as extreme pain in or close to the uterus. This may be misdiagnosed as abruptio placentae or acute appendicitis, depending on the position of the pain. It is generally recommended that fibroids should not be removed from the pregnant uterus because of the risk of severe and uncontrollable haemorrhage.

The procedure for removal of a myomatous polyp is described in Chapter 5.

Indications for myomectomy

The sole purpose of myomectomy is to improve fertility; it should never be used as a surgical exercise, nor to preserve the uterus in the mistaken belief that such an act will maintain the femininity or sexuality of the patient. Unfortunately, more than two-thirds of women who have had myomectomy are at risk of developing menstrual irregularities or menorrhagia.

Instruments

The gynaecological general set described in Chapter 2 is required, with the addition of two other valuable items:
1 *Myoma screw*; this device is rather like a large corkscrew with a wide spiral which can be inserted into particularly large fibroids in order to assist in manoeuvring the tumour.

2 *Bonney's myomectomy clamp*; this is often of great help in reducing the amount of bleeding during the procedure. It is applied across the base of the uterus at the junction of the body and cervix uteri, softly occluding the uterine arteries as they pass up the lateral side of the uterus.

Preoperative preparation

As well as the general preparation of the patient for an abdominal operation, it is often worthwhile carrying out an ultrasound examination to differentiate between fibroids and ovarian pathology. An intravenous urogram (IVU) is also of value in determining if there is any evidence of displacement or obstruction to the ureters by the fibroids.

It is important to have adequate blood crossmatched prior to the procedure, as there is a considerable risk of bleeding both during the operation and in the immediate postoperative period.

Anaesthesia

No special anaesthetics are required.

The operation

Opening the abdomen
The incision is made as described in Chapter 6.

Clearly, if the fibroid to be removed is very small, having been previously identified and measured at laparoscopy, then a low transverse incision may be appropriate. It is *possible* to remove even the most enormous fibroid through a transverse or Pfannenstiel incision, but it is more a mark of the surgeon's desire to make the operation unnecessarily difficult rather than any innate surgical skill. If the operation is likely to be a 'tour de force' then the procedure is best carried out with adequate access via a subumbilical mid-line incision.

Delivery and inspection of the uterus
The uterus having been delivered as far as possible out of the abdominal cavity, the size and position of the tumour or tumours should be studied (noting the number as far as may be possible at this stage) to determine if enucleation is feasible and, if so, where best to place the incision or incisions.

Tumours situated in the anterior or lateral walls of the uterus are more suitable for enucleation than those in the posterior wall.

Anterior cervical myomas are well suited for enucleation, but posterior cervical tumours are much more inaccessible and the bed which remains after their removal may be difficult to reach. Central cervical myomas usually enucleate very readily but their removal leaves an immensely elongated supravaginal cervix, which may be more difficult to deal with satisfactorily.

The uterus should be palpated very carefully in order to detect seedling tumours, which, if overlooked, would jeopardize the final success of the operation. This step is best postponed until the larger tumours have been disposed of or until the uterine cavity has been explored, as this makes detection much easier. Professor Joel-Cohen advocates routine opening of the uterine cavity via an anterior incision; this greatly simplifies the procedure, giving an excellent view of the cavity and allows easy access to the posterior wall fibroids.

Haemostasis during the procedure
The principal objection to myomectomy in the past was the bleeding over which the operator had little or no control. Myomectomy to be ideal requires to be almost bloodless, for profuse oozing from the bed of the tumour so hampers the operator that there is not sufficient time for the removal of the smaller tumours and a neat reconstruction of the uterus afterwards before there are signs of severe blood loss. By the use of the clamp devised by Bonney, myomectomy can be performed on an almost bloodless uterus, so that not only can the operator work as deliberately as he chooses, but also, if in the end he should find it impossible to terminate the myomectomy satisfactorily, the patient, having lost little or no blood, is in a perfectly good condition for hysterectomy.

The clamp is usually applied from the pubic end of the abdominal wound with the angle between the blades and the shanks opening downwards to grip the round ligaments (Fig. 9.1); otherwise, as the blades are closed, they will slip down past the cervix on to the upper end of the vagina and the uterine vessels will no longer be controlled. In some instances the instrument fits better in reverse, i.e. with the angle between the blades and the shanks opening upwards. By the use of this clamp the blood flowing through the uterine vessels and the cervix is arrested.

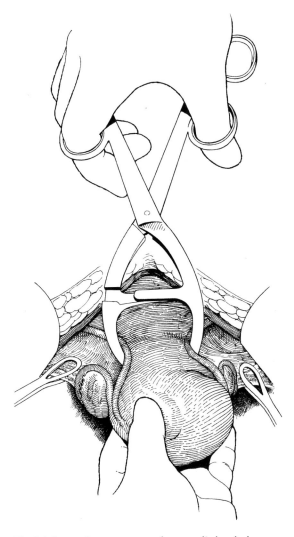

Fig. 9.1 Bonney's myomectomy clamp applied to the lower uterus.

The vessels themselves are not injured, being too well protected by the tissues in which they are embedded. The flow of blood through the ovarian vessels is arrested temporarily by ring forceps; all the vessels going into the uterus being thus occluded, it is rendered almost bloodless. When the clamp and forceps are removed, on completion of the operation, the uterus flushes up, but on returning to the abdominal cavity the flush soon passes off, and if the slight oozing from the suture holes does not then cease it can be stopped with the application of pressure with a swab or small pack for a few minutes, or an additional suture or two, inserted where required. Figure-of-eight sutures of Vicryl are ideal for this purpose.

A tumour low down in the body of the uterus or in the cervix prevents the clamp being applied. In such a case the tumour must be enucleated first and the clamp applied afterwards. The intravenous injection of 0.25 mg of ergometrine by the anaesthetist as the surgeon opens the abdomen promotes uterine contractions in the non-pregnant as well as the pregnant uterus, and reduces the vascularity so completely that a clamp is often not required. When the Bonney myomectomy clamp is not available, a rubber catheter can be attached around the cervix to achieve the same result.

Whether a clamp or a tourniquet is used, it should not be left in position for periods of more than approximately 20 min without being released. If necessary, after its temporary release, it can be reapplied following compression of the uterus in a hot towel. The reason for this release is that during an extended myomectomy with its associated trauma, however gentle the surgeon may be, there is a considerable accumulation of histamine-like substances which are suddenly released into the general circulation in large quantities after the clamp is removed. This is undoubtedly one of the reasons why postoperative shock has in the past been more of a sequel to myomectomy than to hysterectomy. If the clamp is temporarily released during the course of a long operation, these waste products will not accumulate and in most cases the body will be able to deal with them satisfactorily. Moreover, the patient is under close supervision by the anaesthetist during and after the first release.

The primary incision in the uterus

The lower the incision is made in the uterus, the stronger will be the subsequent scar. The relative strength of a lower segment caesarean section scar compared with that of a classical caesarean section scar provides a reasonable comparison with the strength of the uterus following myomectomy through a supracervical incision and one in the fundus. Whenever feasible, therefore, the incision should be made in the mid-line of the anterior wall of the uterus as low down as is possible with adequate exposure of the tumour. It is a useful preliminary procedure to mobilize the peritoneum of the uterovesical fold and reflect the bladder down sufficiently in the mid-line to facilitate a low incision of approach to the tumour and to provide a peritoneal fold which at the end of the operation can be used to cover the incision. Professor Joel-Cohen has also advocated not opening the uterovesical fold, simply folding the loose peritoneum over the uterine wall scar and tack-suturing it in place at the end of the procedure. This useful procedure reduces the risk of intraperitoneal postoperative bleeding and adhesion formation. When an incision has to be made into the posterior wall of the uterus (and this should be avoided wherever possible), postoperative oozing increases the risk of the small intestine becoming adherent to the incision and causing obstruction at a later date. For this reason, when a fibroid is deep in the posterior wall of the uterus, it is preferable to approach it through the uterine cavity after opening this anteriorly.

Whichever incision of approach is used, it is important at the end of the operation to make sure that the uterus is left in a well anteverted position; for this reason, the round ligaments should be shortened where necessary to suspend the uterus in a good position before closing the abdomen.

Removing a solitary fibroid
Figure 9.2 shows the incision over the dome of a protruding fibroid; the incision is carried down to the point at which the fibroid clearly bulges into the incision. At this stage the false capsule can be clearly identified and, running the handle of the scalpel around the plane, the whole fibroid can be 'shelled' out. Small bleeding points in the base of the cavity are individually tied or diathermied.

Obliterating the cavity
The cavity should be obliterated methodically using a series of circular mattress sutures, laid one on the other until the whole space has gone (Fig. 9.3). This serosa should then be closed using a small number of interrupted sutures. Vicryl is usually recommended as the material of choice, since modern synthetic absorbable sutures are very tough and may cut through the delicate myometrium. If the uterine cavity has been entered it is not necessary to close the mucosa as a separate layer.

As an alternative, the whole cavity can be obliterated using large, full-thickness through-and-through sutures.

Bonney's techniques for closure of the cavities For historical purposes, the drawings produced by Bonney of the closure of a complicated cavity in the myometrium are reproduced in the original, and the method of closure after removal of a very large fibroid using the 'hood' technique is shown in Figs 9.4–9.11.

Complications and postoperative problems

It is clear that with a careful operative technique and meticulous attention to haemostasis, excellent results can be achieved. However, the major immediate complication of the procedure is haemorrhage which persists in spite of many attempts to achieve haemostasis. The unfortunate end result of this is that the patient loses her uterus and, with it, all chance of a pregnancy. Therefore, it is important that all patients embarking on myomectomy should be warned of this possibility.

Menorrhagia will persist if submucous fibroids are missed at operation or there is endometrial hyperplasia, or even if there is coincidental dysfunctional bleeding. Opinion about the true incidence of this problem varies considerably but the figure of 66% of patients developing menorrhagia or having persistent menorrhagia is close to the truth.

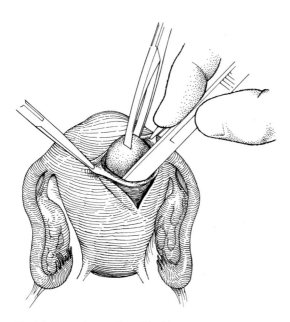

Fig. 9.2 Removing a solitary fibroid.

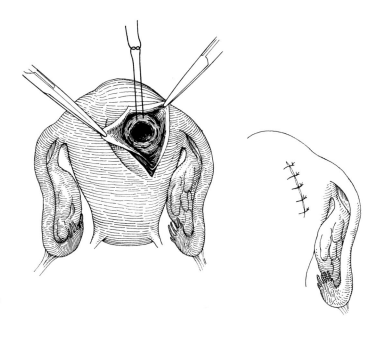

Fig. 9.3 Obliterating the cavity in the uterine wall.

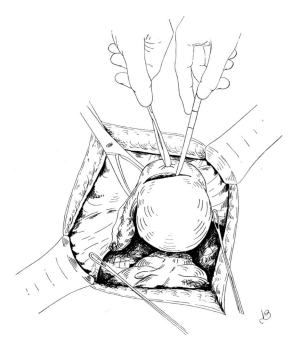

Fig. 9.4 Myomectomy by Bonney's 'hood' operation: making the transverse incision.

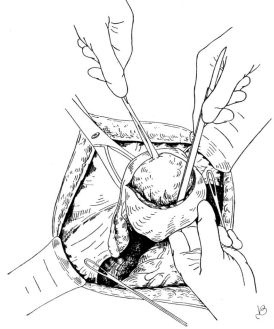

Fig. 9.5 Myomectomy by Bonney's 'hood' operation: enucleating the tumour.

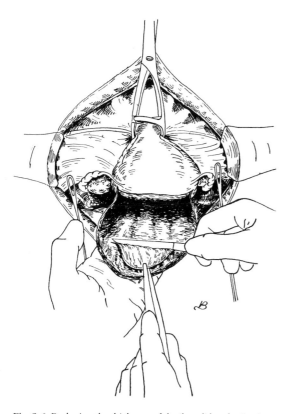

Fig. 9.6 Reducing the thickness of the 'hood' by planing it.

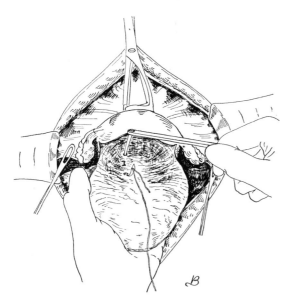

Fig. 9.7 Inserting the first tier of sutures to bring the 'hood' over the top of the uterus.

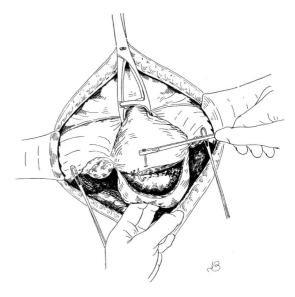

Fig. 9.8 Continuing the suture of the 'hood'.

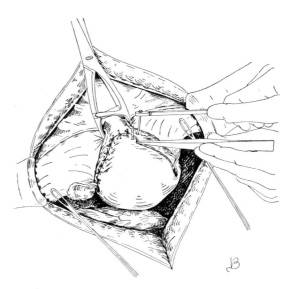

Fig. 9.9 The 'hood' finally sutured on the front of the uterus.

Pregnancy following myomectomy

The major concern for both the patient and her obstetrician is that the uterus will not rupture during subsequent pregnancy and labour. It has generally been the experience of gynaecologists that there is little danger of the uterus rupturing during the pregnancy but it is

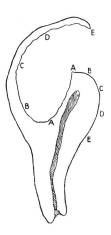

Fig. 9.10 The capsule left after the enucleation.

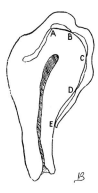

Fig. 9.11 The 'hood' in place.

usually recommended as a prudent measure that where the myomectomy has been an extensive procedure and the cavity has been opened, that a prophylactic elective caesarean section should be performed.

Fibroids in pregnancy

There are three complications of fibroids which may occur in pregnancy:
1 Red degeneration (necrobiosis).
2 Torsion of a pedunculated fibroid.
3 Mechanical problems causing either retention of urine or impaction of the pregnant uterus in the pouch of Douglas.

Red degeneration

This complication is due to bleeding into the substance of the fibroid associated with a degenerative process. The patient presents with a pain in the abdomen which is localized to the uterus and which moves with the uterus; indeed, this is a useful test to apply if the diagnosis is in doubt. The pain is rarely severe but can cause considerable discomfort. A moderate fever is not uncommonly associated with these changes. These symptoms are associated with a general malaise.

Examination of the patient frequently reveals a tender firm area on the surface of the uterus, the size of which varies with the size of the fibroid. Uterine activity—even Braxton Hicks contraction—can cause considerable discomfort.

The *differential diagnosis* of acute appendicitis, urinary tract infection, antepartum haemorrhage, strangulated hernia and torsion of an ovarian cyst have all to be considered. The most important diagnostic test is to demonstrate clearly that the pain is emanating from the wall of the uterus and moves with the uterus. There is a possible role for ultrasound in the differentiation of the complication from ovarian lesions.

Treatment of the condition, once a firm diagnosis is made, is *conservative* with bed rest, mild sedation and analgesia being the mainstays.

In such cases there is no indication for operation, and even when a laparotomy is performed no attempt to remove the fibroid should be made; otherwise, disastrous haemorrhage may ensue.

Torsion of a pedunculated fibroid

This is a very rare condition in the non-pregnant state and is even rarer during pregnancy; its only importance is that it must be differentiated from red degeneration. The symptomatology tends to be more acute with vomiting being a more prominent feature.

The pain and discomfort tends not to settle with conservative treatment. Consequently, laparotomy is required, particularly if there is a possibility of an ovarian mass being twisted through torsion.

This condition is the only one where it is reasonable to operate on a fibroid in pregnancy.

Mechanical complications

Acute retention due to the presence of a large cervical

fibroid is extraordinarily rare and most unlikely to occur because of the infertility which would inevitably be associated with the condition. If there are difficulties in relieving the retention by passage of a catheter, it is often easier and safer to insert a suprapubic catheter which can be retained until it is decided how the fibroid is to be dealt with.

The operation

If the fibroid is paracervical, it may be feasible to perform a myomectomy, thus preserving the pregnancy. However, greatly increased vascularity will be experienced and the patient may well end up with a hysterectomy. Similarly, a true cervical fibroid will present the clinician with the difficult choice of an interval myomectomy or a pregnancy hysterectomy. If the patient is adamant that she wishes to preserve the uterus at all costs, it will be in her interests to terminate the current pregnancy, have a myomectomy and then attempt to become pregnant again.

If the retention has occurred later in pregnancy it may be possible to tide the patient over until the fetus is viable by retaining the suprapubic catheter until such time as a caesarean section can be performed.

An impacted fundal fibroid in a retroverted uterus will usually manifest itself early in pregnancy, the patient having experienced large bowel symptoms previously. The problem is usually solved by disimpaction under a light general or epidural anaesthetic. The fingers are inserted into the posterior fornix and the fibroid liberated from the pelvis by light pressure.

Fibroids obstructing labour
This complication is rare because even though a fibroid may appear to lie low down in the uterine cavity in the non-pregnant or early pregnancy state, as pregnancy develops, the fibroids are elevated along with the growth of the uterus.

The choices available to the clinician are:
1 *Caesarean section and subsequent myomectomy.* This is the treatment of choice for those patients who desire further pregnancies. It is regarded by the editor as putting patients unnecessarily at risk to embark on a myomectomy at the same time as the Caesarean section. Myomectomy is much simpler and safer in the fully involuted uterus.

2 *Caesarean hysterectomy.* This procedure has considerable attractions for the patient who has completed her family. The chances of the fibroid uterus producing problems which may require hysterectomy in the future are high.

Another major indication is when there has been an intrapartum catastrophe such as a tear of the cervix into the lower part of the uterus, which may be associated with the obstructing fibroid or due to attempts to deliver the child past the obstruction.

A fortunately rare indication for this procedure is when the obstruction and prolonged labour have resulted in gross infection of the uterus, particularly when there is gas formation due to *Clostridium welchii* or associated septicaemia and endotoxic shock.

Even in patients where it appears that the shock is so profound that death is imminent, it is important to attempt to remove the cause of the problem, since remarkable recoveries are well documented after removal of the offending organ.

The authors do not regard a need for sterilization or a past history of minor menstrual upsets as an indication for hysterectomy. There are a surprising number of women who will volunteer their uteri to the surgeon's knife; the surgeon must beware of acquiescing to the patient's whims.

Further reading

As in a number of other chapters, the editor would refer the student to older editions of textbooks such as Bonney and Te Linde for comprehensive cover of this subject. It seems that myomectomy has fallen in popularity in the last two decades in Western medicine. This may be due to the fact that women are completing their childbearing years and if a fibroid uterus is found subsequently, then a hysterectomy is looked upon as the simplest management method. Therefore, there are few new references to myomectomy after 1970:

Neuwirth RS. A new technique for and additional experience with hysteroscopic resection of submucous fibroids. *Am J Obstet Gynecol* 1978;131:91–4.

Others review past experience of major establishments, such as Loeffler FE, Noble AD. Myomectomy at the Chelsea Hospital for Women. *J Obstet Gynaecol Br Commonwealth* 1970;77:167–70.

10 Vaginal hysterectomy and radical vaginal hysterectomy (Schauta and Coelio-Schauta procedures)

Vaginal hysterectomy

Whilst the main indication for vaginal hysterectomy is in the treatment of genital prolapse, it is a frequently used alternative to abdominal hysterectomy for other conditions. The objection to the procedure in the absence of prolapse have been on the grounds of limited access, but with good technique this objection can be overridden.

More practical contraindications are:
1 A uterine size larger than the equivalent of a 12-week pregnancy.
2 Endometriosis or pelvic inflammatory disease.
3 A narrow subpubic arch.
4 A long, narrow vagina.
5 Where it is essential that the ovaries are removed, such as in the management of corpus cancer (although vaginal hysterectomy may be the management of choice in grossly obese women).

Although a large uterus can be removed vaginally, either by splitting the uterus in two or by fragmentation of the uterus (morcellation), it is more simply managed abdominally. It is important that vaginal hysterectomy should be achieved simply and easily without considerable trauma or the need for excessive force.

Endometriosis and pelvic inflammatory disease are sometimes encountered during the course of a vaginal approach and can usually be overcome; however, if diagnosed preoperatively they generally indicate a preference for an abdominal approach. The last two relative contraindications (endometriosis and pelvic inflammatory disease) restrict access and render the vaginal route potentially difficult and more hazardous.

The indications for a vaginal hysterectomy are usually benign, such as dysfunctional uterine bleeding or a small fibroid uterus. The procedure is often favoured by those who advocate hysterectomy as one method of sterilization. Premalignant conditions of the cervix may, in the relatively rare circumstances where hysterectomy is indicated, be preferentially dealt with using the vaginal route. This is particularly important when there is a wide abnormal transformation zone, especially when it extends on to the vaginal fornices, and in those circumstances when abdominal access may be difficult, increasing the risk of leaving behind premalignant tissue. Malignant conditions of the cervix and corpus uteri when surgical treatment is chosen can be dealt with by the more radical vaginal procedures. However, the commonest indication for the use of vaginal hysterectomy is in patients where there is gross abdominal obesity and the production of an abdominal wound may render postoperative recovery more complex.

The advantages of vaginal hysterectomy are as follows:
1 There is no abdominal wound.
2 There is no transgression of the abdominal peritoneum.
3 There is no significant disturbance of the intestines.
4 There is usually less postoperative discomfort, easier mobilization and very commonly earlier discharge from hospital.
5 There is no risk of an abdominal wound infection.

The disadvantages of vaginal hysterectomy are:
1 A markedly increased risk of pelvic infection which, although low is significantly greater than that found with the abdominal procedures.
2 A theoretical risk of prolapse in the longer term.

The principles of the procedure

These are similar to those of abdominal hysterectomy. There are three main pedicles on each side of the uterus to be secured:
1 The tubo-ovarian, including the round ligaments.
2 The uterine vessels.
3 The cardinal and uterosacral ligaments.
The pelvic peritoneum is opened anterior to the uterus and posteriorly in the pouch of Douglas, and although in the past it has been reconstituted after removal of the uterus and strenuous attempts have been made to make sure that the pedicles are extraperitoneal, this is generally not now performed.

As with the abdominal hysterectomy care with the handling of the bladder and an appreciation of the position of the ureters must be made.

Instruments

Vaginal operations are more simply performed with two assistants but this is not always possible and one assistant and the occasional help of a scrub nurse can be sufficient.

Although in the past narrow-bladed vaginal retractors have been used, it is the authors' preference to utilize a broad Sims' speculum which can be further assisted by the use of right-angle vaginal retractors (Landon retractors). These retractors can be managed easily and it is important to instruct the assistants not to push too deeply with these retractors as this simply pushes the operative site further away from the surgeon.

The personal choice of suture materials varies enormously. In general catgut is no longer used, with most clinicians preferring either Vicryl or Dexon. Some clinicians utilize simple pedicle needles, others clamp the tissues and then use stitch ligatures. It is the authors' preference to use cutting needles at all times in surgery, which some other experts would regard as anathema. Whatever system is used, it is the accurate placing of sutures which is more important than the particular material or stitch system.

Preoperative preparation

This should follow the normal procedure for gynaecological operations. The patient being brought into hospital shortly before surgery, having had appropriate preoperative assessment performed. It is now standard to use antibiotics intraoperatively using either a single agent which will cover *Bacteroides*, or in some circumstances combinations of antibiotics. The antibiotic should cover the full period of the surgical procedure. It is normally given intravenously at induction by the anaesthetist. It is not necessary to perform extensive cleansing of the vagina and cervix prior to the patient coming to theatre.

Anaesthesia

The use of epidural or caudal anaesthesia either alone or in addition to a light general anaesthetic is very helpful in reducing minor bleeding and is often used to relieve early postoperative pain, but this may not be absolutely essential. Simpler techniques such as the use of postoperative rectal analgesic suppositories will obviate the need for maintaining epidural catheters.

Vaginal hysterectomy, however, is an operation which lends itself perfectly to being performed under regional anaesthesia, which once more is an advantage for the grossly obese patient, or in the patient who has significant lung impairment.

Position of the patient

It is important that the normal lithotomy position is used with both the hips and the knees being hyperflexed. It is very tempting, particularly with some of the modern operative tables that are available, to have the legs elevated but stretched out virtually straight with only a small angle at the hips. This unfortunately reduces good access and can make a simple operation significantly more difficult. It is also very important to make sure that the buttocks are right at the end of the table but not hanging over, as once more this can make the performance of the surgery significantly more difficult.

The operation

As all patients should have emptied their bladder prior to being taken down to theatre it is not necessary to perform catheterization at the beginning of the procedure. It is important to check the size and mobility of the

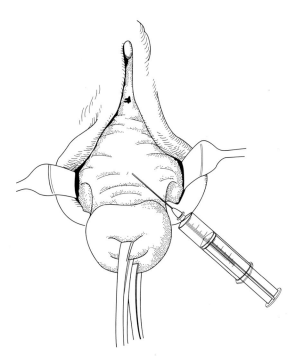

Fig. 10.1 Infiltration of subepithelial tissues.

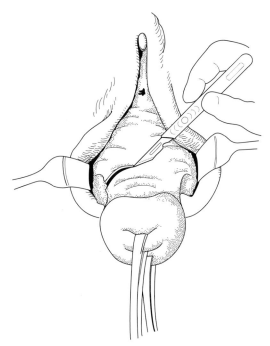

Fig. 10.2 Incision around the cervix.

uterus by performing a bimanual examination as this is an ideal opportunity to make sure there is no unexpected pathology.

Most surgeons use some form of subepithelial tissue infiltration. It is the authors' choice to use approximately 20 ml of 1 in 400 000 adrenaline in saline. This helps to define tissue planes and reduce minor bleeding. In order to facilitate this process, the cervix is grasped by either two volsellum forceps or two Littlewood's forceps. The cervix is drawn down to put the vaginal tissues on tension and the infiltration is placed circumferentially approximately 2–3 cm above the cervical os into the soft tissues anterior to the bladder, around the cervix and into the soft tissues of the posterior fornix (Fig. 10.1).

The incision
The incision is carried circumferentially around the cervix over the area which had been infiltrated by the 1 in 400 000 adrenaline (Fig. 10.2). This incision may require development anteriorly into a tear drop shape if

an anterior prolapse is present and correction of the prolapse is required. As the incision is made, the infiltrate very clearly allows definition of the subepithelial layers and the epithelium can easily be lifted up by a tooth forceps in the surgeon's left hand; with angled scissors in the right, the subcutaneous tissues can then be incised vertically down on to the anterior part of the cervix. It is important not to angle the scissors upwards as identification of the anterior surface of the cervix will make sure that no trauma occurs to the bladder base.

Division of the cervicovesical ligament
One of the assistants draws down the cervix using the attached tissue forceps. The surgeon lifts the anterior vaginal wall in his left hand with the toothed dissectors and this allows definition of vertically running tissue (the cervicovesical ligament). This ligament is divided with the Monaghan's scissors (Fig. 10.3) and the bladder can now easily be deflected off the anterior part of the cervix either using the scissors themselves or

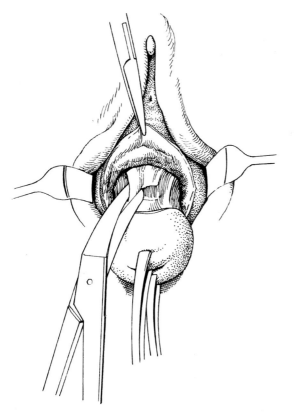

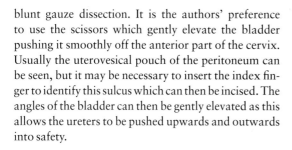

Fig. 10.3 Division of the cervicovesical ligament.

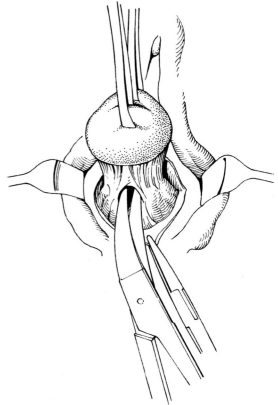

Fig. 10.4 Opening the pouch of Douglas.

blunt gauze dissection. It is the authors' preference to use the scissors which gently elevate the bladder pushing it smoothly off the anterior part of the cervix. Usually the uterovesical pouch of the peritoneum can be seen, but it may be necessary to insert the index finger to identify this sulcus which can then be incised. The angles of the bladder can then be gently elevated as this allows the ureters to be pushed upwards and outwards into safety.

Opening the pouch of Douglas
The cervix is now elevated and the forceps handed to one of the assistants, and once more using the tissue forceps in the left hand the epithelium of the posterior fornix can be drawn down, putting the tissues behind the cervix on tension. Then, by boldly cutting up towards the back of the cervix the pouch of Douglas is opened (Fig. 10.4).

Division of the cardinal and uterosacral ligaments
With the cervix drawn downwards and over to one side the surgeon can now place the index finger of the left hand through the opening into the pouch of Douglas. Lying in front of his finger as he draws it down will be the uterosacral and anterior to that the cardinal ligaments. These can be put on stretch tension by the left hand and a strong clamp placed over this pedicle (Fig. 10.5). This first clamp will include the uterosacral ligament and a significant part of the cardinal ligament. The tissues can be divided on the medial side of the clamp. It is important not to be overambitious and to include too much tissue in this clamp as the risk of slippage is considerable and may generate a large number of postoperative problems. The clamp may be tied at this point using a stitch ligature technique (Fig. 10.6). The same procedure is performed on the opposite side and at this point, if the anterior peritoneum has not

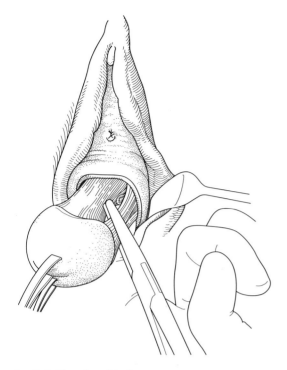

Fig. 10.5 Clamping of the ligament.

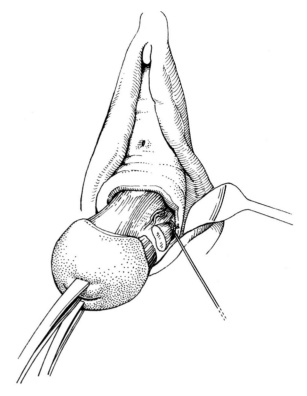

Fig. 10.6 Ligation of divided pedicle.

already been opened it is possible to perform this procedure easily (Fig. 10.7).

It is now clear that the upper part of the cardinal ligaments becomes readily accessible alongside the cervix. A further firm clamp is placed close to the uterus to include the remaining part of the cardinal ligament —at this point the cervix is obviously elongating and the uterus being gently drawn down through the introitus.

Division of the uterine vessels
The uterine vessels are now lying just above the last clamped pedicle. If the uterus is small, the descending branch of the uterine artery may already have been included in the last clamp. It is important to make sure that the next clamp to lie alongside the uterus will include the uterine vessels as they pass at right angles to the uterus and then branch and run up alongside the uterine body (Fig. 10.8). It is sometimes helpful to put

the finger of the left hand behind this pedicle to make sure that it is clearly identified and the softer area of the broad ligament noted above the clamp.

It is important to note that if the uterus is small it may be possible to take the uterosacral and cardinal ligaments in one clamp and the uterine vessels in the next clamp. Once the uterine vessels have been divided they can be carefully sutured together with the uterosacral and cardinal pedicles; it is normal to put these pedicles on long ties in order to deal with them at the end of the procedure.

Division of the tubo-ovarian pedicles
All that remains supporting the uterus in the abdomen is the peritoneum of the broad ligament and the tubo-ovarian pedicles, which will include the round ligaments as well as the infundibulopelvic ligaments. At this point, the anterior part of the uterus may be delivered from the vagina leaving the pedicles visible

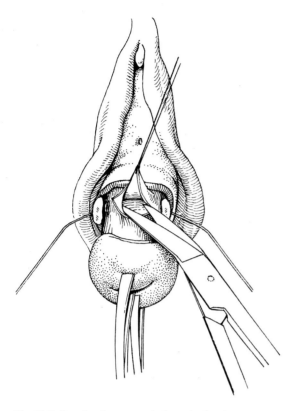

Fig. 10.7 Opening the uterovesical pouch of peritoneum.

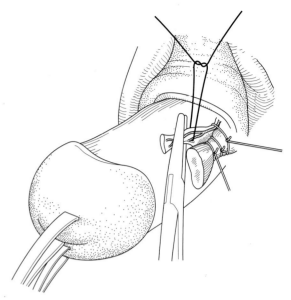

Fig. 10.8 Transfixion of the ligated and clamped uterine vessels.

(Doderlein's manoeuvre). A firm clamp with longitudinally running grooves can be applied at this point (Fig. 10.9). Once the uterine side of the clamp has been divided, the opposite side clamp can be easily applied under direct vision. In other circumstances with a narrow vagina it may be only possible to remove the body of the uterus once the pedicles have been completely divided. Once the pedicles have been divided, the uterus can be completely removed from the vagina leaving behind only the long clamps (Zeppelin) which are holding the outer part of the infundibulopelvic and round ligaments. These are usually tied. Some surgeons would use a transfixion stitch at this point but the danger of traumatizing small veins is significant and the author prefers simply to tie with Vicryl. Sir Rustram Feroze in the last edition showed in Fig. 10.10 the various techniques available for tying pedicles. The editor feels that a simple tie system with a single knot is adequate.

Closure of the vagina

In the past, significant efforts have been made to draw together the various pedicles into a bunch at the top of the vagina with a view to reducing the risk of prolapse. There is no significant evidence of the value of this technique and similarly the meticulous closure of the peritoneal edges is also now no longer practised. All that is required at this point is to close the vaginal vault, normally in an anteroposterior manner using a series of mattress sutures. It is not normal to drain the retroperitoneal space and it has been the author's practice to end the procedure to use an indwelling catheter for the first 12 h postoperatively and a light vaginal pack soaked in Acriflavin.

Complications

Complications are uncommon if the technique is meticulous. The commonest complication is that of a collection of small haematomas above the vaginal vault, which at best may cause a mild pyrexia for a few days, but at worst may cause a significant pelvic infection with marked morbidity. It is said that some pyrexia will occur in approximately 20% of vaginal hysterectomy patients. It is significantly less for abdominal procedures.

100

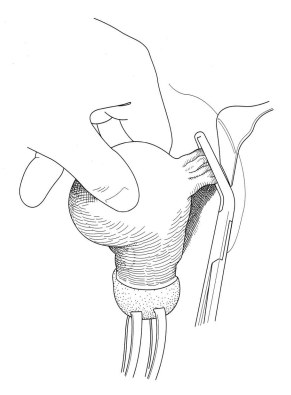

Fig. 10.9 Clamping the tubo-ovarian pedicles.

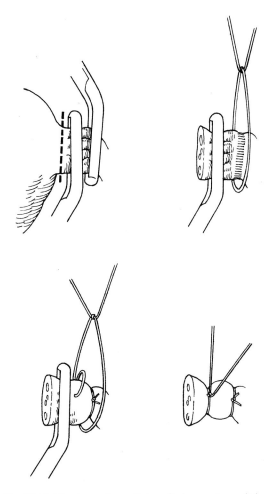

Fig. 10.10 Ligation and transfixion of tubo-ovarian pedicles.

Radical vaginal hysterectomy

In previous editions of *Bonney's Gynaecological Surgery* the radical vaginal hysterectomy, or Schauta's procedure, was described as being of more historical interest than practical use. During the 1990s this operation was resurrected and now forms an important part of the care of the patient with early stage cervical cancer. When Schauta developed his radical vaginal operation in the early 1900s it met the great need to reduce the significant infective morbidity and sometimes mortality associated with the radical abdominal procedure developed by Wertheim. The operation also met the needs of operating on the very obese and rather unfit patient.

The main failure of the Schauta procedure was that there was no way to deal with the possibility of involved pelvic lymph nodes. As this became recognized as an obligatory part of the treatment of cervical cancer, the

Schauta operation fell into disuse, except where other operations were developed to deal with the need for a lymphadenectomy. For example, the Mitra operation was developed to perform an extraperitoneal lymphadenectomy combined with the radical vaginal hysterectomy. Unfortunately, this neat operation did not achieve widespread utilization and since the development of adequate anaesthetics, blood transfusion and particularly antibiotics, the Wertheim procedure has held sway for most of the 20th century.

The main reason for the resurrection of the Schauta procedure has been the development of satisfactory laparoscopic extraperitoneal lymphadenectomy and laparoscopic transperitoneal lymphadenectomy, outlined by Daniel Dargent. Dargent has utilized the modifications of the Schauta technique, developed by the Austrian school of Amreich, together with all the modern developments of laparoscopic minimal access surgery so that it is now possible to perform a full radical hysterectomy vaginally after a minimally invasive laparoscopic procedure, removing all the pelvic, and sometimes if appropriate, para-aortic lymph nodes as well.

I will describe the radical vaginal hysterectomy as developed by the editor following the guidance of Daniel Dargent in recent years. The laparoscopic element will be described separately.

The principles of the procedure

As with the radical abdominal hysterectomy utilized for early cancer of the cervix, the radical vaginal procedure aims to remove the entire uterus and, if appropriate, the tubes and ovaries, together with an adequate amount of vaginal, paravaginal and parametrial tissues. The amount of parametrial tissue, in particular the cardinal ligaments, that can be removed in the vaginal operation is very impressive and is usually categorized as being equivalent to the Piver or Rutledge type II and III procedures.

Anatomical considerations

When the abdominal approach is used for the radical hysterectomy, the uterine artery crosses medially from its take off point on the anterior division of the internal iliac artery to cross over the roof of the ureteric tunnel before dividing into an ascending and descending branch to supply the uterus. The ureter runs around the cervix under the uterine artery in a tunnel of loose connective tissue, the upper part of which must be released in order to remove the uterine artery and the lymphatic drainage associated with it. In the vaginal operation the uterus is drawn downwards into the vagina and the bladder retracted upwards with the result that the uterine vessels now run downwards and medially, while the ureter, because of the tension from the uterine vessels, is caused to also run downwards and then appears to turn upwards to enter the bladder. Thus, a ureteric loop is created, the bend of which is called the ureteric knee by vaginal surgeons. Under this loop runs

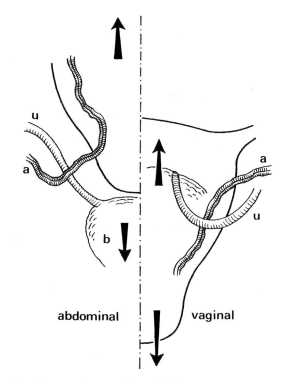

Fig. 10.11 Preparation of vaginal cuff.

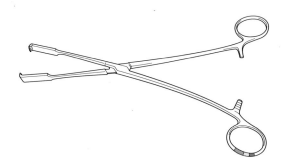

Fig. 10.12 Chrobach clamp.

the uterine vessels passing first above and then beneath the ureter (Fig. 10.11).

It is important to understand this concept that the change in apparent position of the uterine artery from clearly being above the ureter to appearing to lie below and medial to it, is entirely due to tension on the uterus.

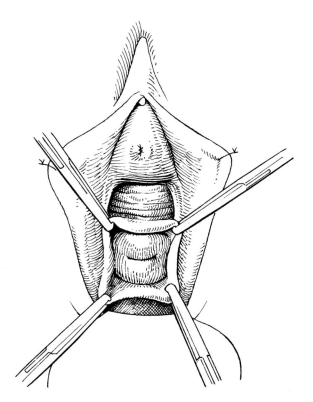

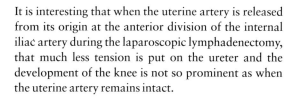

Fig. 10.13 Preparation of vaginal cuff.

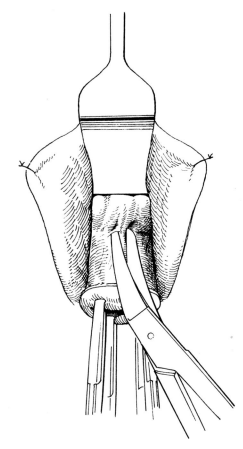

Fig. 10.14 Vaginal incision.

It is interesting that when the uterine artery is released from its origin at the anterior division of the internal iliac artery during the laparoscopic lymphadenectomy, that much less tension is put on the ureter and the development of the knee is not so prominent as when the uterine artery remains intact.

Instruments

Similar instruments to those required for the vaginal hysterectomy are necessary. However, it is important to add a narrow-bladed Wertheim's retractor approximately 1.25 cm wide together with long-toothed tissue forceps developed by Chrobach (Fig. 10.12), a Czechoslovakian gynaecologist working in Vienna at the same time as Wertheim. These important clamps are used to grasp the vaginal cuff which is developed at the beginning of the procedure. The Schauta element of the

laparoscopic lymphadenectomy and radical vaginal hysterectomy (Coelio-Schauta) is normally performed after the laparoscopic lymphadenectomy is completed. At the laparoscopic lymphadenectomy, the patient may be lying prone, or may already be in lithotomy position. It is essential during the Schauta procedure for the patient to be placed in lithotomy, if not already in that position, and once more the hips should be flexed as much as possible with the buttocks right on the end of the table. It is also helpful to have access to a video camera which will film the vaginal element of the procedure so that the assistants may see the procedure themselves on the television monitors, markedly improving the quality of assistance.

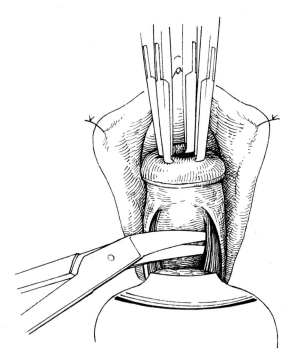

Fig. 10.15 Dissection of rectum from posterior vaginal wall.

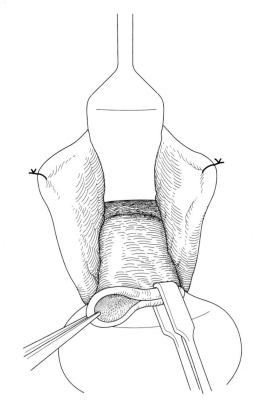

Fig. 10.16 Closure of vaginal cuff.

Anaesthesia

Usually a general anaesthetic is used, sometimes with additional or alternative epidural or caudal anaesthesia. Blood loss is usually minimal with this operation but it is normal to crossmatch 2 units.

The operation

Preparation of the vagina cuff

As this operation is normally performed for early stage cervical cancer it is common that only a small part of the cervix is infiltrated by the tumour. The cervix should be gently drawn down by grasping a healthy part of the cervix and infiltrating the vaginal tissues above and around it. Using Littlewood's or Kocher's forceps the vaginal tissue to be removed is defined. This is normally some 2–3 cm of vagina. It is important not to remove too long a length as this can produce debilitating shortening of the vagina. Once the edge of the vagina has been defined and drawn down (Fig. 10.13), infiltration is completed as for a vaginal hysterectomy

and at this point the vagina is incised just above the position of the Littlewood's forceps. As the vagina is incised the vaginal edge is drawn forwards off the cervix to lie in a position to cover over the cervical tissue. The incision is carried circumferentially around the vagina, taking care not to cut too deeply: because of the increased length of vagina being removed there is a risk to the bladder anteriorly (Fig. 10.14). Posteriorly the pouch of Douglas can be simply entered in the upper part of the posterior fornix (Fig. 10.15).

Closure of the cuff of the vagina

It is important now to draw the elongated edges of the vagina over the cervix covering over the carcinoma so that it is completely protected from contact for the remainder of the procedure. Utilizing the Chrobach clamps and beginning at one edge, the anterior and posterior vaginal edges are drawn together over the cervix and the Chrobach clamps applied serially.

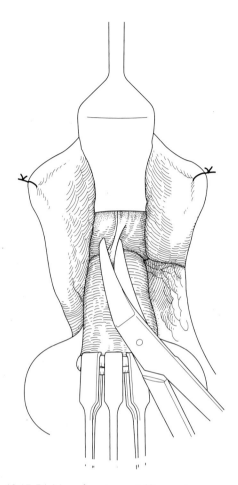

Fig. 10.17 Division of cervicovescial ligament.

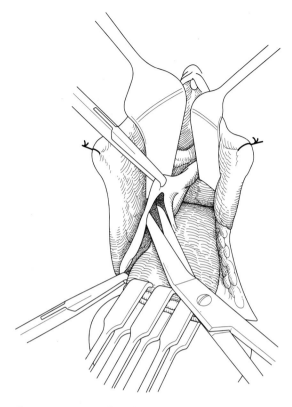

Fig. 10.18 Opening the right paravesical space.

Normally four clamps will hold the whole vaginal edge and allow manipulation of the vagina, cervix and uterus, utilizing three or four points of attachment (Fig. 10.16).

In the past, other clinicians have sewn the vaginal edges together and maintained a number of threads which can be used to manipulate the cervix and uterus.

The Schuchardt incision
I will only mention this incision to note that in the past it has been used, but in the editor's experience it is unnecessary and causes significant postoperative discomfort and scarring. The incision when made is really a large left lateral episiotomy incision widening the entrance to the vagina to give greater access (see Chapter 15, page 163).

Elevating the bladder
As the edges of the vagina have been drawn together, the tissues lying immediately above the vaginal cuff can now be gently incised in order to make the bladder as safe as possible (Fig. 10.17). The editor gently dissects downwards rather than upwards on the anterior part of the cervix in order to determine accurately the lower border of the bladder. Once the bladder edge has been defined it can be gently elevated with the back of the scissors, pushing it upwards, cutting the cervicovesical ligament, but making sure that the peritoneum anteriorly is not opened. At this point the medial side of a broad pillar of tissue including the base of the ureteric tunnel is demonstrable on either side of the mid-line.

105

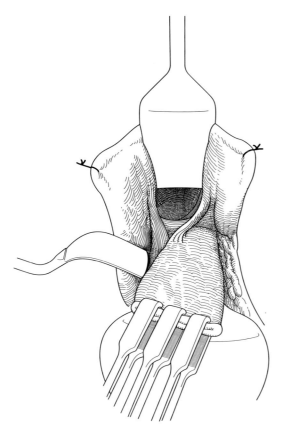

Fig. 10.19 Joining the paravesical and pararectal spaces. Horizontal fascia exposed.

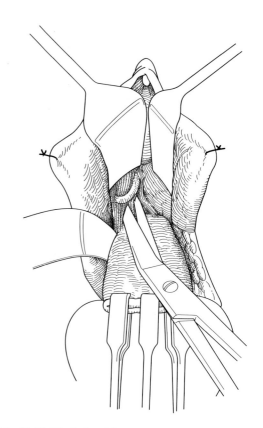

Fig. 10.20 Displaying right ureter.

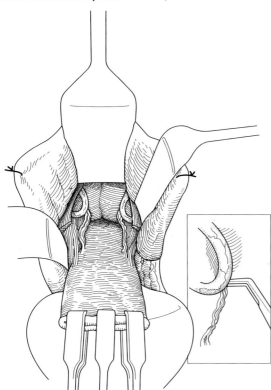

Fig. 10.21 Ligation and display of left uterine vessels.

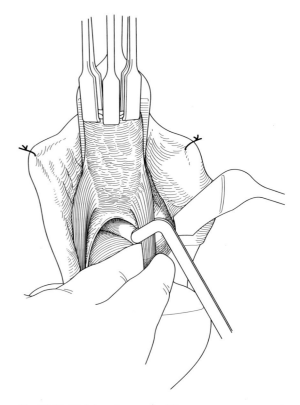

Fig. 10.22 Division of uterosacral ligaments.

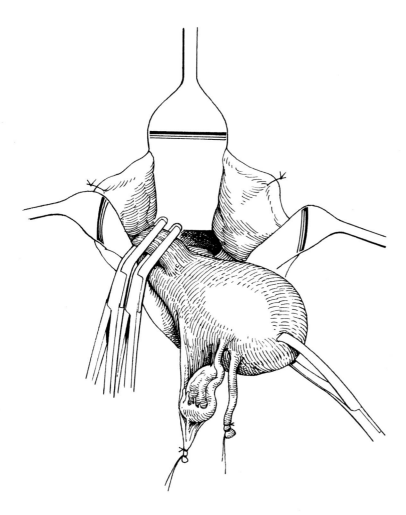

Fig. 10.23 Division of cardinal ligaments.

Opening of the right paravesical fossa
One of the assistants takes the Chrobach clamps and draws the cervix over to one side, and the proximal lateral edge of the cut vagina is grasped with a straight tissue forcep. At this point the angled Monaghan scissors can be inserted at right angles to the edge of the vaginal skin, upwards and laterally, gently opening the scissors as they advance but taking care not to close them in the space, and in this way each paravesical fossa can be simply and accurately accessed (Fig. 10.18). This space is then developed further by placing the narrow curved Wertheim retractor (Fig. 10.19) into the space. The angled Wertheim's retractor fits neatly around the pubic ramus opening up the space completely. On the medial side of the space which has been so developed

lies a pillar of tissue, bordered on its lateral side by the Wertheim's retractor and the paravesical space, and on its medial side by the open area which has been separated as the central part of the bladder has been drawn upwards. With the Wertheim's retractor in place and the index finger below the bladder lying on the cervix the ureter can be palpated within the ureteric tunnel and a 'click' can be felt as the firm ureter is rotated against the Wertheim's retractor. This gives the surgeon a good idea of the position of the ureter and how far up the pillar it lies. It is now necessary to divide the pillar in order to demonstrate the ureter.

Dissection of the ureters
With one assistant maintaining tension on the

107

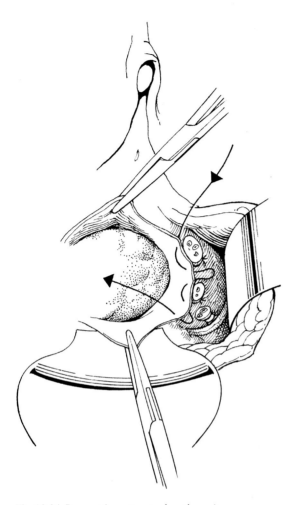

Fig. 10.24 Purse-string suture to close the peritoneum.

Chrobach clamps, the other assistant holding the Wertheim's retractor in the paravesical space, the surgeon can then gently divide by blunt dissection the lower part of the ureteric pillar. By gently dividing what is, in effect, the floor of the ureteric tunnel and occasionally noting the position of the ureter knee within the ureteric pillar, the ureter can be identified and gently elevated. As the ureter is elevated (Fig. 10.20) on its medial and inferior side will be seen the descending branch of the uterine artery lying in the soft tissue on the anterolateral part of the uterus. The descending branch of the uterine artery can then be clamped and divided. It is the author's preference to place a small Navratil right angle clamp below the uterine artery to elevate it (Fig.

10.21), and following the laparoscopic division of the uterine artery by gently teasing the artery down it will be possible to see the small clip which has been placed on the medial part of the artery where it has been divided close to the internal iliac. In the standard Schauta procedure, which is not combined with the laparoscopic division of the uterine artery, the uterine artery can be divided at a high level by gently drawing it down and then dividing it having clamped it with the right angle clamp.

This process of identifying the uterine artery is performed in a gentle and cautious manner, gently teasing it down with a forcep and pushing the ureter away, upwards and laterally.

Dividing the uterosacral ligament and identifying the cardinal ligaments

As the ureter has now been elevated and pushed away and the uterine artery divided, the finger can be inserted into the opening in the pouch of Douglas and the uterosacral ligaments hooked by the finger. These may be divided and ligated, or in some circumstances may simply require being cut (Fig. 10.22). The next element to be identified is the broad band of the cardinal ligament. This is clearly seen running at right angles to the cervical tissue and by placing the index finger around it, the ureter can be elevated well above it, and a long length of cardinal ligament identified. These can be grasped with a Zeppelin clamp at a chosen point to include a significant part of the parametrial tissue (Fig. 10.23). The ligament is divided and the lateral ends are sutured and released. At this point there is nothing holding the uterus into the abdomen apart from the peritoneum which runs across the uterovesical fold, and unless a pure Schauta procedure is being performed the round ligaments and uterine pedicles will already have been dealt with laparoscopically. The uterovesical fold can be identified, by running the index finger around the side of the uterus then incised and the entire uterus drawn down simply cutting the remaining peritoneum. At this point all that is left to be dealt with is the peritoneum of the pelvis, if that is to be closed, and the vaginal vault.

Closure of the vault

It is the authors' practice to simply close the vaginal vault making sure not to foreshorten the vagina too much. Once more a pack is placed into the vagina and a catheter in the bladder, and the procedure is complete.

Some author's prefer to close the peritoneum, but this is not absolutely essential (Fig. 10.24).

If a laparoscopic procedure has already been performed, at the end of the whole operation a check of the intra-abdominal area can be made for haemostasis. There are usually minimal problems and the ureters can be observed as they function, and any minor clot removed.

Postoperative care

It has been the author's experience that the modern variation of the Schauta procedure is significantly less damaging to the bladder than has been previously noted. In virtually all patients, the catheter in the bladder can be maintained for 3 days and is then removed and normal function occurs. More prolonged bladder catheterization may sometimes be necessary until normal bladder function resumes. Recovery is rapid. The average time in hospital in the editor's series of patients is just under 5 days. This compares very favourably with the 10 days of the Wertheim's procedure. (Forty-five cases of Coelio-Schauta versus over 1000 cases of Wertheim's hysterectomy.)

Mobilization is rapid as the patient has only four small abdominal wounds. To date, no patient has required blood transfusion and there has been no trauma in the author's series to bladder or ureter.

Further reading

When the editor was asked to edit this text, one of his earliest thoughts was to ask Sir Rustam (Mole) Feroze to write this chapter. He was the acknowledged British master of the procedure. I have now gained a considerable experience of the Schauta Procedure and feel comfortable in describing my own experience (JMM).

Students should also re-examine older editions of *Bonney's Gynaecological Surgery* for the variations of technique illustrated there.

For years, the argument between vaginal and abdominal hysterectomy raged; to a large extent, this has now disappeared but it may interest the student to read Copenhaver EH (1965) Hysterectomy: vaginal versus abdominal. *Surg Clin North Am* 45: 751–763.

11 Radical hysterectomy and pelvic node dissection

Carcinoma of the cervix is currently the second most common female cancer worldwide and remains the commonest cancer in women in developing countries. Although it is estimated that there are over 370 000 new cases a year worldwide, it has become a rare tumour in England and Wales with only 2740 cases registered in 1997. The reason for this low incidence has been the introduction of the national programme for regular cytological screening in 1988, which has reduced the incidence by over 40%.

Persistent infection with the human papilloma virus (HPV) has been identified as having a causal role in cervical cancer and its DNA can be identified in almost 100% of tumours. Current work on vaccines against HPV as a means of preventing cervical cancer appears promising. Smoking and prolonged use of the oral contraceptive pill have also been recognized as risk factors.

Traditionally, treatment of cervical cancer has been with either surgery or radiotherapy, the latter being used to treat all stages of the disease, with radical surgery reserved for early stage disease especially in younger women. Adjuvant radiotherapy following surgery has been used in the 15–30% of surgical cases where the pelvic lymph nodes were found to contain metastatic disease.

The major advantage of surgery over radiotherapy in younger women is the possibility of preserving the ovaries and the reduction in vaginal morbidity. Radiotherapy invariably results in ovarian failure and the vagina is often irreparably damaged with shortening and narrowing.

However, since the last edition of this textbook there has been increasing use of concomitant chemoradia- tion both in the primary and adjuvant setting for all stages of the disease because of apparent survival advantages over radiotherapy alone. In the surgical management, the laparoscopic approach has gained in popularity and has several advantages over the open approach. Morbidity is less and it provides increasing variation in management including fertility-sparing operations such as cervical trachelectomy.

History

Radical hysterectomy for the treatment of carcinoma of the cervix consists of the removal of the whole uterus, at least the upper one-third of the vagina, the parametrium and paracolpos to the pelvic side wall. The pelvic lymph nodes are dissected up to and in- cluding the common iliac nodes. However, in North American practice it is now more usual to extend the node dissection to include the lower para-aortic lymph nodes up to the renal vessels.

W.A. Freund, in 1878, was the first to advocate ab- dominal hysterectomy for the treatment of cancer of the uterus, but it is to Reis of Chicago that the honour of developing the radical operation is given. In 1895, he demonstrated by operations on dogs and the human cadaver that it should be possible to remove the uterus, its appendages, the cellular tissue of the pelvis and the lymphatics up as far as the common iliac vessels with- out killing the patient. Clark, in 1896, put this sugges- tion into practice on a living woman at the Johns Hopkins Hospital and was quickly followed by others, while Thring of Sydney independently began to prac- tise a similar procedure. The establishment of the radi- cal technique as an accepted procedure was, however, due to Wertheim of Vienna, who performed the first of his extensive series in 1898.

In the first half of the 20th century, the operation was used extensively to treat almost all stages of cancer of the cervix. During this period, however, it became increasingly clear that radiotherapy was superior to surgery in treating all later stage disease and of at least equal potency in treating earlier disease. Also, the risks of surgery, in an era where there was no blood transfusion service and antibiotics were not available, were enormous.

The primary mortality from the operation as performed by Wertheim was initially 30%, later reduced to 10%. Bonney, in his series, produced similar figures reducing his primary mortality from 20% to 11% in the last 200 of his first 500 cases. Although these figures are horrific by modern-day standards (the editor had not had a single operative death in his first 300 cases), they must be taken in the context of a time of no antibiotics and no blood transfusions. Nowadays the emphasis has moved from mortality towards morbidity and great efforts must be made continually to reduce this to the absolute minimum.

Preoperative assessment

Before treatment can commence, a histological diagnosis must be made. If an invasive lesion of the cervix is suspected, colposcopy should be performed and an adequate biopsy performed. Any diagnostic biopsy should be greater than 5 mm in depth for histology to confirm International Federation of Gynecology and Obstetrics (FIGO) stage Ib disease requiring more radical surgery but should not be excessive. Large cone biopsies add little to the diagnosis, induce a marked inflammatory response and compromise assessment of tumour size by both histology and preoperative MRI. A small diagnostic loop or wedge biopsy is ideal and conization should only be considered as a therapeutic option for complete excision of a small lesion. Examination under anaesthesia (EUA) is not essential if pelvic examination assessed whilst awake is deemed to be adequate. However, one should have a low threshold for performing an EUA if there is any doubt.

The tumour is examined to determine its full extent and any spread within the pelvis. This is best achieved by performing a *bimanual examination*. Firstly, the vagina is examined using two fingers of the right hand; this gives information about the cervix and the size and shape of the tumour. It also indicates whether there has been any spread to the fornices or into the mid or lower vagina. The vaginal examination is not of great value in assessing the extent of spread towards the pelvic side wall. This is best determined by carrying out a bimanual examination with one finger of the right hand in the rectum and the left hand on the abdomen. Using this technique the rectovaginal septum, the uterosacral ligaments, the parametrium and the pelvic side wall can be accurately assessed. Some teachers recommend the use of the combined examination whereby the index finger is inserted into the vagina and the second finger is inserted into the rectum. The authors do not feel that this technique adds significantly to the information from the bimanual examination.

We have found routine cystoscopy singularly uninformative for most small tumours less than 4 cm and reserve it for large tumours and those small tumours encroaching onto the anterior vaginal fornix. The kidneys should be investigated for hydronephoses by IVU, ultrasound or MRI as ureteric obstruction stages the tumour as at least stage IIIb. However, as with cystoscopy, an abnormal finding is extremely rare with stage Ib1 tumours.

Once the cancer has been staged, the most appropriate form of treatment can be discussed with the patient, taking into account the stage, her age and the treatment methods available. Surgery may be by an open abdominal approach or laparoscopic/vaginal and it may be possible to preserve fertility.

For a radical abdominal hysterectomy the patient should be admitted the day before surgery and prepared as for a major abdominal procedure (see Chapter 3).

Anaesthesia

The authors use a technique of epidural or spinal analgesia combined with general anaesthesia and are convinced that there are major advantages in terms of reduced blood loss due to less intraoperative ooze. Where facilities are available the epidural can be used for effective postoperative analgesia.

Surgery

It is the authors' practice to operate from the right side of the patient and this should be taken into account when reading the surgical description.

When a surgeon is undertaking a major operation for a gynaecological cancer he must not be compromised by having only one assistant. A second assistant is required as a 'dynamic retractor' that needs to be adjusted at various times during the operation. This is particularly the case with a radical hysterectomy where the 'third' blade is sited at different points during the operation.

Instrumentation
The gynaecological general set as described in Chapter 2 is required with the addition of a disposable automatic blood vessel clip ligator.

Preparation
The patient is initially placed in the lithotomy position and the vulva and vagina are washed and prepared. The bladder is catheterized with a self-retaining catheter with a small 5 ml balloon and is attached to a drainage device.

An Amreich retractor is now inserted into the vagina and, using the packing forceps, the vagina is firmly packed using a dry 3 metre vaginal gauze roll. The patient's legs are then taken down from lithotomy position. The end of the pack should be left long and placed between the patient's legs, with the packing forceps attached to the end so that the pack can be easily removed during the procedure.

The abdomen is now washed, prepared and draped appropriately for the incision to be used.

Incision
The authors favour a mid-line subumbilical incision that can be extended above the umbilicus as necessary. This gives excellent access to the pelvis as well as to the lower para-aortic area. However, in obese women with a short distance between the umbilicus and pubic symphysis and a large pannus the authors favours a Maylard or Cherney incision that can provide excellent access. The abdomen is opened as described in Chapter 6.

Inspection
It is essential to inspect the pelvis fully to confirm the operability of the tumour. The parametrium is palpated for infiltration with tumour and the pelvic side walls for enlarged lymph nodes. The upper abdomen is inspected for evidence of metastatic disease and para-aortic lymphadenopathy.

Primary tumour (radical hysterectomy)

The authors' preference is to perform the radical hysterectomy first followed by the lymphadenectomy though many surgeons perform the operation in the reverse order. The choice is based on the surgeon's preference and on the philosophy as to whether one should abandon surgery for the primary if there is obvious metastatic disease in the pelvic lymph nodes that will require adjuvant therapy. Our practice is to remove enlarged lymph nodes as they are more likely to be radioresistant followed by removal of the primary tumour to reduce the risk of central recurrence.

The operation

Operative position and packing of the intestine
The patient should be placed in a steep Trendelenburg position allowing the intestines to be easily packed away from the pelvis. This is usually achieved with one large moist pack marked by an arterial clip at the end of the tape. It is sometimes necessary to incise the peritoneum along the lateral side of the sigmoid colon at the pelvic brim to mobilize and elevate the sigmoid out of the pelvis.

Forceps to uterus
The uterus is grasped with two medium tissue forceps at the uterine cornu incorporating the round and ovarian ligaments as well as the tubes (see Chapter 7).

Round ligament
The right round ligament is grasped with medium tissue forceps in its lateral half and cut.

Uterovesical fold
At the same time, the first assistant lifts the loose peritoneum over the bladder with a toothed forceps and the surgeon runs his scissors under the uterovesical fold separating the soft fascia. The peritoneum is then incised along the fold across to the left round ligament.

Infundibulopelvic/ovarian ligaments
If the ovaries are to be removed, the pelvic peritoneum lateral and along the ovarian vessels is cut to mobilize the infundibulopelvic ligament. The left index finger now elevates the ovary and tube, and thrusts through the thin peritoneum of the posterior leaf of the broad

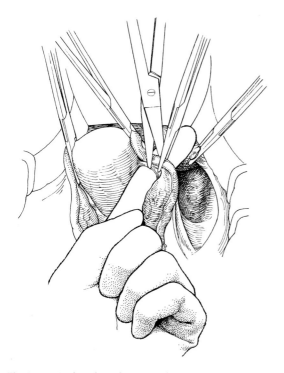

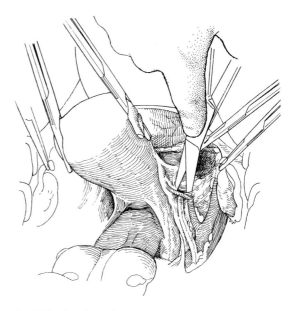

Fig. 11.2 Identifying the uterine artery close to the pelvic side wall.

Fig. 11.1 Dividing the right ovarian ligament.

ligament medial or lateral to the ovary depending on whether it is to be preserved or removed. The infundibulopelvic or ovarian ligament is then clamped with a medium tissue forceps with the tip in the defect created by the index finger. Prior to cutting the ligament it may be appropriate to adjust the uterine clamp with its tip in the peritoneal defect to prevent a back flow of blood. The ligament can now be cut (Fig. 11.1).

The round and infundibulopelvic ligaments can now be tied or may remain held by the clamps until the end of the operation as this facilitates the maintenance of tension on the tissues, which is required at certain times in the operation. However, using this technique often requires one or other of the assistants to be constantly holding the clamps to prevent them entering the pelvis.

The same procedure is now performed on the left side.

Identification of ureter, identification and ligation of uterine artery

The uterine clamps are now handed to the first assis-

tant, who draws the uterus over towards himself. The second assistant controls the clamps on the round and infundibulopelvic ligaments (if used), and maintains traction on the Morris retractor. If the assistants maintain this slight tension, the space alongside the uterus is immediately available.

The surgeon now separates the soft areolar tissue of the opened broad ligament down to the level at which the anterior division of the internal iliac artery becomes visible. Using the Monaghan's scissors, the ureter, uterine artery and the obliterated hypogastric artery are readily identified. The uterine artery is cleared in front and behind so that it is completely separated from the ureter which it overlies (Fig. 11.2). The ureter is separated from the peritoneum for a short distance and a Meigs' forceps is inserted below the uterine artery. This forceps is then lifted up, gently putting the artery on the stretch. If the forceps is opened, all the areolar tissue below the artery is separated and the ureter can be seen to be completely clear. A straight tissue forceps is now placed between the open jaws of the Meigs' forceps and the artery clamped (Fig. 11.3). The Meigs' forceps is now removed and, using the straight forceps to elevate the artery, the vessel can be accurately clamped close to

113

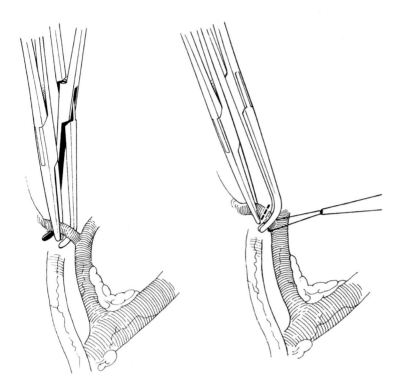

Fig. 11.3 Dividing the right uterine artery at its origin.

its origin at the internal iliac artery with the Meigs' forcep. The vessel is now cut close to the Meigs' forceps and ligated. It is here that the Meigs' forceps are of such enormous value: they are long, the tip or the heel can be used to loop the tie around, yet they are delicate enough not to leave a large mass of tissue behind in the ligated pedicle.

The same procedure is performed on the opposite side.

In obese women with a deep pelvis where access may be limited, it is sometimes easier to ligate the uterine artery using the arterial liga clips rather than applying a Meigs and tying around it. The medial end of the uterine artery can still be held with a straight tissue forceps, which provides traction whilst dissecting the ureteric tunnel.

Occasionally, small veins close to the ureter or the artery bleed; this can produce a confusing picture to the trainee surgeon. It is important not to clamp any structure in this area until it is clearly identified; therefore, the editor would recommend the insertion of a swab into the space to stem oozing and to return to the area after a few minutes. (The scrub nurse must be informed that a swab has been inserted and the fact

marked on the count board.) Upon returning to the area it will be found that the structures are easily identified and the dissection can be proceeded with.

Reflection of bladder

The authors recommend leaving this stage until after the ureters and the uterine artery have been isolated, as there is frequently troublesome bleeding from small vessels which are damaged. Separation is easily achieved by pushing down the uterovesical fold with a swab folded over the finger. The smooth surface of the packed upper vagina is readily recognized and small fibres of tissue can be divided. If there is difficulty in finding this tissue plane, a light stroke with the scalpel across the width of the upper vagina with traction on the bladder and uterus will reveal the correct level. Frequently, engorged veins are found lying in the lateral part of this dissection. These should be handled gently; otherwise, the profuse haemorrhage which can occur will cause problems in the next steps.

If the finger or the back of Monaghan's scissors are pushed into the lateral part of this dissection, the ridge of tissue which is formed gives a clear indication of the site of the ureteric tunnel; occasionally, the ureter in the last 2 cm of its course is visible at the bottom of this dissection.

The lateral dissection should be performed one side at a time because of potential for venous bleeding.

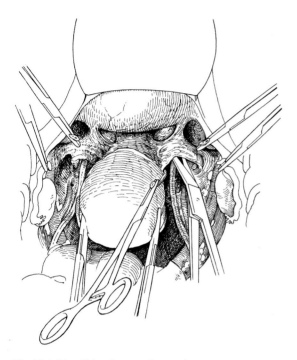

Fig. 11.4 Identifying the ureteric tunnel.

Development and incision of the roof or the ureteric tunnel

The roof of the ureteric tunnel can often be well demarcated by placing the Morris retractor centrally and applying an upward pull countered by the uterus being gently pulled cranially.

The tissue forceps on the uterine artery is drawn medially over the top of the ureter, and Monaghan's scissors are inserted over the top of the ureter along its tract to open out the ureteric tunnel (Fig. 11.4). If the opened scissors are elevated, the ureter can be seen along its tract, completely separated from the roof of the tunnel (Fig. 11.5a,b). With the scissors protecting the ureter, a straight tissue forceps is placed along the tunnel roof and clamped. The roof is cut medial to the forceps exposing the ureter as it enters the bladder. The pedicle is now firmly tied.

Occasionally, the division of the left ureteric tunnel can be facilitated by performing some of the dissection from the medial aspect of the tunnel.

Separation of the ureter from the upper vagina

Using Monaghan's scissors, the ureter is separated from the upper vagina and dislocated laterally; this reveals the cardinal ligament passing downwards and laterally. The ureter is completely separated from the peritoneum in the lower part of the pelvis but remains in contact in the upper part. In the authors' view it is not necessary to strip the ureter to its full length in the pelvis.

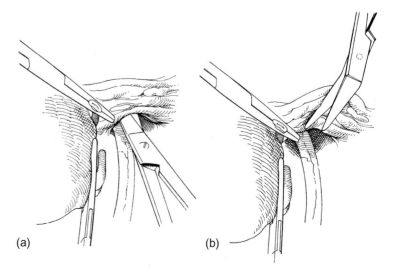

Fig. 11.5 (a, b) Separating the ureter from the roof of the ureteric tunnel.

(a)   (b)

115

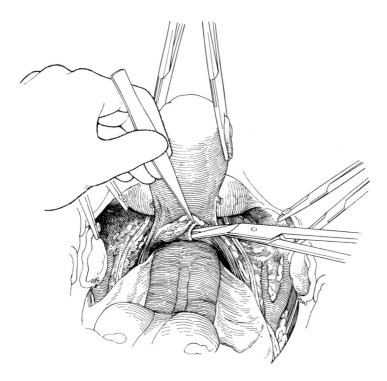

Fig. 11.6 Opening the space between the rectum and the vagina.

Opening of the rectovaginal space

It has been the authors' recent practice to perform this step prior to the dissection of the ureteric tunnels. This is because bleeding from the vaginal veins during the preparation and dissection of the tunnels may be difficult to control whilst the uterus is *in situ*. As a result, the surgeon may often rush this step of the operation in a hurry to remove the uterus. In contrast, the opening of the rectovaginal space is bloodless and the reflection of the rectum off the vagina and the development of the uterosacral ligaments can be performed precisely and at ease before proceeding to the ureteric tunnels.

The Morris retractor is now removed and the uterine clamps are handed to the second assistant, who elevates the uterus at the front of the abdominal incision. This brings into view the whole of the pouch of Douglas. The peritoneum immediately below the cervix is now grasped with a pair of toothed dissectors held in the left hand and the surface is cut with Monaghan's scissors. The scissors are then introduced into the space and opened, revealing the soft areolar tissue running down between vagina and rectum (Fig. 11.6). This incision across the peritoneum is now completed posteriorly in a transverse manner, keeping the ureter under direct vi-sion at all times. The incision runs over the surface of the uterosacral ligaments; it is important not to cut into these ligaments but to merely separate the peritoneum from their surface.

Placing a swab over the first three fingers of the left hand, the rectum is swept from the vagina using an extension movement of the hand; at the same time, the peritoneum is separated from the uterosacral ligaments, revealing them as an arched structure (Fig. 11.7).

Sharp dissection can also be used to identify and skeletonize the uterosacral ligaments further.

Placement of clamps, and incision

At this point in the dissection the surgeon can put the final touches to this part of the procedure by checking that the ureters are free from the vagina and cardinal ligaments and that the bladder is reflected down far enough to expose the requisite length of vagina.

The uterosacral ligaments run posterolaterally from the cervix. They can be palpated by hooking the index finger around them. The Zeppelin tissue forceps are now placed midway along the ligaments, which are divided using the scissors. It is unnecessary to place

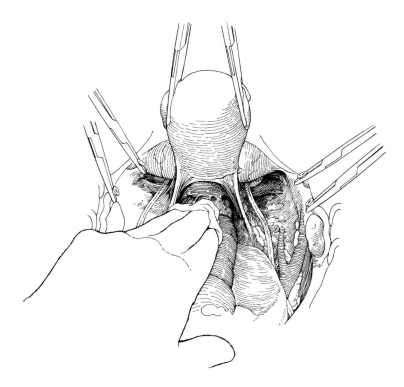

Fig. 11.7 The rectum separated from the vagina showing the arch of the uterosacral ligaments.

the clamps as far laterally as possible except when dealing with a large primary tumour.

A second set of Zeppelin clamps are placed on the cardinal ligaments, again, the lateral extent being based on the size of the primary lesion. The ligaments are divided and the vaginal pack is now removed and a third set of clamps, more angled than the previous, is placed on the paracolpos which are excised (Fig. 11.8).

Incision of vagina
The anterior wall of the vagina is incised with a scalpel and the incision is extended through the posterior wall whilst lifting the uterus upwards and cranially to protect the rectum from injury.

Ligation of pedicles
Some bleeding occurs as the vagina is incised and a small swab can be pressed against the incised edge while the Zeppelin clamps are individually stitch ligatured. Great care is taken to have the ureter fully visible at this time. Some authorities recommend pulling the ureters away from the field with coloured vascular loops but the authors do not recommend this,

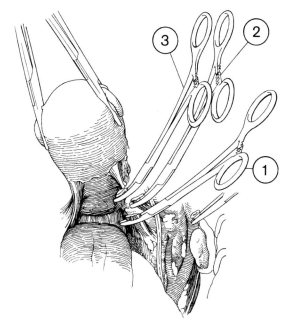

Fig. 11.8 The position of the tissue clamps on the uterosacral and cardinal ligaments and the paracolpos.

117

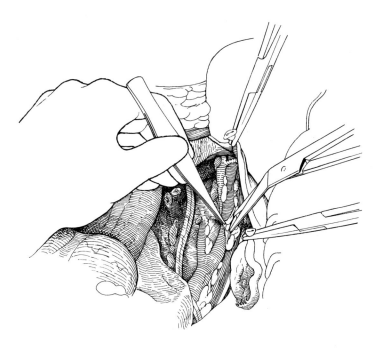

Fig. 11.9 Beginning of the pelvic node dissection.

preferring the ureter to lie naturally within the operation field.

Oversewing vaginal edge

After the pedicles are secured with a Vicryl stitch, the rim of the vagina is sutured using a continuous stitch as a haemostat. This should be locked on the posterior edge and run continuously on the anterior edge to help evert the rim making the taking of the next 'bite' easier. The surgeon should hold the thread of the suture himself to provide the correct tension required.

Once all bleeding is controlled, the pelvis can be left and the node dissection carried out.

Lymphadenectomy

Some authorities feel that the pelvic lymph nodes should be dissected prior to the radical hysterectomy phase; the authors have practised both and feel that the dissection is much simplified if the uterus has been removed first.

The extent of the node dissection varies between surgeons but should consist of the removal of all visible pelvic lymph nodes from the bifurcation of the common iliac artery caudally. If there are any enlarged

nodes identified during the procedure, dissection should extend cranially to include the common iliac lymph nodes. Any enlarged common iliac or para-aortic nodes should be sampled.

Taking the two clamps which are attached to the round and infundibulopelvic ligaments and drawing them apart, the external iliac artery and vein are revealed. The second assistant places the Morris retractor over the artery and retracts firmly under the inguinal ligament. The fascia over the iliopsoas muscle is now picked up in toothed dissectors and incised along the line of the artery (Fig. 11.9), taking care not to damage the genitofemoral nerve. This incision is carried up to the retractor, and the lateral external iliac nodes lying under the inguinal ligament are drawn down across the vessels. Individual lymphatic channels are meticulously clipped using small metal artery clips (Auto suture or liga clips); occasionally, small blood vessels are severed and should also be clipped (Fig. 11.10).

The line of dissection now continues along the length of the external iliac artery, developing a sheet of fascia and nodal tissue which will leave the arteries clean from the bifurcation of the common iliac artery to the inguinal ligament. If tension is maintained on this fascia with the left hand, and separation and dissection performed using the Monaghan's scissors in the right,

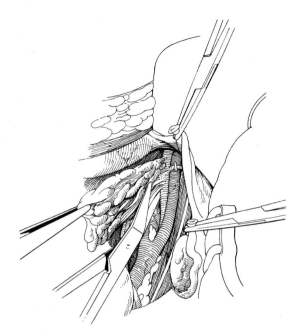

Fig. 11.10 The complete block of lymph nodes being removed from the external iliac vessels.

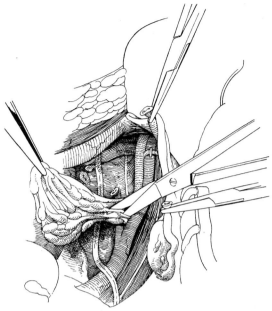

Fig. 11.11 Completing the pelvic lymph node dissection in the obturator fossa.

it is possible to roll the vessels round so that all nodal tissue is removed *en bloc*. At the upper end of the dissection the sheet of tissue separated is continued down the internal iliac artery (Fig. 11.11), taking great care to keep an eye on the ureter and the obturator nerve. Finally, this dissection dips below the external iliac vein so that the obturator fossa can be emptied of all nodal material, resulting in a block of tissue lying close to the tied uterine artery. The mass is lifted out and may be separated into its constituent parts. Bleeding is surprisingly little, especially if small vessels and lymphatics are clipped with the metal clips as the dissection proceeds.

Closure of the abdomen

At the end of the lymphadenectomy the pelvis should be checked for haemostasis and any bleeding controlled. In the past, it was felt that drainage of the pelvic space was required to prevent the formation of lymphocysts. However, the authors have shown that as long as the pelvis is not re-peritonized, there is no benefit to drainage. For this reason a drain should only be inserted if there is any concern regarding haemostasis.

In premenopausal women where the ovaries are conserved, consideration should be given to transpose the ovaries outside the pelvis in case adjuvant radiotherapy to the pelvis is required. The inferior margins of the ovaries can be marked with metal artery clips to assist the radiotherapist with planning treatment.

If a suprapubic catheter is to be inserted, this can be inserted by direct vision before the abdomen is closed. The bladder is filled by inserting 400 ml of saline through the transurethral catheter facilitating insertion of the suprapubic catheter. The authors have found these to be superior to transurethral catheters in allowing the patients to initiate passage of urine spontaneously. They also facilitate bladder training and assessment of residual urine volumes without the need for frequent catheterization with all its attendant risks. Most patients will pass urine spontaneously during the first 10 days postoperatively, but up to 30% will require longer periods of drainage to allow for bladder recovery.

The abdomen can be closed by mass closure or in layers as described in Chapter 6.

Table 11.1 Complications of radical hysterectomy

Intraoperative	Postoperative	Long term
Haemorrhage and vascular trauma	Ileus	Bladder dysfunction
Ureteric, bladder, bowel and nerve trauma	Infection	Ureteric and bladder fistulae
	Thromboembolic disease	Lymphocyst and leg oedema
	Ureteric and bladder fistulae	
	Lymphocyst	

Table 11.2 Sites associated with a high risk of haemorrhage

Ureteric tunnel
Paracolpos and vaginal edge
External iliac artery and vein
Obturator fossa
Bifurcation of the common iliac artery

Recommended plan of management

There is considerable debate about the correct management for carcinoma of the cervix. There is increasing use of chemoradiation over radiation alone for primary treatment in all stages of disease as well as for adjuvant therapy after surgery. The use of neoadjuvant chemotherapy prior to surgery for bulky stage Ib2 and IIb tumours is also currently being evaluated.

Complications of radical hysterectomy

Complications may be subdivided into intraoperative, postoperative and long term, and are summarized in Table 11.1.

Haemorrhage
Haemorrhage during a radical hysterectomy is a significant risk, especially at certain anatomical sites during dissection (Table 11.2).

Bladder dysfunction
Following radical hysterectomy and node dissection, the commonest complication is bladder dysfunction, manifesting itself as difficulty in initiating micturition and fully emptying the bladder. Catheterization is essential in the postoperative period but is often unnecessary for a prolonged time.

Attempts at nerve-sparing techniques have been adopted by some surgeons, especially in Japan (Sakamoto, Yabuki), to try and reduce bladder dysfunction. These techniques have recently been replicated in Western patients (Trimbos).

All patients who have had radical hysterectomies should have the urethral catheter removed at 5 days or the suprapubic catheter turned off, and be allowed to initiate spontaneous micturition. If the patient cannot void or can only pass small volumes, then catheter drainage should be reinstated for a further 48 h. When the patient is able to void, the residual urine volume should be assessed on the evening of the first day. If the residual urine volume is greater than 100 ml, then another period of 48 h of catheterization should be instituted. Women who are unable to pass urine spontaneously at the time of discharge from hospital should be taught intermittent self-catheterization.

Ureteric dysfunction
Most patients (87%) show ureteric dilatation 48 h after the operation, usually with complete recovery by 6 weeks. At the end of the first week, 20–30% of postoperative IVUs are abnormal: dilatation of the upper renal tract is seen whereas the distal one-third may be normal or narrowed.

In almost all patients these changes will have disappeared by the end of the first year after surgery. When irradiation has been used preoperatively, devascularization of the ureter can be critical, resulting in fistula formation or at least fibrosis, stricture and loss of peristalsis in the affected segment.

The incidence of ureteric fistula appears to be decreasing in the reported literature. It is probably most influenced by the routine use of prophylactic antibiotics, better pelvic drainage and a reduction in the use of preoperative radiotherapy.

Ureteric stricture is very rare following radio therapy alone and relatively rare following surgery but occurs more commonly after combination surgery and radiotherapy. If there is an obvious external cause for the stricture, such as a lymphocyst or local recurrence of tumour, appropriate steps must be taken to deal with this problem. If the obstruction does not clear or cannot be simply resolved, a urinary diversion must be made.

Vesicovaginal fistula

This complication is less common than uretero-vaginal fistula in most reported series. It usually follows intraoperative trauma to the bladder, most commonly in the mid-line and at a high level in the bladder. Consequently, management should be all about masterly inactivity and continuous bladder drainage. Most fistulae heal spontaneously if the bladder is effectively drained, the exceptions being when the patient has had pre- or postoperative radiotherapy.

Urinary tract infection

Febrile morbidity occurs in 30–50% of patients following radical hysterectomy, the most common cause being urinary tract infection.

It is important to use a sterile technique when inserting the urethral catheter and to maintain a high urine output in the postoperative period. In addition, catheter specimens of urine should be collected if there is a pyrexia and at the time of removal of the catheter.

Pelvic lymphocysts

The incidence of lymphocysts detected by ultrasound is approximately 15–20% with between 1 and 4% being identified clinically. The lymphocyst appears a few days after operation and may grow steadily for the next few months. Thereafter, in most cases, steady resolution occurs as the fluid contained in the cyst is reabsorbed, probably due to the growth of new lymphatics and the expansion of existing channels. On rectal examination they are palpable as a smooth, tense mass attached to the pelvic side wall and must be distinguished from tumour recurrence and infection. This differentiation is most easily carried out by ultrasonography.

Lymphocysts require active management when they produce pain, obstruction or become infected.

1 Pain may be a sign of infection, pressure on a viscus or vascular channel or directly on nerves. Symptomatic relief must be given but the major aim of the treatment must be to remove the cause of the pain.

2 Partial or, rarely, total bowel obstruction can occur and requires drainage of the lymphocyst to relieve the compression. More commonly, tenesmus is experienced which can be very debilitating. Occasionally, these cysts drain spontaneously via the vagina or rectum.

3 Venous obstruction can be a very significant problem with a high morbidity and mortality. It is vitally important to differentiate the leg oedema which can temporarily occur following lymphatic dissection from that produced by secondary deposits in the lymphatics and that due to venous obstruction by a lymphocyst. The lymphocyst and venous obstruction is best diagnosed by ultrasound.

4 Infection is the most frequently encountered problem complicating lymphocysts. The actual bacterial agent concerned may not be known and therefore it is essential to use broad-spectrum multiple-agent therapy to ensure elimination of infection. Persistent or recalcitrant disease is an indication for surgical drainage.

Nerve damage

The nerve damage most likely to occur is to the genitofemoral and the obturator nerves during node dissection on the pelvic side wall. It is not unusual for the genitofemoral nerve to be present as a number of thin strands rather than a single nerve bundle; these strands may be mistaken for lymphatics and dissected out by the operator. Damage to the nerve results in loss of sensation over a small part of the anterior surface of the upper thigh and the labia of the vulva. The obturator nerve may be damaged when removing the obturator nodes, which lies along the length of the nerve. Damage to this nerve may produce palsy of the adductors of the inner thigh or pain of the muscles or skin in the inner thigh.

Prevention is best achieved by carefully identifying the nerves before continuing with the dissection.

Rather less commonly, deep dissection of the pelvis may produce some sciatic nerve damage, usually manifesting itself as sciatica, but it is much more common to have this type of pain following infiltration of the perineural lymphatics by tumour micrometastases.

Peroneal nerve damage is a risk whenever any patient is put into lithotomy poles.

Further reading

At the present time, the editor would recommend to the reader who wishes to learn more about radical hysterectomy and its role in the management of carcinoma of the cervix the monograph by Hugh Shingleton and James Orr entitled *Cancer of the Cervix: Diagnosis and Treatment* published by Churchill Livingstone in 1983. This book comprehensively covers the problem of the patient with carcinoma and, in particular, discusses the indications for primary surgery in the management of this disease and the role of lymph node dissection.

The editor's colleague John Shepherd—in Chapter 5 of *Clinical Gynaecological Oncology* by Shepherd and Monaghan, 1985, Blackwell Scientific, Oxford—clearly describes the technique of Wertheim's hysterectomy in the management of early carcinoma of the cervix.

Both this chapter and Shingleton and Orr's monograph are extensively referenced.

The editor would also recommend Chapter 14 of Byron J Masterson's *Manual of Gynecologic Surgery* published in 1979 by Springer-Verlag, New York. This chapter by James Daly is a beautifully illustrated account of the procedure, particularly of the para-aortic node dissection.

Cherney LS. A modified transverse incision for low abdominal operations.

Sakamoto S, Takizawa K. An improved radical hysterectomy with fewer urological complications and with no loss of therapeutic results for invasive cervical cancer. *Baillières Clin Obstet Gynecol* 1988;2:952–62.

Trimbos JB, Maas CP, Deruiter MC, Peters AAW, Kenter GG. A nerve-sparing radical hysterectomy: Guidelines and feasibility in Western patients. *Int J Gynecol Cancer* 2001;11:180–6.

Yabuki Y, Asamoto A, Hoshiba T, Nishimto H, Satou N. A new proposal for radical hysterectomy. *Gynecol Oncol* 1996;62:370–8.

Of major historical interest to the reader are the landmark papers of Freund and Wertheim: Freund WA Method of complete removal of the uterus. *Am J Obstet Gynecol* 1879; 7:200; and Wertheim E Zur Frag der Radikaloperation beim Uteruskrebs. *Arch Gynak* 1900;61:627.

Some years later, Bonney published his own impressive series: Bonney V (1935) The treatment of carcinoma of the cervix by Wertheim's operation. *Am J Obstet Gynecol* 30:815. This personal series of almost 500 patients is a tremendous testament to the great man's skill.

Mattingly RF (1980) Surgical treatment of cervical cancer — factors influencing cure, in *Controversies in Gynaecological Oncology*, pp. 39–68 (published by the RCOG, London). In this excellent paper, the late Dick Mattingly presents the accumulated knowledge of a lifetime as a gynaecological oncologist, bringing his own brand of quality writing to the subject.

12 Pelvic exenteration

The procedure of pelvic exenteration was first described in its present form by Brunschwig in 1948. It has been used mainly in the treatment of advanced and recurrent carcinoma of the cervix. Its primary role at the present time is in the management of that relatively high number of patients who will develop recurrent cancer of the cervix following primary radiotherapeutic treatment. It has been estimated that between one third and one half of patients with invasive carcinoma of the cervix will have residual or recurrent disease after treatment. Approximately one quarter of these cases will develop a central recurrence which may be amenable to exenterative surgery. However, pelvic exenteration as a therapy for recurrent cancer of the cervix has not been widely accepted and many patients will succumb to their disease having been through the process of radiotherapy followed by chemotherapy and other experimental therapies without being given the formal opportunity of a curative procedure.

In the early years, high operative mortalities and relatively low overall survival (20% 5-year survival in Brunschwig's series) resulted in few centres taking up the surgery. The more recently published results of exenterative procedures show an acceptable primary mortality of approximately 3–4% and an overall survival/cure rate of between 40 and 60%. The procedures may also be applicable to a wide range of other pelvic cancers including cancer of the vagina, vulva and rectum, both for primary and secondary disease. It is relatively rarely applicable to ovarian epithelial cancers, melanomas and sarcomas because of their tendency for widespread metastases.

The surgery involved is extensive and postoperative care complex; as a consequence, the operation has become part of the repertoire of the advanced gynaecological oncologist working in a centre with a wide experience of radical surgery. The procedure demands of the surgeon considerable expertise and flexibility as virtually no two exenterations are identical. Also considerable judgement and ingenuity are required during the procedure in order to achieve a comprehensive removal of all tumour. A degree of tailoring of surgery can be carried out as it may well be that with small recurrences a more limited procedures can be carried out with a degree of conservation of structures in and around the pelvis. Where extensive radiotherapy has been carried out, complete clearance of all organs from the pelvis (total exenteration) together with widespread lymphadenectomy may be essential in order to achieve a cure. There is now considerable evidence that even in those patients with pelvic node metastases at the time of exenteration a significant salvage rate can be achieved.

Selection of patients for exenterative surgery

Exenterative surgery should be considered for locally advanced primary pelvic carcinoma as well as recurrent disease. Many patients will be eliminated from the possibility of surgery at an early stage because of complete fixity of the cancer to the bony structures of the pelvis. The only exception to this rule is the rare circumstance where a vulva or vaginal cancer is attached to one of the pubic rami, when the ramus can be resected and a clear margin around the cancer obtained.

Palliative exenteration

In general terms exenterative surgery should not be used as a palliative measure except perhaps in the presence of malignant fistulae in the pelvis, when it may significantly improve the quality of the patient's life without any significant extension to that life. The patient and her relatives must be made fully aware that the surgery is not being carried out with a curative intent.

Patient assessment

The average age of patients who are subject to exenteration lies between 50 and 60 years, but the age range is wide from early childhood through to the eighth or ninth decade. Advanced age is not a bar to success in exenterative surgery.

It is frequently difficult following radiotherapeutic treatment to be certain that the mass palpable in the pelvis is due to recurrent disease and not to radiation reaction, persistent scarring associated with infection or the effects of adhesion of bowel to the irradiated areas.

In recent years CT scan and MRI have been used extensively in the preoperative assessment of patients for many oncological procedures. The considerable difficulties and uncertainties that are generated for the radiologist assessing the CT or MRI scan where patients have had preceding surgery or radiotherapy, is rarely more problematic than when patients are being assessed for exenteration. Some clinicians feel that the scan is an integral part of preoperative assessment, whereas the editor has not found the level of reliability of CT scan in particular to be acceptable. A tissue diagnosis is essential prior to embarking on exenterative surgery and the use of needle biopsy, aspiration cytology or frequently open biopsy at laparotomy will need to be performed. As distant metastases tend to occur with recurrent and residual disease, it is sometimes helpful to perform scalene node biopsies and radiological assessments of the pelvic and para-aortic lymph nodes together with fine-needle aspiration or biopsy to assist with the assessment. The mental state of the patient is also vital, but should not in itself be a bar to surgery.

Absolute contraindications to exenteration

If there are metastases in extrapelvic lymph nodes, upper abdominal viscera, lungs or bones there appears to be little value in performing such major surgery. However, there is evidence that patients with pelvic lymph node metastases may well survive and have a high quality of life in a small but significant percentage of patients.

Relative contraindications to exenteration

Pelvic side wall spread. If the tumour has extended to the pelvic side wall either in the form of direct extension or nodal metastases the prospects of a cure are extremely small and the surgeon must decide whether the procedure will materially improve the patient's quality of life. The triad of unilateral uropathy, renal nonfunction or ureteric obstruction together with unilateral leg oedema and sciatic leg pain is an ominous sign. The prospects of a cure are poor. Perineural lymphatic spread is not visible on CT and can be a major source of pain and eventual death.

Obesity. This is a problem with all surgical procedures producing many technical difficulties as well as postoperative respiratory and mobilization problems. The more massive the surgery, the greater are these problems. Barber in 1969 noted the very high risk associated with obesity in their series.

Types of exenteration

In North America the majority of exenterations performed are total (Fig. 12.1b). In the authors' series approximately half of his exenterations have been of the anterior type (Fig. 12.1a) removing the bladder, uterus, cervix and vagina, but preserving the rectum. For small, high lesions around the cervix, lower uterus and bladder it may be possible to carry out a more limited procedure (a supralevator exenteration) retaining considerable parts of the pelvic floor. Posterior exenteration (abdominoperineal procedure) is relatively rarely performed by gynaecological oncologists as these tend to be the area of activity of the general surgeon.

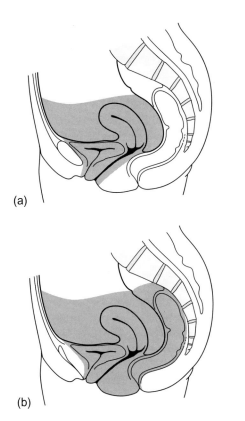

Fig. 12.1 The limits of resection for (a) an anterior and (b) a total exenteration.

Preoperative preparation

It is important that the surgeon and his team of nurses and ancillary workers must be confident in their ability to manage not only the extensive surgery involved, but also the difficult, testing and sometimes bizarre complications that can sometimes occur after exenteration.

Probably the most important part of the preoperative preparation is the extensive counselling which must be carried out to make certain that the patient and her relatives, particularly her partner, understand fully the extent of the surgery and the marked effect is will have upon normal lifestyle. Of particular importance is discussion about the removal of normal sexual function when the vagina has been taken out. It is essential, too, to discuss the possibility of reconstructive surgery of the vagina and bladder, and the necessary transference of urinary and bowel function to the chosen type of diversionary procedure which will be performed, and to communicate honestly the significant risks of such extensive surgery. During the course of this counselling, the patient should be seen by a stomatherapist. Where it is possible, the senior nurse specialist will arrange for psychosexual counsellors skilled in cancer treatment to make preliminary contact with the patient.

At this very traumatic time it is important not to overwhelm the patient and her family with too much information. A fine judgement has to be made about the pace and volume of information imparted. To aid this communication, the author finds it ideal for the patient to meet with other patients who have had the procedure to discuss on a woman-to-woman basis the real problems of and feelings about exenteration.

Most preoperative investigations are now performed in the outpatient setting and will include a full blood analysis, heart and lung assessments including chest X-ray, ECG, echocardiography and appropriate tests dependent on the patient's fundamental condition.

The patient is usually admitted to hospital 2 or 3 days prior to the planned procedure to obtain high-quality bowel preparation. With modern alternative liquid diets and antibiotic therapy, complete cleaning of the small and large bowel can be achieved very rapidly. The anaesthesiologist responsible for the patient's care will see the patient and explain the process of anaesthesia. The author prefers to carry out all radical surgery under a combination of epidural or spinal analgesia together with general anaesthetic. Cardiac and blood gas monitoring is essential. Although the majority of patients do not require intensive care therapy, its availability must be identified prior to the surgical procedure. Prophylaxis against deep venous thrombosis is usually organized by the ward team utilizing a combination of modern elastic stockings and low dose heparin which is initiated immediately following surgery. High risk patients may require fractionated heparin.

The operation

The final intraoperative assessment

The final decision to proceed with the exenteration will not be made until the abdomen has been opened and assessment of the pelvic side wall and posterior abdominal wall has been made utilizing frozen sections where necessary. In the author's practice the procedure is performed by a single team. If the patient has decided that a plastic surgical procedure such as the formation of a neovagina is to be carried out, then a second plastic surgical team will carry out any necessary operation at the same time as the diversionary procedures are being performed by the primary team.

Once the patient has been anaesthetized and placed in the lithotomy position in the operating theatre, the final assessment can begin with pelvic examination followed by catheterization of the bladder with an indwelling size 14 Foley catheter. If it is thought likely that an anterior exenteration will be performed it is useful to pack the vagina firmly with a long gauze roll (Fig. 12.2). The patient is returned to the supine position and the abdomen is opened either utilizing a longitudinal mid-line incision extending above the umbilicus or a high transverse (Maylard) incision (Fig. 12.3) cutting through muscles at the interspinous level. Exploration of the abdomen will confirm the mobility of the central tumour mass and thereafter dissection of para-aortic lymph nodes and pelvic side wall nodes will be carried out (Fig. 12.4) and sent for frozen section. At the time of this initial intraoperative assessment, the experienced exenterative surgeon will have assessed the pelvic side

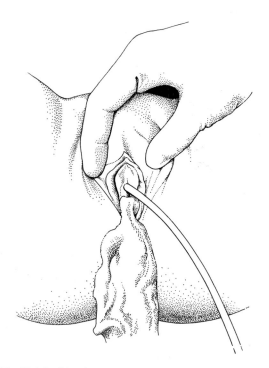

Fig. 12.2 Packing the vagina.

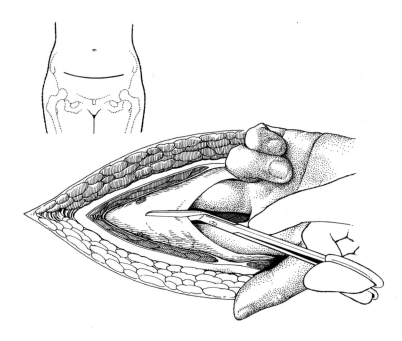

Fig. 12.3 A Maylard or high transverse incision.

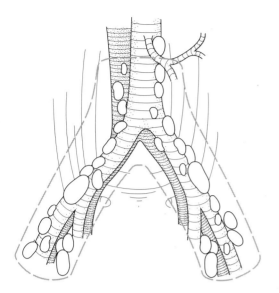

Fig. 12.4 Pelvic and para-aortic node assessment.

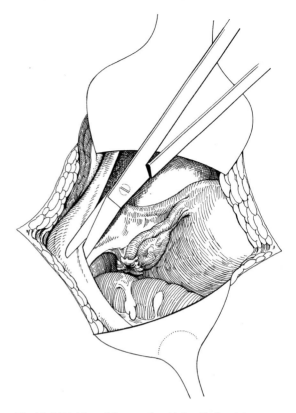

Fig. 12.5 Division of the round and infundibulopelvic ligaments and the beginning of the lateral pelvic dissection.

wall by dividing the round ligament, drawing back the infundibulopelvic ligament and opening up the pelvic side wall (Fig. 12.5). This manoeuvre will have opened tissue planes, including the paravesical, pararectal and presacral spaces, to a deep level (Fig. 12.6) allowing the surgeon to familiarize himself with the full extent of the tumour. These dissections can be carried out without any significant blood loss. If it is considered not possible to proceed with the operation due to fixity of the tumour, the abdomen may be closed at this stage as no significant trauma has been carried out by the surgeon. Considerable experience and judgement is required to make this decision. It is sometimes helpful to remove any suspicious tissue from the pelvic side wall and obtain further frozen sections. Time spent here may really mean 'life or death' for the patient. Often the most difficult decision is actually to stop operating. Very occasionally with some vulval cancers, resection of pubic bones may be necessary, but in general terms if there is bony involvement by tumour the procedure should be abandoned.

After the comprehensive manual and visual assessment of the pelvis and abdominal cavity has been made, a line of incision for removal of the entire pelvic organs will begin at the pelvic side wall, over the internal iliac artery and will pass forward through the peritoneum of the upper part of the bladder meeting with the similar

lateral pelvic side wall incision at the opposite side (Fig. 12.7). The sigmoid colon will be elevated and at a suitable point will be transected; the peritoneal incision will be carried along around the brim of the pelvis identifying the ureter as it passes over the common iliac artery and meeting up with the similar incision on the opposite side. Having divided and tied the round ligaments and opened the pelvic side wall space, the infundibulopelvic ligament can also be identified, divided and tied. The incision is continued posteriorly and the ureters separated and identified. If an anterior exenteration is to be performed, the peritoneal dissection will be brought down into the pelvis to run across the anterior part of the rectum, just above the pouch of Douglas; this will then allow a dissection from the anterior part of the rectum passing posteriorly around the uterosacral ligaments to the sacrum releasing the entire anterior contents of the pelvis. For a total exenteration

127

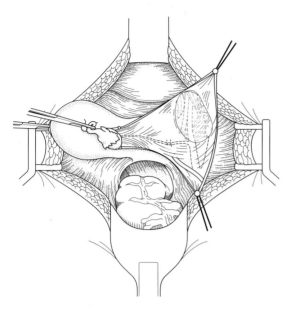

Fig. 12.6 Deepening the lateral pelvic dissection to reveal the pelvic spaces.

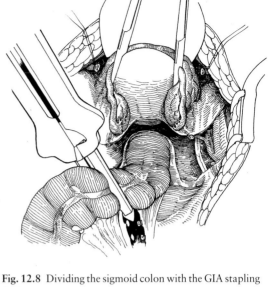

Fig. 12.8 Dividing the sigmoid colon with the GIA stapling device.

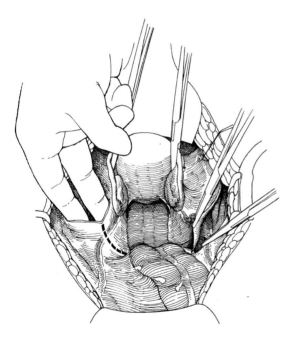

Fig. 12.7 The pelvic incision for an anterior exenteration.

the dissection is even simpler; the mesentery of the sigmoid colon is opened and individual vessels clamped, divided and tied. The colon is divided usually utilizing a gastrointestinal anastomosis (GIA) stapling device which allows the sealed ends of the colon to lie, without interfering with the operation (Fig. 12.8). A dissection posterior to the rectum is then carried out from the sacral promontory, deep behind the pelvis; this dissection is rapid and simple, and complete separation of the rectum from the sacrum will be allowed. This permits complete and usually bloodless removal of the rectal mesentery including lymph nodes. Anteriorly the bladder is dissected with blunt dissection from the cave of Retzius resulting in the entire bladder with its peritoneal covering falling posteriorly. This dissection is carried right down to the pelvic floor isolating the urethra as it passes through the pelvic floor (perineal diaphragm). As the dissection is carried posteriorly into the paravesical spaces, the uterine artery and the terminal part of the internal iliac artery will become clearly visible. By steadily deepening this dissection the anterior division of the internal iliac will be isolated, the tissues of the lower obturator fossa identified and, at this point, large exenteration clamps may be placed over the anterior division of the internal iliac artery and its veins (Fig. 12.9 and 12.10). The ureter by this time will have

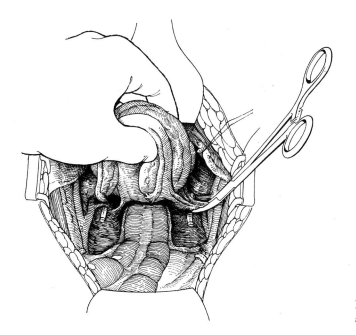

Fig. 12.9 Exenteration clamps applied to the anterior division of the internal iliac arteries.

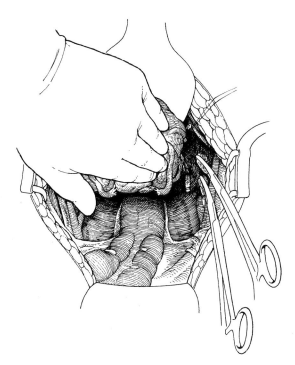

Fig. 12.10 Mobilizing the central mass of tissue.

been divided a short distance beyond the pelvic brim. The pelvic phase of the procedure is at this point completed and the perineal phase is now to be carried out.

The patient is placed in extended lithotomy position and an incision made to remove the lower vagina for an anterior exenteration and the lower vagina and rectum in a total exenteration (Fig. 12.11). Anteriorly the incision is carried through above the urethra just below the pubic arch to enter the space of the cave of Retzius which has been dissected in the pelvic procedure. The dissection is carried laterally and posteriorly, dividing the pelvic floor musculature, and the entire block of tissue is then removed through the inferior pelvic opening. Small amounts of bleeding will occur at this point, usually arising from the edge of the pelvic floor musculature. These can be picked up either by isolated or running suture which will act as a haemostat.

Once the perineal dissection has been completed and haemostasis achieved, the surgeon has choices available depending on the preoperative arrangements made with the patient. If in the preoperative assessment period it has been decided by the clinician and the patient that a neovagina should be formed then at this point either the surgeon or his plastic surgery colleague will initiate the development of a neovagina. This may be in the form of a myocutaneous graft such as the

129

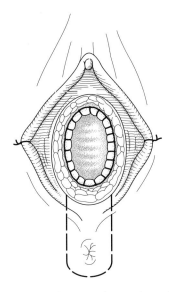

Fig. 12.11 The perineal incisions for anterior and total exenterations.

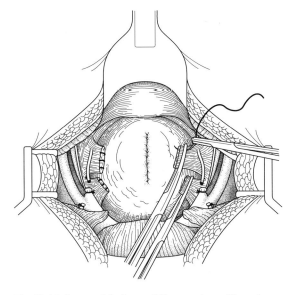

Fig. 12.12 Suture of the internal iliac arteries and lateral pelvic pedicle.

vagina formed using the gracilis muscle, a Singapore graft from alongside the vulva, or techniques which revolve around the development of a skin graft placed within an omental pad or the technique of transposition of a segment of sigmoid colon to form a sigmoid neovagina. These individual techniques will not be dealt with in this chapter, but may be seen elsewhere (see Chapter 14). For many patients, however, the desire to have a new vagina is a very low priority and it is surprising how frequently the patients will put off these decisions until well after the time of exenteration. Survival of the cancer appears to be the uppermost desire that they are determined to achieve. To this end, the careful closure of the posterior parts of the pelvic musculature, a drawing together of the fat anterior to that and a careful closure of the skin is all that is required. It is usually possible to preserve the clitoris, the clitoral fold and significant proportions of the anterior parts of the labia minora and labia majora so that when recovery is finally made the anterior part of the genitalia has a completely normal appearance. On some occasions patients will be able to have a neovagina formed some significant period of time following the exenteration. This is now becoming the predominant pattern in the editor's experience of some 89 cases.

Once the perineal phase is finished, the legs can be lowered so the patient is once more lying supine and at-

tention can be addressed to dealing with the pedicles deep in the pelvis. All that remains following a total exenteration will be the two exenteration clamps on either side of the pelvis and a completely clean and clear pelvis. The pelvic side wall dissection of lymph nodes can be completed before dealing with the clamps and any tiny blood vessels that require haemostasis are ligated. As the exenteration clamps are attached to the distal part of the internal iliac arteries it is important that comprehensive suture fixation is carried out (Fig. 12.12). This is usually readily and easily done, although occasionally the large veins of the pelvic wall can provide difficulties and the use of mattress sutures may be necessary to deal with these complex vascular patterns. Having completed the dissection of the pelvis, the clinician now moves to produce either a continent urinary conduit or a Wallace or Bricker type ileal conduit and if the procedure has been a total exenteration, as the majority are, a left iliac fossa stoma will be formed; the individual techniques of these procedures are dealt with elsewhere (see Chapter 26 and 28).

Dealing with the empty pelvis

A problem which must be avoided is that of small bowel adhesion to the tissues of a denuded pelvis. This is particularly important when patients have had preceding radiotherapy as the risk of fistula formation in these circumstances is extremely high. There have been a variety of techniques utilized to attempt to deal with this potentially life-threatening complication including the placing in the pelvis of artificial materials such as Merselene sacks, Dacron and Gortex sacks even using bull's pericardium. Stanley Way in the 1970s described a sack technique in which he manufactured a bag of peritoneum which allowed the entire abdominal contents to be kept above the pelvis. This resulted in an empty pelvis, which from time to time became infected and generated a new problem—that of the empty pelvis syndrome. Intermittently over the years patching with the peritoneum has been used, but the most successful approach appears to be the mobilization of the omentum from its attachment to the transverse colon leaving a significant blood supply from the left side of the transverse colon and allowing the formation of a complete covering of the pelvis forming a soft 'trampoline of omentum' which will then stretch and completely cover and bring a new blood supply into the pelvis. Occasionally, procedures such as bringing in gracilis muscle flaps into the empty pelvis have been carried out to deal with the difficulty of a devitalized epithelium due to previous radiation.

It is the editor's current preference to utilize an omental graft mobilizing the omentum from the transverse colon using a Powered Ligating and Dividing Stapler (PLDS) (Fig. 20.5). This allows a broad pedicle to be left at the left hand end of the transverse colon maintaining an excellent blood supply to the omentum. This is brought down to the right side of the large bowel, dropping into the pelvis immediately to the left side of the ileal conduit which is anchored just above the sacral promontory. By careful individual suturing around the edge of the pelvis and sometimes by refolding the peritoneum upon itself, a complete covering of the true pelvis with a soft central trampoline area can be generated (Fig. 12.13). A Redivac drain is inserted below the omentum which when activated will draw the omentum down into soft contact with the pelvic floor. The small bowel can thus come into contact with an area with a good blood supply obviating the risk of adherence and subsequent fistula formation. At the end of the procedure, the bowel is carefully orientated to make sure that no hernia can develop and the abdomen is closed with a mass closure. The stomas are dressed in theatre and their appliances put in place. The patient

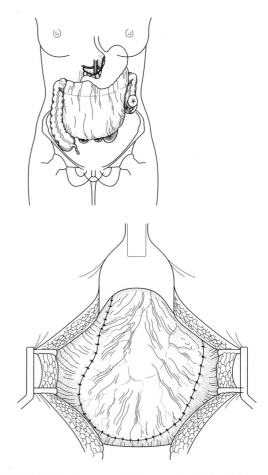

Fig. 12.13 Development of the 'omental pelvic floor': (a) omental incision; (b) soft trampoline area.

leaves the operating theatre and is then transferred back to the ward at the appropriate time.

Postoperative care

The postoperative care of exenterations is straightforward, maintaining good fluid balance, good haemoglobin levels and ideally a significant flow of urine between 2.5 and 3.5 L/day. Bowel function often returns at the usual time of 2–4 days following the procedure and a nasogastric tube, which is the author's preference, can be removed at 3–4 days and the patient returned to oral intake beginning with simple fluid on the third day. During and following the procedure, prophylactic antibiotic cover is maintained as is subcutaneous heparin cover as a deep vein thrombosis prophylaxis. Mobilization should be rapid and the patient is most often discharged between 10 and 15 days postoperatively once she is used to dealing with her stomas and the ileal conduit tubes have been removed.

Results of exenteration

Most series show that the 5-year survival following exenteration is of the order of between 40 and 60%, depending very largely upon selection of patients (Robertson et al. 1994).

A figure which is rather more difficult to obtain is the exact number who have been assessed for exenteration but have then failed at one of the many hurdles that the patient must pass before finally having the procedure carried out. It is therefore likely that the final, truly salvageable figure is an extremely low percentage. Recently, the value of carrying out exenterations in patients who have positive lymph nodes has been shown to be low but significant and it is now many clinicians' practice to carry on with an exenterative procedure even in the circumstances where one or two lymph nodes are involved by tumour.

References

Barber HRK. Relative prognostic significance of preoperative and operative findings in pelvic exenteration *Surg Clin North Am* 1969;49(2):431–7.

Brunschwig A. Complete excision of the pelvic viscera for advanced carcinoma. *Cancer* 1948;1:177.

Crawford RAF, Richards PJ, Reznek RH *et al.* The role of CT in predicting the surgical feasibility of exenteration in carcinoma of the cervix. *Int J Gynecol Cancer* 1996;6:231–4.

Disaia PJ, Creasman WT. *Clinical Gynecologic Oncology; Cancer of the Cervix, Pelvic Exenteration*, Chapters 2–8, New York: Mosby, 1981: pp. 82–8.

Robertson G, Lopes A, Beynon G, Monaghan JM. Pelvic exenteration: a review of the Gateshead Experience 1974–1992. *Br J Obstet Gynaecol* 1994;101:529–31.

Shingleton HM, Orr JW. In: Singer A, Jordan J, eds. *Cancer of the Cervix, Diagnosis and Treatment*. Edinburgh: Churchill Livingstone, 1983: p. 170.

Stanhope CR, Symmonds RE. Palliative exenteration—what, when and why? *Am J Obstet Gynecol* 1985;152:12–16.

Symmonds RE, Webb MJ. In: Coppleson M, ed. *Pelvic Exenteration, Gynecologic Oncology*. Edinburgh: Churchill Livingstone, 1981: pp. 896–922.

Symmonds RE, Webb MJ. In: Coppleson M, ed. *Pelvic Exenteration, Gynecologic Oncology*. Edinburgh: Churchill Livingstone, 1992: pp. 1283–312.

Way S. The use of the sac technique in pelvic exenteration. *Gynecol Oncol* 1974;2:476–81.

13 Operations on the vulva

Vulvar biopsy

Biopsy of the vulva is a simple procedure not requiring general anaesthesia, special preparation or complicated instruments. It must be performed with precision in order to provide the pathologist with an adequate and representative sample of the vulvar abnormality. It is the most important determinant of malignancy. No matter how expert and experienced the operator, a biopsy of a vulvar lesion is mandatory prior to radical surgery. The use of colposcopy with dilute acetic acid or the application of toluidine blue is of value in identifying areas to be biopsied, especially the preinvasive lesions.

The biopsy may be performed by excising the lesion or by using a dermatologist's (Keyes) punch; either technique will give a full-thickness biopsy of the vulvar skin, allowing adequate comment to be made by the pathologist on the nature of the lesion. Analgesia is required for both techniques and is best produced by infiltrating below and around the lesion with 1 or 2% lidocaine with added adrenaline to extend the period of analgesia and to reduce vascularity.

The Keyes punch is used for removing a circular plug of tissue, the depth of which is controlled by the pressure exerted by the operator while rotating and cutting with the punch. The plug of tissue cut is then grasped and separated at the base, using a disposable scalpel (Fig. 13.1). The hole remaining is small and will occasionally require a stitch, although for many cases a styptic pencil or Monsel's solution will stop the bleeding.

Excision or incision biopsy may be performed using the same technique of analgesia followed by the cutting of an elliptical strip of tissue, taking care to remove the full thickness of the dermis. Excision biopsy is appropriate for very small or localized lesions such as naevi, and incision biopsy for larger areas when a specimen should be removed from the growing edge.

The defect can then be closed using a fine absorbable suture on a cutting needle. Although Dexon and Vicryl may be used, these will require removal as their natural pace of resolution is slow and may produce local irritation.

Simple vulvectomy

Indications

Simple removal of the vulvar tissues is most commonly performed for the treatment of extensive vulvar intraepithelial neoplasia (VIN), or at the end of failed medical treatment for vulvar dystrophies. Other indications include massive hypertrophy of the clitoris or labia, intractable pruritus vulvae or Paget's disease. The removal may be total or partial depending on the extent of the disease; important sexual structures such as the clitoris may be preserved if not involved in the pathological process.

Patient preparation

No special preparation is necessary except to shave the vulva. It is useful to colposcope the vulva preoperatively in those cases where VIN is present to outline the full extent of the lesion or lesions, remembering that this problem is frequently multifocal. The vulva can be washed with toluidine blue to identify the areas

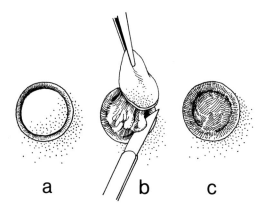

Fig. 13.1 Vulvar biopsy using the Keyes punch.

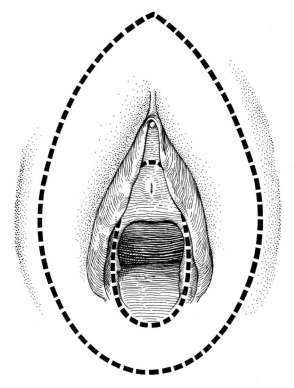

Fig. 13.2 The incision for simple vulvectomy.

involved; from personal experience the editor would recommend the use of dilute (3%) acetic acid, as used in cervical colposcopy, the most important caveat being that frequently the acetic acid must be applied for a longer period of time before the characteristic changes appear.

Anaesthesia

A general anaesthetic is usually used although, for removal of small parts of the vulva, local infiltration techniques may be appropriate.

Instruments

The general gynaecological set is required (see Chapter 2).

The operation

The patient is placed in lithotomy position and colposcopy performed where indicated to outline the lesion.

The incision is shown in Fig. 13.2; it should be elliptical to include the clitoris, both labia and the fourchette. The inner limits are usually the vaginal mucocutaneous junction and a point a short distance above the urethral orifice. The exact limits will vary depending upon the extent of the lesion or lesions to be removed.

If the anterior part of the skin to be removed is grasped with a Littlewood's forceps and drawn down, the incisions can be deepened to the deep fascia. The

entire vulva is then removed by peeling and cutting simultaneously in a posterior direction (Fig. 13.3).

Three major bleeding areas will be found: the first when the clitoral vessels are cut, and the second and third when the terminal branches of the internal pudendal arteries are cut on either side of the fourchette. These vessels may be clipped and dealt with by inserting a crossed or square mattress suture which will pick up all the small vessels, especially around the base of the clitoris. Surprisingly few other vessels require individual treatment.

Resuturing requires a good eye in order to produce a symmetrical closure. The anterior part of the incision should be brought together using an interrupted vertical mattress suture in order to remove dead space below the skin. This area should be sutured down to a point a short distance above the urethral orifice so as not to hood the opening. Thereafter, the remainder of the vulva can be covered by apposing the two cut edges, taking care to sew evenly so that 'dog ears' are not produced (Fig. 13.4). Rarely, difficulty may be found in

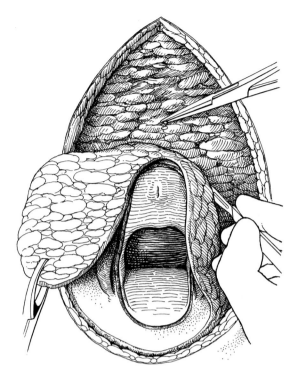

Fig. 13.3 Removing the vulval skin.

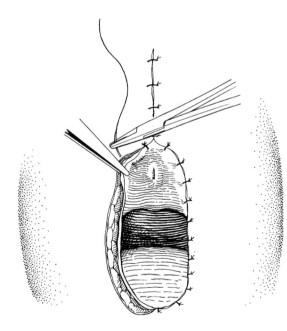

Fig. 13.4 Suturing the cut edges.

bringing the edges together; this can be obviated either by using short releasing incisions posteriorly alongside the anus, as in the radical vulvectomy operation, or by incising horizontally across the vagina and thereby releasing the tension.

Variations

These are legion, from partial procedures through hemivulvectomy to skinning vulvectomy whereby only the epithelium is removed. This latter procedure has been performed using the CO_2 laser and is described later. The authors have used a combination of simple vulvectomy to the vulva and laser surgery to the peri-anal area in the treatment of widespread multifocal VIN with excellent results.

At the end of the procedure it is usual to insert a catheter into the bladder and maintain it for the first 3 days; this helps to keep the vulva dry in the immediate postoperative period.

Postoperative management

The patient must be rapidly mobilized and encouraged to bathe and use the bidet frequently. It is important to dry off the vulva after bathing and not to use creams or talc. It is superfluous to insist on the patient drying herself with a hairdrier after bathing but this has been advocated by some clinicians.

Usually, the wounds heal well and sutures can be removed after 7 days. Occasionally, haematomas may develop and should be treated conservatively unless they are large and painful, when drainage and tying of the vessels involved is necessary. Infection should be carefully watched for and guarded against by meticulous nursing and frequent vulval swabbing with a simple antiseptic substance.

For the patient who has suffered chronic pruritus vulvae the nights after operation come as a blessed relief.

Treatment of Bartholin's cysts

Excision

Preparation of the patient
As for vulvovaginal operations.

Instruments
Two Allis's or Littlewood's tissue forceps, toothed dissecting forceps, fine dissecting scissors.

135

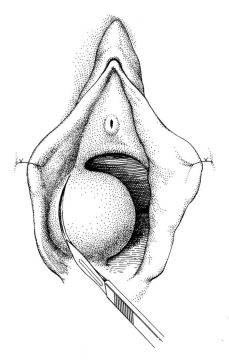

Fig. 13.5 Incising the Bartholin's cyst.

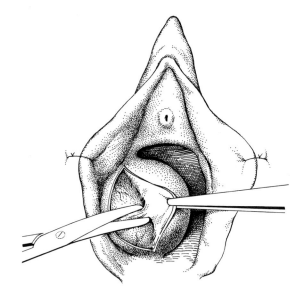

Fig. 13.6 Enucleating the cyst.

The operation
Skin incision The incision should run along the long axis of the labium majus, and be so placed that there is no risk of dyspareunia when healed (Fig. 13.5). The skin will draw naturally apart, revealing the tense surface of the cyst.

Enucleation of the cyst The tissue plane around the cyst is now developed using a separating action of the scissors; occasional strands of fascia may need to be cut. If the gland has been involved in previous episodes of infection this dissection may not flow smoothly and more sharp dissection will be required (Fig. 13.6). Tiny blood vessels will be cut and should be dealt with by fine ties or diathermy.

The gland duct is resected and the entire cyst removed (Fig. 13.7).

Obliteration of the cavity It is essential to completely close the cavity as venous oozing frequently occurs if a space is left, producing a haematoma which may be the nidus for infection and will significantly delay healing.

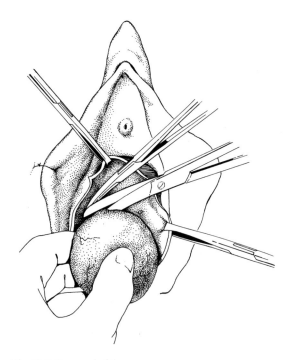

Fig. 13.7 Removal of the cyst.

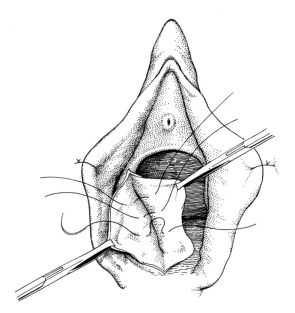

Fig. 13.8 Obliteration of the cyst cavity.

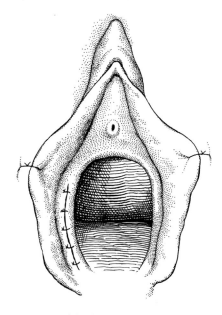

Fig. 13.9 Closure of the skin.

Using interrupted catgut, Dexon or Vicryl sutures the cavity is obliterated; two layers will usually suffice (Fig. 13.8).

Skin closure The cut edges of the wound are now apposed using interrupted sutures (Fig. 13.9). Continuous or subcuticular sutures are appealing but should be avoided so that any serous or sanguinous ooze can escape. A drain is not usually necessary but may be inserted and recorded if the procedure has been unusually bloody.

Marsupialization

This popular alternative procedure allows some continuing function of the glandular tissue.

The procedure is very similar to that already described except that the incision is carried through into the cyst, releasing its contents. The edge of the cyst cavity is then opened widely and the cyst wall is sutured using interrupted stitches to the skin edge so as to saucerize the cyst, allowing free drainage of its secretions to the exterior. During healing, the edges have a tendency to fuse, increasing the risk of new cyst formation.

Bartholin's gland abscess
If the gland is infected at the time of surgery it is wise to open, drain, send the contents for culture and treat the patient with an appropriate antibiotic. Drainage is maintained by inserting a gauze wick. Frequent vulval toilet is carried out and the patient encouraged to use the bath and bidet from the second postoperative day. The vulva should be carefully dried after each visit.

Radical surgery for carcinoma of the vulva

It is now generally accepted that the optimum basic management for carcinoma of the vulva is to carry out a radical vulvectomy and groin node dissection. There is no evidence that direct extension of vulval carcinoma to the pelvic nodes occurs without first passing through the groin nodes. The pelvic nodes should only be dissected when the carcinoma reaches the femoral canal.

It is not justifiable to dispense with the groin node dissection except when the carcinoma invades for less than 1 mm or in the exceptional circumstances where the patient is unfit for the more radical procedure.

Anatomical distinction between different levels of

nodes in the groin is surgically unimportant as the aim of the technique is to remove all the groin nodes *en bloc*.

The operation should be carried out in departments with a considerable surgical, anaesthetic and nursing experience of the operation; this will result in high operability rates (97% in the editor's series) and excellent long-term survivals. In a series of over 760 cases the editor has an overall actuarial 5-year survival of 72%. When the groin nodes are negative this rises to 94.7% and falls to 62% when they are positive, with an operative mortality of 3%.

Patient preparation

The patient should be admitted 2 days prior to surgery for intensive cleansing of the vulval region by antiseptic bathing as well as routine preoperative preparation.

Sentinel node identification

The concept of there being a single, or a small number, of sentinel nodes identifiable as the first lymph node group to be involved when cancer spreads from the vulva to the groin nodes has been mooted for many years. Disaia in 1979 first commented on the possibility of performing a sentinel node dissection in order to determine the necessity for carrying out a full groin node dissection.

Until the work of Levenbach was carried out in the late 1990s it was extremely difficult to achieve high levels of accuracy in identification of sentinel nodes. Levenbach and his colleagues used vital blue dyes which, when injected in the leading edge of a cancer of the vulva, would spread by the lymphatics and could be identified in the first lymph node involved in the lymphatic chain close to the medial side of the superficial nodes in the groin.

However, although this simple technique in both concept and performance was investigated extensively there remained a small proportion of patients where it was not possible to identify a sentinel node, and therefore the technique's application to most patients with vulval cancer was deemed too inaccurate to be acceptable.

In more recent times, following work done in breast cancer the use of the Neoprobe, a scintillation counter which will measure 'hot spots' generated in lymph nodes following the injection of technetium into the leading edge of tumours has demonstrated a very high level of accuracy in the identification of the sentinel node or nodes. This technique has now been widely investigated in Britain, America, Holland and Italy, and is reaching the point at which clinicians are comfortable to perform a sentinel node biopsy and, based upon the determination of the status of that lymph node in terms of metastatic disease, to either dispense with or continue to perform a groin node dissection. In the fullness of time a greater experience of this technique will be necessary to provide complete confidence. However, the technique, if it is applicable, will conserve the groin nodes in a high proportion of patients, reducing markedly the unhappy consequence of leg oedema and discomfort generated following dissection of the groin lymphatics and the associated nerve bundles lying close to the nodal mass.

The operation

The patient is positioned lying supine with the feet approximately 25 cm apart and supported by ankle rests to elevate the calves from the table. Some authorities recommend the 'ski' position so that two, or even three, teams can operate simultaneously. This is a recipe for confusion and does not significantly speed up the operation. Slight Trendelenburg is sometimes necessary to facilitate access to the groins, especially if the patient is obese.

Skin incision
An incision curving down towards the groin is made from the anterior superior iliac spine to a mid point over the symphysis pubis, followed by an incision from the anterior superior iliac spine to a point 8 cm below the public tubercle with a curve towards the groin fold. A third incision is now made from this last point, curving upwards and medially, to meet the crural fold (Fig. 13.10). The skin removed from the groin will be minimal, a narrow band less than 0.5 cm wide, with a narrow releasing incision over the line of the upper part of the saphenous vein. The vein is isolated, ligated and cut at the apex of this releasing incision.

Defining the fascial planes
The band of skin in the groin is picked up using Lane's tissue forceps so that the block of tissue in the groin can be manoeuvred during the dissection. By putting slight tension on the upper and lower edges of the skin incisions, undercutting can be achieved down to the

aponeurosis of the external oblique muscle above the groin (Fig. 13.11) and to the fascia over the sartorius muscle which forms the lateral boundary of the femoral triangle. This fascia is now incised longitudinally from the anterior superior iliac spine to the apex of the femoral triangle. The medial edge of the fascia is now picked up using two small Spencer Wells clips and elevated (Fig. 13.12). The strands of the femoral nerve can now be seen in the soft tissue at the medial side of the sartorious muscle. Some of these fibres are now cut as the femoral artery is defined and meticulously cleaned from the apex of the femoral triangle to the inguinal ligament. The condensation of fascia lateral to the artery along the inguinal ligament is separated with scissors to leave the external oblique aponeurosis clean.

Removing the groin nodes from the femoral vessels

On the medial side of the femoral artery the femoral vein can be seen; it is cleaned from the inguinal ligament distally, the saphenous vein is clamped, cut and ligated as it enters the femoral vein, and the whole block of tissue containing the groin nodes is turned medially (Fig. 13.13). On the medial side of the femoral vein the fascia over the adductor muscles is incised longitudinally and, having cut through the fat at the apex of the femoral triangle, the fascia is stripped from the adductor muscles as far medially as the gracilis aponeurosis. The round ligament is picked up as it leaves the inguinal canal and divided and ligated. The subfascial dissection

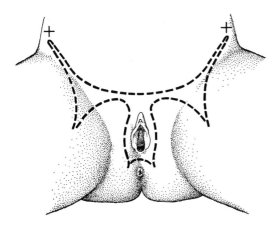

Fig. 13.10 Butterfly skin incision.

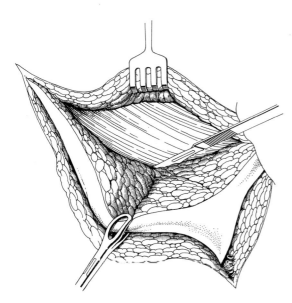

Fig. 13.11 Cutting the upper incision to the external oblique aponeurosis.

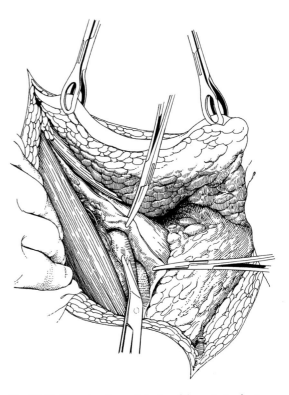

Fig. 13.12 Elevating the medial edge of the sartorius fascia and cleaning the femoral artery.

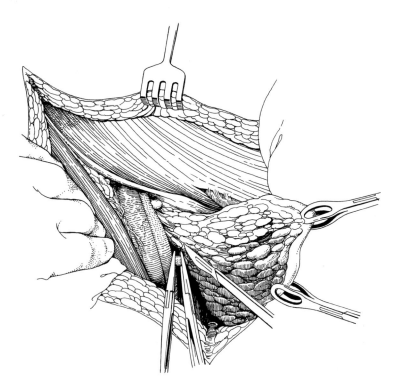

Fig. 13.13 Clamping and dividing the saphenous vein below the cribriform fascia.

is then completed through to the pubic symphysis. The entire groin nodes have been removed *en bloc* (Fig. 13.14).

Pelvic node dissection

The pelvic nodes are now approached by incising through the external oblique muscle approximately 2 cm above the inguinal ligament, beginning above the femoral canal and extending superolaterally for 8 cm. The internal oblique muscle is then incised along the line of its fibres exposing the transversalis fascia and peritoneum. Using the fingers, the peritoneum is swept from the outer pelvis exposing the external iliac vessels. The exposure is completed by extending the medial end of the wound down to the femoral canal, applying large Spencer Wells clips to the inferior epigastric arteries (Fig. 13.15).

Through this incision the external iliac vessels can be cleaned of nodes up as far as the common iliac vessels, and in direct continuity with the groin node dissection. Although Cloquet's node is said to be constant, the lateral and medial external iliac nodes are a more regular feature (Fig. 13.16).

Closure of the abdomen

This is achieved by a continuous Vicryl suture, beginning at the medial end over the femoral canal, travelling laterally, and then returning to the medial end to complete the closure of the external oblique muscles. At this point the femoral canal is reconstituted by suturing the medial part of the external oblique incision to the fascia of the pectineal line, so that the femoral canal admits a finger tip and pressure is not put on the femoral vein (Fig. 13.17).

Closure of the skin and drainage of the groin

Using the linear and releasing incisions, closure of the skin presents no problems and can be carried out without tension either using interrupted Vicryl suture or skin staples for extra speed. Drainage of the space left in the groin is mandatory as up to 300 ml of fluid can collect on each side per day. Drainage is carried out by either vacuum or low-pressure continuous drainage through large diameter drains. The authors feel that the old practice of sartorious muscle transplant to cover the femoral vessels is not necessary, as the risk of disruption appears to be more theoretical than real.

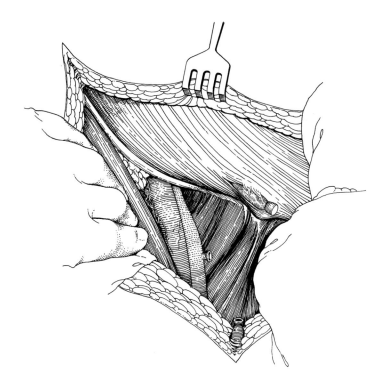

Fig. 13.14 The completed groin dissection.

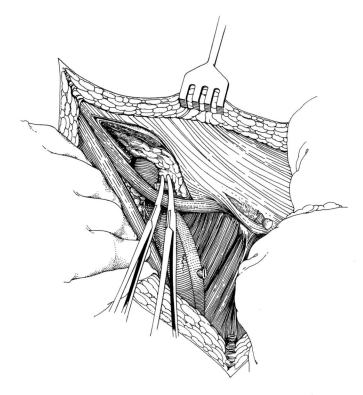

Fig. 13.15 Clamping the inferior epigastric
artery. Paupart's ligament.

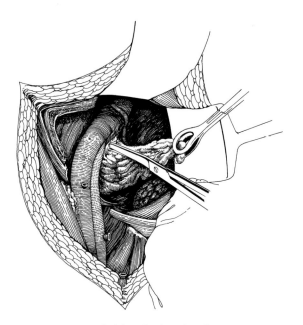

Fig. 13.16 Removal of the pelvic lymph nodes.

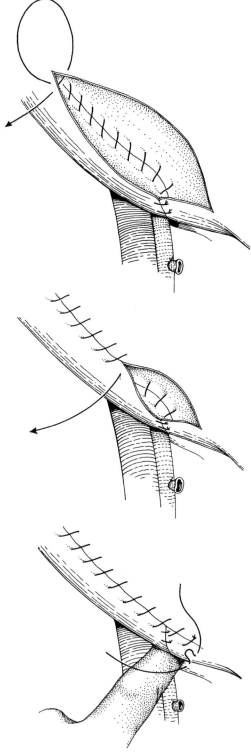

Fig. 13.17 Repair of the inguinal ligament.

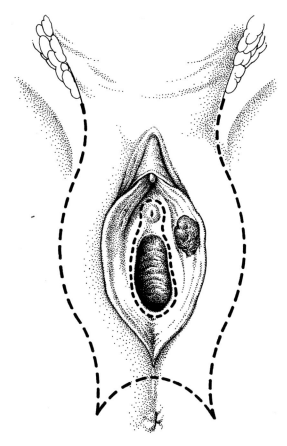

Fig. 13.18 The vulvar incision.

A similar procedure is now performed on the opposite side.

Removal of the vulva

The patient is now placed in the lithotomy position.

The vulval incision must be varied according to the size and position of the carcinoma. The basic principles of removal are:

1 A wide margin of normal skin must surround the carcinoma.

2 The margin must be adequate both laterally and medially.

3 All dystrophic skin must be removed with the specimen.

The incision that was carried into the crural fold is now extended laterally to the vulva to end alongside the anus, the anus is skirted by a curved incision, and a similar incision is made on the opposite side (Fig.

13.18). The urethra and vagina are now encircled by the inner incision; if the lesion extends close to the urethra it may be necessary to remove the lower half of the urethra.

The lateral incisions are now deepened down to the deep fascia and periosteum and the entire vulva removed. Free bleeding occurs at this time from three sites in the main: the ends of the two internal pudendal arteries and the vascular tissue around the base of the clitoris. Square mattress sutures are of great value in dealing with these points.

Primary closure of these wounds is easily achieved and the patient leaves theatre lying flat with suction drains in the groins and a catheter in her bladder (Fig. 13.19).

Variation in technique

It has been mooted for many years that it may be possible to carry out this operation without the need for continuity of tissue between the vulva and the groin. If carcinoma of the vulva spreads by lymphatic embolization and not by permeation of the lymphatic channels it is reasonable to perform separate groin node incisions. Since 1985 the editor has been using a three-incision technique. The lines of incision are shown in Fig. 13.20. This technique is very simple: the groin dissection is performed as described in this chapter and the dissection is completed by removing the block of tissue at the point where the round ligament appears from the inguinal canal.

The skin is closed using a Dexon suture to bring the mid points together and the remainder is apposed using a stapling device. There is no tension in the wounds and the primary healing rate is excellent.

Postoperative care

The epidural catheter is removed at the end of the procedure and the patient is then started on subcutaneous heparin 5000 units twice daily for 10 days. As the patient's legs are no longer immobilized, she is encouraged to commence active movements at a very early stage; it is probably this factor as much as the subcutaneous heparin which has contributed to the disappearance of thromboembolic disease in the postoperative period.

Post-operative prophylactic antibiotics are not routinely used although they should be rapidly prescribed if there is any sign of systemic infection.

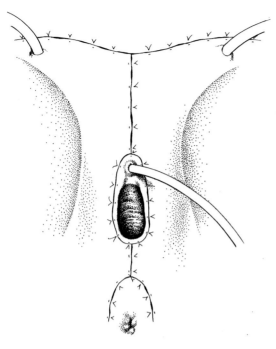

Fig. 13.19 Completed repair of the vulvar wound.

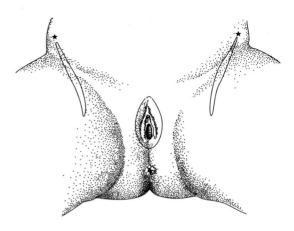

Fig. 13.20 The three-incision technique for radical vulvectomy and groin node dissection.

Primary healing is now achieved in the majority of patients.

Complications

Wound breakdown is still the major complication, and should be treated by meticulous local cleansing. Wound healing after breakdown can be promoted by the use of honey dressings and artificial sea water baths.

Other complications include secondary haemorrhage, thromboembolic disease, femoroinguinal lymphocysts, leg oedema and occasionally hernias and prolapse vaginae.

The recent changes made in the incisions have resulted in an increase in primary healing, rapid mobilization, a reduction in thromboembolic disease, and a shortening of the time spent in hospital.

Further reading

Textbooks

The editor has been especially fortunate to be able to work

in the regional department of gynaecological oncology in Gateshead which has traditionally attracted a vast number of patients with carcinoma of the vulva. He has built on the department's experience under Mr Stanley Ways so that around 35 new cases are seen each year. The distillate of this experience has been published in Chapter 8 of *Clinical Gynaecological Oncology* by Shepherd and Monaghan (1985) published by Blackwell Scientific, Oxford.

Also, for a comprehensive and beautifully presented review of the whole of vulvar disease, the editor would recommend Eduard Friedrich's *Vulvar Disease* (1983) published by W.B. Saunders, Philadelphia. This delightful book is illustrated throughout and annotated in a truly personal style, demonstrating a lifetime of interest and careful thought by Professor Friedrich.

The editor's series has now passed 760 cases in a 28-year period in Gateshead. During that time major changes have been made in the design of incisions with a high degree of individualization of care. The extent of surgery and particularly the use of adequate margins has defined further management to a very high degree. In more recent times the development of sentinel node identification has resulted in even better individualization. If the student reads through references in date order, he will note the steady move towards individualization of treatment with better preoperative assessment of the patient.

References

For those readers with an interest in the landmark references the editor would recommend:

Taussig FJ. Primary cancer of the vulva, vagina and female urethra: five-year results. *Surg Gynecol Obstet* 1935;60:477.

Taussig FJ. Cancer of the vulva: an analysis of 155 cases (1911–1940). *Am J Obstet Gynecol* 1940;40:764–69.

Way S. The anatomy of the lymphatic drainage of the vulva, and its influence on the radical operation for carcinoma. *Ann R Coll Surg Engl* 1948;3:187.

An example of the move towards individualization of treatment for carcinoma of the vulva is seen in one of the better papers on the subject by Hacker NF, Berek JS, Lagasse LD, Nieberg RK, Leuchter RS. Individualization of treatment for stage I squamous cell vulvar carcinoma. *Obstet Gynecol* 1984;63:155–62.

The editor has summarized his own views in *Die Lymphonodektomie in der gynakologischen Onkologie—Indikation, Technik und Konsequenzen fur die Therapie-planung*, Hepp, Scheidel, Monaghan (eds), published by Urban and Schwarzenberg, Munich, 1985.

14 Operations on the vagina

Vaginal cysts

Most cysts found in the vagina are embryological remnants, usually Wolffian. They are most commonly situated either in the anterior part of the lower vagina or in the lateral part of the upper vagina. They vary in size and are usually noticed because they interfere with intercourse or the insertion of tampons or surgical instruments. They rarely produce symptoms and even more rarely become infected. Cysts throughout the length of the posterior part of the vagina are commonly inclusion dermoids developing after childbirth, trauma or vaginal surgery.

It is important to determine the size and position of the cyst prior to surgery as some may extend for a considerable distance towards the pelvic side wall, and what begins as a minor procedure may well turn into a major one. If the cyst is found to have a long communicating tract, it is better to allow the cyst to drain into the vagina and then to identify the tract using radiology or by inserting dye at the beginning of a procedure where facilities for opening the abdomen are available.

Instruments

The gynaecological minor set instruments described in Chapter 2 are adequate with the addition of a small number of malleable probes.

Patient preparation

If the full extent of the cyst is known to be small no special preparation is required. If there is any likelihood of the abdomen being opened, however, the patient should be fully prepared and an appropriate consent form signed.

Anaesthesia

If the cyst is small and accessible the procedure may be performed under local analgesia; however, for the majority of cysts it is much easier for the operator and kinder to the patient to use a general anaesthetic.

The operation

Position
The patient is placed in lithotomy position and the vulva prepared and draped. If the cyst is on the anterior vaginal wall an Auvard's speculum is inserted; for cysts in other positions the area is exposed by the assistant holding a lateral vaginal retractor.

Skin incision
The tissue overlying the cyst is grasped with Allis's tissue forceps at the upper and lower ends of the cyst and an ellipse of skin is removed without cutting into the cyst. The cyst may then be enucleated by dissecting the surrounding tissues away using fine dissecting forceps. If the cyst cannot be enucleated it should be opened and the lining peeled away, leaving a clean cavity. Small vessels may bleed and require individual attention.

Precautions
Great care should be taken during the dissection, which should be predominantly 'separate and cut' rather than 'sharp'. Attention to and identification of surrounding structures will pay great benefits.

Closure
If possible, the cavity should be obliterated, closing the skin with interrupted stitches. If the cavity is large or there has been much haemorrhage or previous infection, it is wise to simply suture around the edge of the cavity and allow it to granulate.

Postoperative care

For most cysts no special care is required except meticulous local cleanliness; for those cysts that have been infected, daily dressing with an antiseptic wick may be required.

Procedures for enlargement of the vaginal introitus

Having eliminated congenital causes for apareunia or dyspareunia, the gynaecologist must consider surgical means to facilitate the act of intercourse. This should always include advice on the use of dilatators, beginning with the patient's own fingers and going on to use graduated plastic obturators. Some patients, however, find these techniques too painful or distasteful and the surgeon must consider operative methods.

Fenton's operation

Instruments
Similar instruments to those used for the excision of a Bartholin's cyst will be required.

The operation
Skin incision A pair of Littlewood's or straight Spencer Wells forceps are used to grasp the skin at the junction with the vagina. The skin may be incised or a narrow strip removed with the scissors (Fig. 14.1).

Development of the flap By slightly undercutting the skin on the vaginal aspect of the incision, a short flap can be developed. Care must be taken not to make this flap too long or to 'button hole' the skin (Fig. 14.2).

Perineal incision A vertical incision is now made towards the anus. All structures must be divided except for the external sphincter (Fig. 14.3).

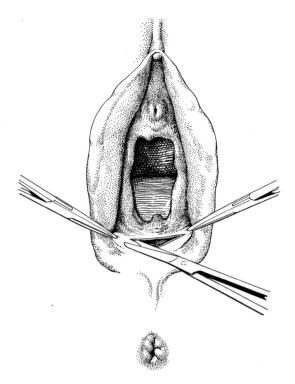

Fig. 14.1 Incising the introital skin.

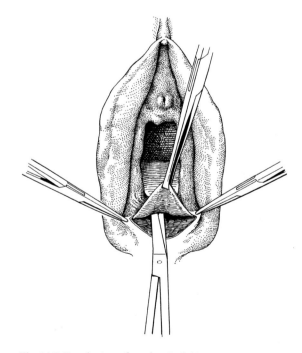

Fig. 14.2 Developing a flap of vaginal skin.

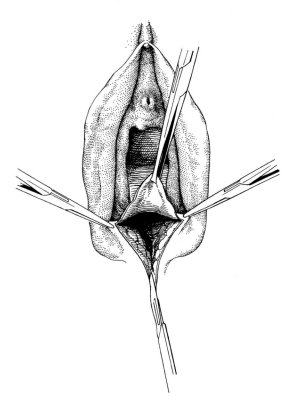

Fig. 14.3 Making the posterior vertical incision.

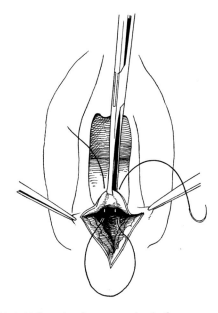

Fig. 14.4 Obliterating the space under the flap.

Division of the hymen If the hymen is thick posteriorly then it must be divided by making two small cuts approximately 1 cm apart. Traction on the two forceps laterally flattens out the flap.

Fixation of the flap and reconstitution of the introitus By passing a Dexon suture into the base of the flap close to the mid-line and anchoring it to the fibromuscular tissue of the perineal incision, two purposes are served. The first is to anchor the flap and keep it in place if the skin sutures are too rapidly absorbed, and the second is to obliterate the space under the flap and reduce the risk of haematoma formation (Fig. 14.4). The skin of the divided perineum is now sutured to the flap (Fig. 14.5) using interrupted stitches so that any ooze beneath the flap can escape. Absorbable sutures such as Dexon or Vicryl may be used for these stitches. Absorption may be incomplete and the patient should be seen 7 days postoperatively for removal of any retained sutures.

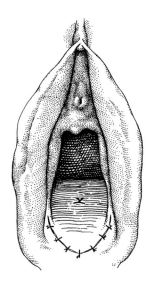

Fig. 14.5 Suturing the skin edges together.

Variation in technique A simplification of the operation is to divide the perineum and lower vagina vertically and then to resuture transversely. This procedure is frequently used where there has been scarring from an episiotomy incision.

Dressing and postoperative care
Scrupulous local cleanliness is essential; local anti-inflammatory agents may be necessary if there is local bruising, but this can be minimized by gentle technique.

The patient should be encouraged to begin to engage in intercourse as soon as the wounds have healed.

Congenital absence and partial development of the vagina

Congenital absence of the uterus or vagina is due to a failure of fusion and canalization of the caudad müllerian ducts. The ovaries, tubes and uterine ligaments are formed but the uterus is present as rudimentary horns and the vagina is absent. Lesser degrees of vaginal atresia also occur, varying from failure of canalization of the lower part to a complete failure of development, but with a normal uterus or uterus didelphys present. In these latter cases cryptomenorrhoea will occur.

Uterovaginal atresia occurs in 1 in 5000 women. The most common presentation is that of a young girl (15 years of age) being brought to see the gynaecologist by her mother because she has failed to begin to menstruate. The girl has normally developed secondary sexual characteristics, including breast, pubic hair and vulval growth. As these girls are usually very nervous, examination in the outpatient department should be limited to the external structures. The mother should be fully informed of the need for a full vaginal and rectal examination of the child under general anaesthetic. An intravenous pyelogram (IVP) is of value as there is an associated urinary anomaly in up to 30% of girls who have maldevelopment of the vagina and uterus.

Under anaesthesia the external genitalia are inspected, the vaginal dimple explored and, most valuable of all, a rectal examination is carried out.

Laparoscopy has made possible a complete assessment of the pelvic structures.

Transverse septum of the vagina (imperforate hymen)

Patients with this problem will present with amenorrhoea but having had many of the signs of menstrual activity, including premenstrual symptoms and intramenstrual discomfort. It is not uncommon to find evidence of endometriosis present on laparoscopy, due possibly to retrograde menstruation. Rarely, the patient will present as an emergency due to obstructive symptoms of the urinary or bowel tract produced by the dilated vagina.

The septum usually lies just above the hymen with the hymenal remnants stretched over it. Occasionally, the septum lies higher in the vagina and is thicker.

The low septum frequently bulges outwards and is discoloured by the dark blood shining through; rectal examination confirms distension of the vagina and uterus.

Instruments
The gynaecological minor set is required.

Patient preparation
No special preparation is needed although it is important to put the patient on broad-spectrum prophylactic antibiotics during and after the procedure.

Anaesthesia
A light general anaesthetic is required.

The operation
The procedure is simplicity itself: the bulging membrane is incised vertically and the retained blood allowed to drain. Once drainage has eased, another incision at right angles is made to form a cross; the edges of the skin flaps are now removed, and any bleeding dealt with by clipping and ligation.

Postoperatively, vulval hygiene is important but vaginal douches must be avoided.

Longitudinal vaginal septum

Patients who are free of dyspareunia may still benefit from excision of a longitudinal vaginal septum, which can cause obstruction at the time of delivery. After emptying the bladder, the septum is held with a clamp, and gentle traction is applied. Attention is required to avoid excess traction as this can draw the urethra, bladder or rectum into the area of excision. The septum is then incised at its inferior and superior attachments from the posterior and anterior vaginal walls, respectively, and the defects repaired using interrupted or continuous absorbable sutures.

Vaginal atresia

A superficial examination of the patient may suggest that the vagina is present but imperforate. The hymen can be seen at the upper part of a small vaginal dimple. However, on rectal examination it is clear that the vagina is not developed and the uterus is present as widely displaced streaks of tissue leading to the ovaries. A diagnostic feature is the ability to trace the uterosacral ligaments uninterruptedly across the front of the rectum. Although the diagnosis is usually made when the girl is in her teens, treatment may be delayed until she wishes to embark on intercourse. The chances of producing a useful communication with the uterus are small and the prospects for procreation infinitesimal. However, a functioning vagina can be made using one of two techniques—McIndoe's and Williams's.

Instruments

The instruments in the gynaecological major set will be required, together with the plastic surgery instruments for cutting the graft (for McIndoe's procedure) and a selection of vaginal moulds (Fig. 14.6).

Patient preparation

The patient is prepared as for any major vaginal procedure; shaving is essential to cut down the risk of infection, and the lower large bowel should be completely empty.

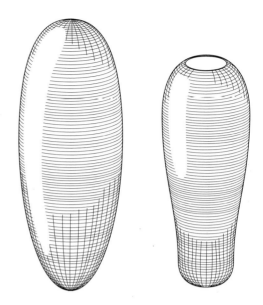

Fig. 14.6 Two types of vaginal mould. On the left the usual shape, on the right the shape used when a functional uterus is present.

Anaesthesia

A general anaesthetic is required.

The operation

McIndoe's operation
The first generally successful procedure to be described for the formation of an artificial vagina was that of McIndoe. The operation involves the formation of a space between the bladder and rectum which is filled with a mould, over which has been placed a skin graft from the patient's thigh.

The operation is usually performed by a gynaecologist and a plastic surgeon working together, the plastic surgeon cutting the grafts and placing them over the mould and the gynaecologist developing the space between rectum and bladder and suturing the mould in place.

Developing the space for the neovagina The patient is placed in the lithotomy position. The skin is incised transversely at the posterior part of the vaginal dimple (Fig. 14.7). This incision is then deepened so that the soft areolar fascia between rectum and bladder is

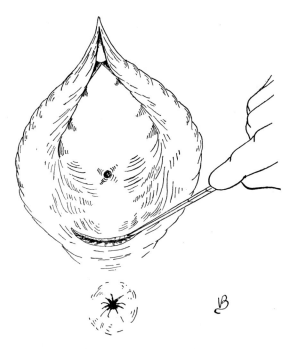

Fig. 14.7 McIndoe's operation: incising the posterior part of the vaginal dimple.

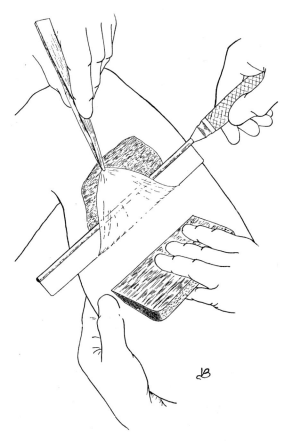

Fig. 14.9 Cutting the graft.

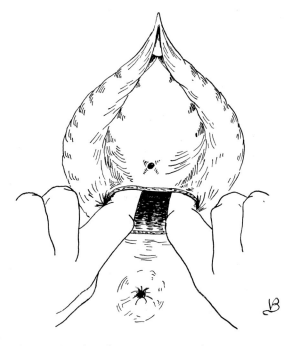

Fig. 14.8 Stretching the cavity anterior to the rectum.

identified. This level is often easier to find if a finger or blunt obturator, such as a large dilatator, is inserted into the rectum. The plane dissects remarkably easily and the peritoneum is rapidly reached.

Using two index fingers, the cavity is developed (Fig. 14.8) so that the chosen mould can fit easily within it. It is important to do this before cutting the graft. Meticulous haemostasis is necessary, although if the correct plane is found there is surprisingly little bleeding.

Cutting the graft This is carried out by the plastic surgeon removing skin from the anterior thigh (Fig. 14.9). The leg is dressed with tulle gras and bandaged. The graft is now draped over the mould in such a way that there is very little overlap; excessive skin should be trimmed away (Figs 14.10 and 14.11).

151

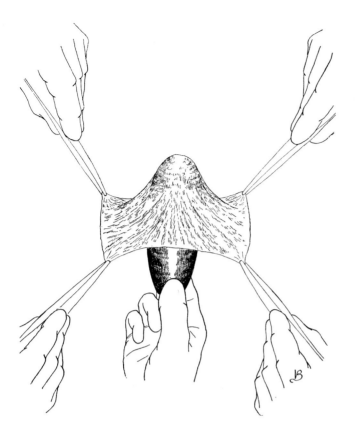

Fig. 14.10 Draping the mould.

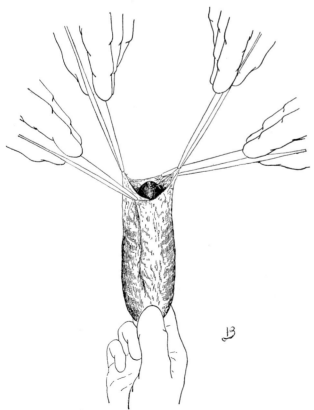

Fig. 14.11 Completing the draping.

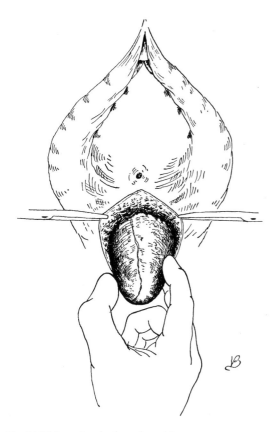

Fig. 14.12 Inserting the draped mould.

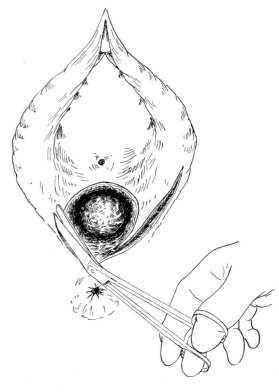

Fig. 14.13 Incising the labia.

Inserting the mould The mould covered by the graft is now inserted into the cavity, where it should lie snugly but without any pressure contact points (Fig. 14.12).

Retention of the mould The mould must now be sutured in place. This is best done by mobilizing the labia via an incision made as shown in Fig. 14.13. The similarities between this incision and that of the Williams's procedure are obvious. The inner edges of this incision are now sutured together so as to form a shelf to retain the mould (Fig. 14.14). This is then reinforced by suturing the outer line of the incision (Fig. 14.15).

The mould is maintained in the new vagina for approximately 3 months; some patients demand that it be removed earlier but this should be resisted. It is important to keep the neovagina open and elastic; if the patient is not regularly practising intercourse she must dilate the vagina frequently using plastic or glass dilators. Any areas of granulation tissue can

be touched with silver nitrate to promote rapid epithelialization.

Williams's operation
Although this operation is of great value to the patient who has vaginal atresia, it is also of enormous benefit to the patient who has shortening or stenosis of the vagina following surgery or radiotherapy. It is a simple procedure producing a pouch of skin lying along the vulva rather than in the axis of the vagina. The postoperative period is short (10 days), and good results are obtained. Arthur Williams first described the operation in 1964 and again in 1976. The authors are grateful to him for permission to reproduce the drawings of the procedure shown in Figs 14.16–14.20.

The patient is draped and catheterized (Fig. 14.16), the incision in the labia is made (Fig. 14.17) and deepened. The inner edges of the incision are now sutured together with interrupted Dexon sutures (Fig. 14.18). An obturator is then placed in the pouch to check the

153

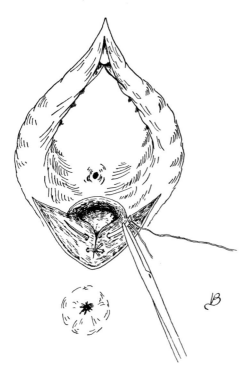

Fig. 14.14 Suturing the inner edge of the incision.

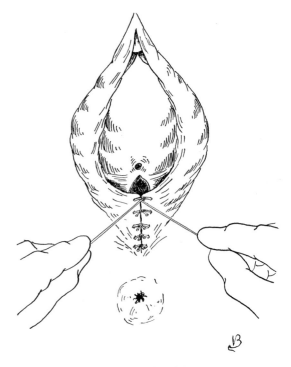

Fig. 14.15 Suturing the outer edge of the incision.

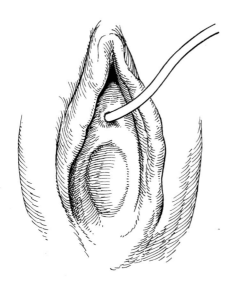

Fig. 14.16 The draped and catheterized vulva showing the vaginal dimple.

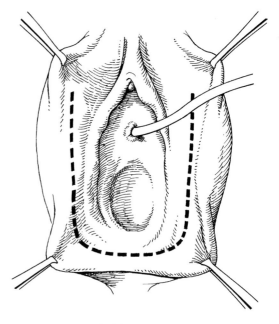

Fig. 14.17 Incising the labia.

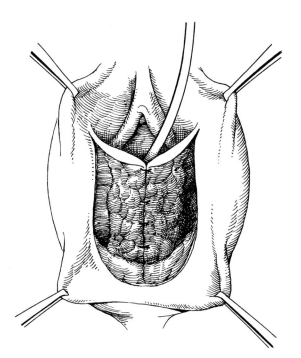

Fig. 14.18 Suturing the inner edges of the labial incision.

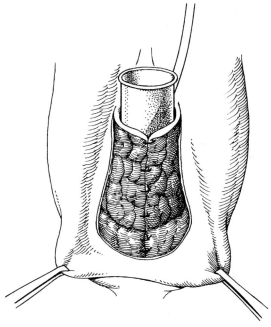

Fig. 14.19 Testing the neovagina's capacity and suturing the levators.

size of the vaginaplasty; if it is satisfactory, the levators are sutured together using two interrupted stitches (Fig. 14.19). The operation is now completed by closing the skin with a series of interrupted stitches; Williams recommended nylon, the authors would use Vicryl (Fig. 14.20).

Vaginectomy, partial and complete

Vaginectomy, or colpectomy, is an operation which is rarely performed but which has very clear indications and very significant benefits. The procedure is most commonly indicated where there is residual vaginal intraepithelial neoplasia (VAIN) in the upper vagina after hysterectomy.

Unfortunately, a considerable number of women will continue to have hysterectomies performed for cervical premalignancy without the benefit of preoperative colposcopy to localize and delineate the disease. As a consequence, in a small number of women there will be incomplete removal of the lesion, resulting in persistently abnormal smears in the postoperative period. If hysterectomy is indicated for cervical intraepithelial

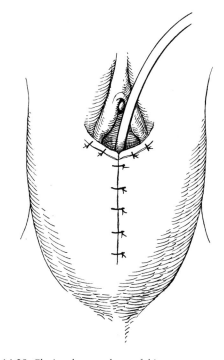

Fig. 14.20 Closing the outer layer of skin.

155

neoplasia (CIN), then ideally this should be performed vaginally in conjunction with colposcopy to reduce the likelihood of the CIN and associated VAIN being incompletely excised. If the lesion or lesions can be seen and fully outlined, then an excisional procedure performed vaginally is the best management method (see below).

If the lesion cannot be fully visualized or it extends into the 'dog ears' at the angles of the vaginal vault then a more extensive surgical procedure via an abdominal approach is the only realistic choice. Some authorities have recommended radiotherapy, but the authors feel that this is not indicated as there is a very significant vaginal morbidity after treatment, often without clearance of the vault lesion, whereas with partial colpectomy there is a good prospect of a reasonable return to normal function.

Colpectomy is not an adequate procedure for invasive carcinoma of the vagina but is of great value in treating microinvasive lesions. In those patients with an upper vaginal lesion and who have a uterus, a hystero-colpectomy is performed—a much simpler procedure than colpectomy after hysterectomy.

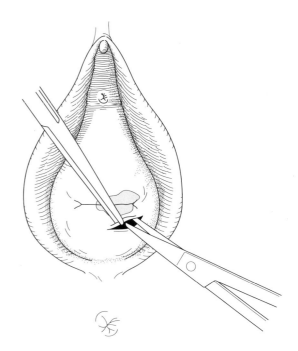

Fig. 14.21 Releasing the vaginal edges.

The vaginal procedure

Instruments
The instruments in the general gynaecology set will be required.

The operation
Identification of the lesion The patient is placed in a lithotomy position, cleansed, draped and the bladder emptied. A bimanual and rectal examination is performed to exclude the possibility of a discrete invasive lesion lying above the suture line at the vaginal vault. A colposcopic assessment of the upper vagina, as described in Chapter 4, is performed followed by mapping of the lesion using Lugol's iodine. Infiltration of the subepithelial tissues with a solution of 1% Xylocaine with adrenaline 1:200 000 helps to define tissue planes and reduce minor bleeding. Access to the vault is best achieved by use of a large Sims' retractor placed in the posterior vagina, with a smaller vaginal retractor placed in the anterior vagina which is moved laterally during the course of the procedure as required.

The incision A 2 cm epithelial incision is made just inferior to the posterior margins of the lesion. A toothed dissector is used to apply traction to the skin flap anteriorly, while the blunted scissors are used to develop the subepithelial plane further towards the vaginal vault and laterally (Fig. 14.21). The skin edges are incised further around the circumference of the mapped lesion as the development of the tissue planes continues. Attention is required not to 'button-hole' the specimen, as this will increase the possibility of leaving diseased tissue remnants behind. Eventually, the incision is completed around the entire lesion, with the only attachment remaining being a thin strip at the vaginal vault with underlying scar tissue. Applying firm traction to the vaginal skin, the attachments at the vaginal vault are now boldly cut from right to left including the 'dog-ears' within the specimen, eventually releasing the entire specimen and without damage to the underlying structures (Fig. 14.22). In leaving the scarred tissue at the vaginal vault and 'dog-ears' till last, the risk of injury to the underlying rectum, bladder and ureters is kept to an absolute minimum, whilst increasing the likelihood of achieving complete excision of the entire lesion with a single specimen.

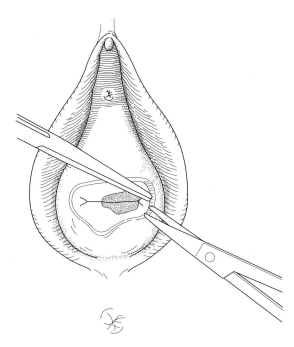

Fig. 14.22 Excising the vaginal skin at the vault.

Dealing with the denuded vault If the peritoneal cavity has been entered at the vaginal vault during the procedure, then this can be either left open or closed using a continuous stitch. Individual vessels can be dealt with using a combination of sutures or diathermy. Once haemostasis is achieved, the denuded tissue at the vaginal vault is left unsutured to regranulate, and a bacterostatic soaked vaginal pack and indwelling transurethral urinary catheter inserted for 24 h.

Postoperative care
No special attention is required, and the patient can be discharged home the following day.

The abdominal procedure

Instruments
The instruments outlined in Chapter 2 for radical hysterectomy will be required.

Preoperative preparation
This should be as for a radical hysterectomy, with the additional procedure of marking the inferior aspect of the lesion with a marker stitch, which will be useful later during the operation to confirm adequate exci-

sion. A firm vaginal pack is essential to facilitate dissection of the vagina from the bladder and the rectum, and an indwelling catheter with a small (5 ml) balloon should be inserted into the bladder.

Anaesthesia
It is a great advantage if this procedure can be carried out under epidural or spinal analgesia as a considerable reduction in small vessel oozing can be achieved.

The operation
Frequently, adhesions from previous surgery have to be cleared before it is possible to visualize the pelvic structures fully. As in the radical hysterectomy procedure, a self-retaining retractor should be used but without the lower blade, which should be replaced by a Morris retractor held by the second assistant. This allows the peritoneum and the bladder to be manipulated to give better vision and access. As a result of the previous surgical intervention, there can be considerable scarring particularly at the angles of the vaginal vault overlying the ureters.

The incision The abdomen is opened via a longitudinal mid-line incision; low transverse incisions give more limited access and should not be used.

Identifying the ureters After clearing obstructions and adhesions from previous surgery, the ureters should be identified as they pass along the pelvic side wall behind the peritoneum. The peritoneum at the brim of the pelvis is opened along a line between the remnant of the round ligament and the infundibulopelvic ligament. Using the fingers, the retroperitoneal space is opened and the ureter identified and separated from the overlying peritoneum (Fig. 14.23).

Dealing with the scar tissue at the angles of the vault The uterine artery should be identified as far laterally as possible and then divided and drawn medially (Fig. 14.24). This will have the effect of identifying the entrance to the ureteric tunnel at its lateral end. This area is often surrounded by dense scarring from the previous surgery; however, if the ureteric tunnel can be accurately defined, the scar overlying it can be cut with confidence and without trauma to the ureter.

Identifying the medial end of the ureteric tunnel Now, the uppermost point of the vagina must be palpated and

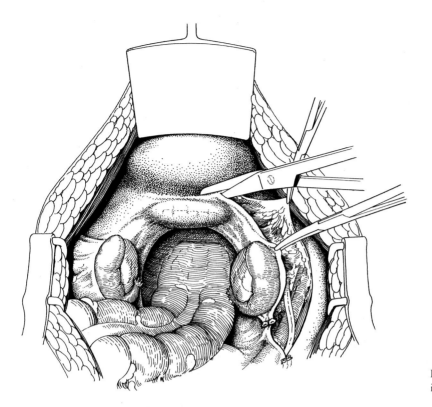

Fig. 14.23 Identifying the ureter in the right retroperitoneal space.

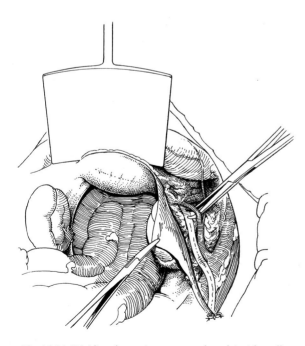

Fig. 14.24 Dividing the uterine artery on the pelvic side wall.

a transverse incision made in the peritoneum so that the bladder can be separated from the anterior surface of the vagina. It may be necessary to use sharp dissection to identify the correct plane. Once this has been identified, the bladder should be pushed down in the midline; this will have the effect of making the scar tissue and the fascia overlying the ureteric tunnel laterally more prominent.

Incising the roof of the ureteric tunnel Frequently, the ureter can be identified as it passes into the bladder. If this is possible, Monaghan's scissors should be gently introduced over the upper surface of the ureter and, using a separating movement without cutting, gently insinuated laterally to appear at the lateral end of the ureteric tunnel. This dissection may be performed from medial to lateral or in the reverse direction. It is important not to kink or to nip the ureter in the edges of the scissors; the simple manoeuvre of lifting the scissors while in the tunnel will allow a good view of the entire length of the ureter. A medium straight tissue forceps is then placed over the scissors and the ureteric tunnel and

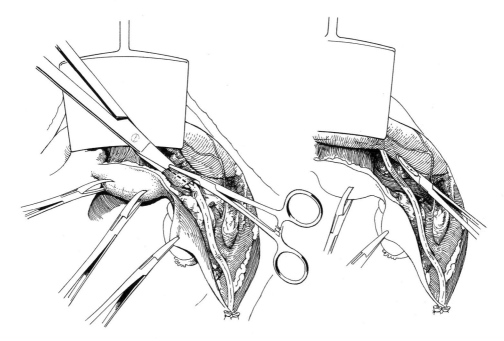

Fig. 14.25 Dividing the roof of the ureteric tunnel.

the scar tissue incised (Fig. 14.25). The pedicle is then tied, as it carries some veins and small arteries to and from the bladder. At this point, there may still be a few strands of fascia passing across the ureter; these should be divided and the tissue plane between the ureter and the vagina identified. The cardinal ligament is now visible below and medial to the ureter. Sharp dissection may still be required if there has been extensive scarring from the previous surgery. The upper vagina is revealed very quickly and the ureters dislocated laterally. The firm pack in the vagina greatly facilitates this dissection.

Releasing the vagina posteriorly An incision is made in the peritoneum at the upper posterior part of the vagina (Fig. 14.26). This incision is then extended laterally over the remnants of the uterosacral ligaments. The rectum is now easily pushed away from the posterior surface of the vagina by passing the fingers down into the rectovaginal space (Fig. 14.27).

Removing the vagina At this point, having released the ureters laterally, the bladder anteriorly and the rectum posteriorly, the surgeon can decide just how much vagina he wishes to remove. The uterosacral and then the

paracolpos is grasped and clamped in Zeppelin clamps and the chosen length of vagina removed (Fig. 14.28). If the requirement is to remove the upper part of the vagina to excise VAIN, no further dissection is necessary and the vagina can be opened at this point to confirm placement of the original marker stitch and adequate excision of tissue. If a total vaginectomy is necessary, the abdominal dissection should be extended down the vagina to the pelvic floor. Thereafter, the patient is put in lithotomy position and the lower vagina dissected free from the urethra and bladder anteriorly and the rectum posteriorly. Great care should be exercised when dissecting below the urethra as the fascia is very dense and the dissection must be very accurate. Having joined up with the abdominal dissection, the entire vagina can be removed. A little bleeding is seen around the pelvic floor but is not of great trouble.

Draining the vagina The space left behind after vaginectomy will vary in size depending on the extent of the procedure. Following partial vaginectomy there is no need for special drainage procedures except to leave the vaginal remnant open. However, after total vaginectomy either a vaginal passive drain or a suction drain should be put in place. This may be augmented by

159

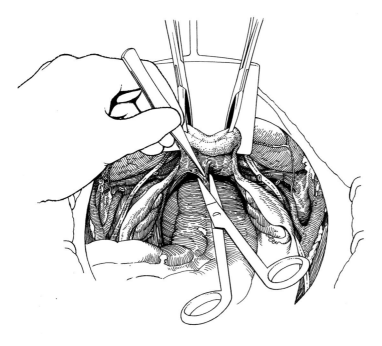

Fig. 14.26 Incising the peritoneum between the uterosacral ligaments.

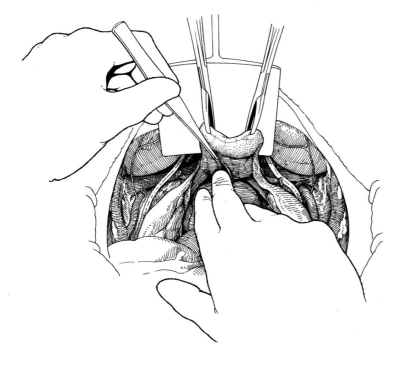

Fig. 14.27 Developing the rectovaginal space.

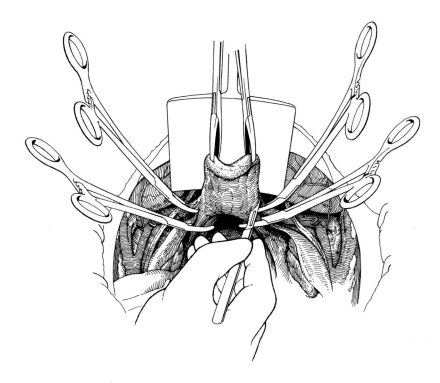

Fig. 14.28 Removal of the vaginal remnant.

a pelvic suction drain brought out abdominally if it has been necessary to perform an extensive dissection in the pelvis.

Complications
The main postoperative problems following this procedure will be similar to those following radical hysterectomy, particularly bladder dysfunction and difficulties in initiating micturition (see Chapter 11).

Postoperative care
The patient should be managed in the same manner as the radical hysterectomy patient, particular emphasis being placed on bladder care, and in the long-term continued surveillance of any remnants of vaginal tissue remaining.

Further reading

Textbooks

Williams has reviewed the whole complex subject in Chapter 1 of *Clinics in Obstetrics and Gynaecology* vol. 5, no. 3, December 1978, 'Gynaecological Surgery' David Lees and Albert Singer (eds), published by W.B. Saunders, London.

References

Since time immemorial unfortunate girls have been born with under- or maldeveloped genitalia. For them, the prospects were appalling until McIndoe and Bannister, in 1938, described their revolutionary operation; McIndoe AH, Bannister JB (1938) An operation for the cure of congenital absence of the vagina. *J Obstet Gynaecol Br Empire* 45: 490. Since this time, many minor procedures have been developed to deal with these unfortunate patients. However, it was not until 1964, when Arthur Williams described his simple procedure, that a further milestone was passed in dealing with this difficult problem; Williams EA (1964) Congenital absence of the vagina. A simple operation for its relief. *J Obstet Gynaecol Br Commonwealth* 71: 511–512.

15 Operations for the correction of urinary fistulae

In the developed world, the majority of urinary tract fistulae will occur following gynaecological surgery, particularly abdominal and vaginal hysterectomy and caesarean section. In underdeveloped areas of the world, fistula formation associated with childbirth remains the most common cause.

The most frequent cause of fistula formation after hysterectomy is failure to dissect the bladder free of the cervix and upper vagina. This problem may be caused by previous surgery, especially Caesarean section, or by the presence of infection, scarring or endometriosis. Fibroids may so distort the uterus that the bladder is drawn up and inadvertently entered. The bladder may also be damaged when the vaginal edge is being sutured because the surgeon fails to recognize the bladder wall.

Even when the bladder is not entered, the damage to the bladder wall may result in avascular necrosis and the appearance of the fistula some 1–2 weeks after the operation.

Patient preparation

Prior to any surgical management, the entire urinary tract should be fully assessed. It is important to do so as it is not unusual to find damage to other parts of the tract which may require concurrent or subsequent management.

An intravenous urogram (IVU) should be performed to evaluate the kidneys and the ureteric areas, and a cystoscopy to determine the relationship of the fistula to the ureteric orifices.

In order to assess the bladder it should be filled with methylene blue dye in solution via a transurethral Foley catheter. If a tampon is inserted into the vagina, any leakage from the bladder will show up as a blue stain on the tampon; however, if leakage is occurring from a ureter the tampon will be wetted with clear urine. Rarely, ureteric reflux associated with a low fistula may confuse the picture.

In general, repair of the vesicovaginal fistula should be delayed for 2–3 months; this occasionally results in spontaneous closure but, most importantly, allows infection to settle and the tissue planes to re-establish themselves.

The exception to this policy of waiting is when the fistula is recognized shortly after it occurs when it is probably best to carry out an immediate repair.

As with most surgical procedures, *the first chance of repair is the best one.*

Prophylactic antibiotics are recommended in the preoperative period, and if the patient is postmenopausal, and there are no contraindications, she should be given oestrogens to improve the quality of the vaginal skin.

Principles of fistula repair

Bonney described six general principles which should be adhered to when repairing any fistula, whether of the urinary tract, alimentary system or any epithelial surface:

1 The tissues to be repaired must be as healthy as possible. In the case of urinary fistulae the urine should be rendered sterile and the area free of infection. Sloughs due to irradiation, trauma or infection must have separated to leave clean healing or healed surfaces.

2 There must be an adequate exposure of the affected area and the tissue surfaces surrounding the defect.

3 There must be no tension on the suture lines when the

fistula is closed. This applies not only at the time of operation but also in the postoperative period. Therefore, adequate drainage of the bladder must be maintained following the procedure.

4 Meticulous haemostasis is essential throughout the operation to avoid haematoma formation and to facilitate healing.

5 Infection must be guarded against as it will seriously jeopardize healing.

6 The final principle applies when a bladder fistula affects the region of the bladder–urethra junction. This is a vulnerable area in relation to urinary control and for this reason it is not only important to close the fistula, but also to reinforce the area with adjacent fascia and muscle, including the anterior fibres of the pubococcygeus muscles when necessary, thus reducing the risk of postoperative stress incontinence. Unless these precautions are taken, stress incontinence, even on walking, will make the patient's life a misery, Also, the insertion of this support will obviate the risk of a new fistula developing if a later attempt is made to correct the stress incontinence.

Repair of the postoperative fistula

Instruments

The instruments in the gynaecological general set, shown in Chapter 2, will be required together with vaginal retractors and Sims' right angle skin hooks. Fine dissecting scissors such as McIndoe's are of great value.

The operation

The best results for repair of vesicovaginal fistulae are obtained when the patient is operated upon by an expert, i.e. a surgeon who has committed his skills, time and experience to caring for these unfortunate women with this distressing condition. The technique described here relies heavily on the experience of others, particularly Chassar-Moir and Sims.

The choice between using a vaginal or abdominal approach will depend to a large extent on the training of the individual: urologists and general surgeons tending to favour the abdominal approach and gynaecologists the vaginal. Occasionally, when the fistula is placed high in the vault, a combined approach will yield the best results.

Exposure

The lithotomy position gives an adequate approach for most vesicovaginal fistulae. The patient's buttocks should be drawn well down the table. Occasionally, the knee–chest position will be needed for an inaccessible fistula behind the pubic arch. A sucker is essential to keep the operative field clear and dry. Tilting the table to lower the patient's head, the so-called lithotomy Trendelenburg position, can be useful.

If the lower vagina is scarred or narrowed, a Schuchardt's releasing incision will give considerably improved access (Fig. 15.1).

Excision of the fistula edges

The edges of the fistula may be made prominent by grasping them and everting using Allis's tissue forceps;

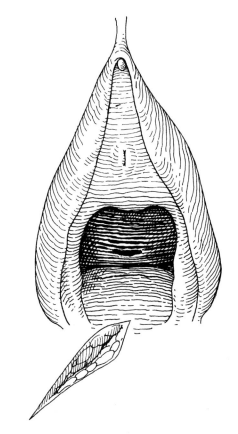

Fig. 15.1 The Schuchardt incision for gaining access to a narrowed introitus.

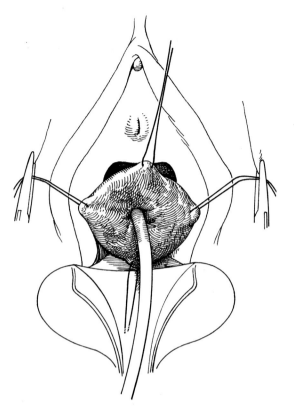

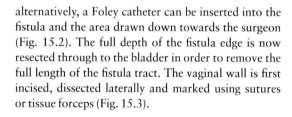

Fig. 15.2 Drawing down the fistula using a small Foley catheter.

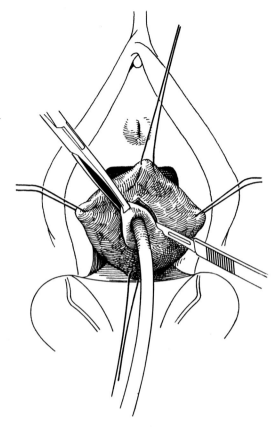

Fig. 15.3 Incising the vaginal skin around the fistula and removing the scarred tissue throughout the full depth of the defect.

alternatively, a Foley catheter can be inserted into the fistula and the area drawn down towards the surgeon (Fig. 15.2). The full depth of the fistula edge is now resected through to the bladder in order to remove the full length of the fistula tract. The vaginal wall is first incised, dissected laterally and marked using sutures or tissue forceps (Fig. 15.3).

Dissection of the bladder muscularis
Next, the muscularis is identified and separated from the vaginal wall for approximately 2 cm around the fistula; any remaining scar tissue around the fistula should now be removed. A purse-string suture is now placed around the edges of the mucosa using a Vicryl stitch on an atraumatic needle (Fig. 15.4). The needle should be so placed that the stitch does not present on the bladder surface of the mucosa.

Closure of the fistula and placing of support sutures
The purse-string suture should now be tied, invaginating the mucosa towards the bladder cavity (Fig. 15.5). This manoeuvre may be aided by looping a suture through the edge of the fistula and drawing it out of the urethra; pulling on this loop assists in invaginating the mucosa and the loop can be simply removed by pulling on one end.

The muscularis is now brought together by placing a number of separate sutures across the defect using an invaginating stitch and drawing the muscularis over the defect (Fig. 15.6). It is important to keep these sutures clear of the mucosa.

Closing the vagina
Finally, the vaginal skin is closed longitudinally using interrupted vertical mattress sutures (Fig. 15.7).

164

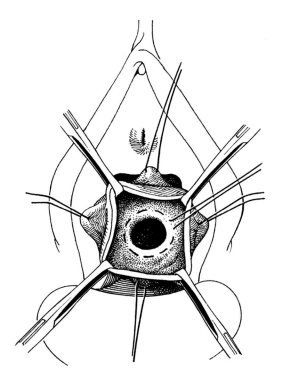

Fig. 15.4 Separating the vaginal skin and the muscularis of the bladder and inserting the purse-string suture around the fistula.

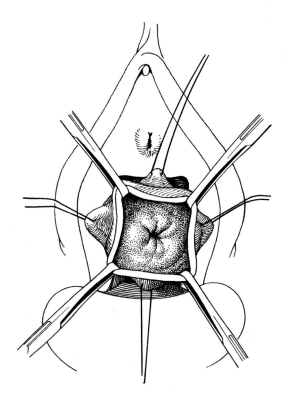

Fig. 15.5 Tying the purse-string suture.

Meticulous haemostasis must be maintained throughout the procedure.

Postoperative management

A Foley catheter is inserted into the bladder and a vaginal pack covered with an antiseptic such as acriflavine is inserted into the vagina. The pack is removed 24 h after operation and the catheter is maintained until there is no evidence of haematuria. Prophylactic antibiotics are prescribed and the patient is usually fit to go home after 8–10 days in uncomplicated cases.

Repair of the obstetric fistula

This type of fistula presents special problems, mainly due to the large area of bladder which may be lost as a consequence of the avascular necrosis that occurred at the time of the injury. If the defect is large, special techniques have to be used to close the gap without tension.

Bladder mobilization downwards will allow the defect to be bridged by drawing the upper freed part of the bladder down to meet the lower relatively fixed section.

Labial fat pads (Martius grafts) are used to support and improve the blood supply of the large defect.

A *gracilis muscle* swinging procedure will also add support and improve the blood supply to those fistulae where tension may be present if they were closed in the traditional manner.

Omental grafts are of help if the fistula is approached from within the abdomen; by preserving the gastroepiploic arteries an excellent new blood supply can be brought to the defect and the repair site.

Repair of fistulae developing after pelvic irradiation

Patients presenting with postirradiation fistulae are the most difficult group to manage, calling for great experience and skill from the surgeon.

165

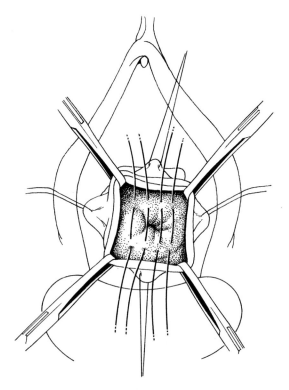

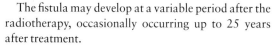

Fig. 15.6 Suturing the muscularis with interrupted invaginating sutures.

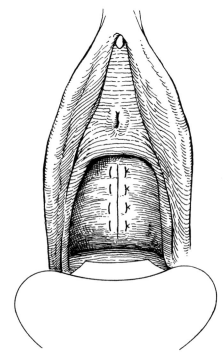

Fig. 15.7 Closing the vaginal skin with a series of interrupted vertical mattress sutures.

The fistula may develop at a variable period after the radiotherapy, occasionally occurring up to 25 years after treatment.

The fistula formation rate is dose-related and is exacerbated by trauma to the area of irradiation, especially by inappropriate surgery.

If the patient has had successful treatment for a carcinoma invading the bladder, fistula formation is almost a natural consequence of successful treatment.

Not infrequently, the vesicovaginal fistula is associated with other fistulae of the gastrointestinal tract also caused by the radiotherapy. It is important to be sure that the fistula has not developed as a consequence of tumour recurrence. In these circumstances the simplest and most effective management may be a diversion of urinary and bowel function using a conduit and/or a colostomy.

The operation

If a repair of an irradiation fistula is to be attempted there must be no evidence of recurrent cancer, and the principles outlined by Bonney must be adhered to.

The surgeon must also decide whether he wishes to retain a functioning vagina or whether, in the interests of simplicity and a more certain result, some form of colpocleisis should be used.

Frequently, the vaginal skin is extremely atrophic with associated radiotherapy changes, including scarring and stenosis, producing grave difficulties with access.

Oestrogens should be used for a short period before surgery is attempted. This will improve the quality of the skin and facilitate healing and the identification of tissue plane. Oestrogens should not be used if the previous carcinoma was of endometrial origin.

The use of Martius grafts, gracilis muscle transplants, bulbocavernosus muscle transplant and omental pedicle grafts will all serve to improve the prospects of cure of the fistula by bringing into the area a much improved blood supply and also allowing the fistula to be closed without tension. Occasionally, the fistula is reduced in size without being completely closed; a second attempt will often be successful.

Unfortunately, a high proportion of patients with postirradiation fistulae will require diversionary procedures to solve their problems.

Further reading

Gynecological and Obstetric Urology by Herbert Buchsbaum and Joseph Schmidt, published by W.B. Saunders, in 1982, has two chapters by Keettal and Laube, and Nanninga and O'Connor in which both the suprapubic and vaginal routes of repair are covered.

References

Very few individual gynaecologists have an opportunity to develop a large experience in the management of vesicovaginal fistulae; one who has is J.B. Lawson. In his working lifetime both in Africa and Britain he has dealt with hundreds of such operations and his writings are worth searching out and reading. They include: Lawson JB. Vesical fistulae into the vaginal vault. *Br J Urol* 1972;44:623–31.

Another master urological surgeon, R. Turner-Warwick, should be read where possible, including Turner-Warwick R. The use of pedicle grafts in the repair of urinary tract fistulae. *Br J Urol* 1972;44:644–56.

Other major landmark references include:

Boronow RC, Rutledge F. Vesico-vaginal fistula, radiation and gynecologic cancer. *Am J Obstet Gynecol* 1971; 111:85–90.

Martius C *Gynaecological Operations* translated by McCall ML, Bolton KA. London: J & A Churchill, 1957.

Moir JC. Personal experience in the treatment of vesicovaginal fistulas. *Am J Obstet Gynecol* 1956;71:476–91.

Moir JC. Vesico-vaginal fistulae as seen in Britain. *J Obstet Gynaecol Br Commonwealth* 1973;80:598–602.

16 Operations for the correction of infertility

John R. Newton

At least 15% of all infertile couples will present with tubal disease. This is either distal tubal disease—the end result of pelvic sepsis—or tubal disease following ectopic pregnancy or ovarian surgery. Often, it is complicated by ovarian or pelvic adhesions. Tubal blockage following sterilization (mid-isthmic or isthmic ampullary portions of the tube) and ascending infection leading to cornual blockage account for the rest of the cases.

Microsurgery, a surgical discipline including magnification, irrigation, complete haemostasis and tissue handling with 'doucement' (gentleness), has dramatically improved the surgical results in recent years.

However, nothing can replace good preoperative investigation of the couple, counselling and the selection of appropriate cases for surgery. In the following sections, discussion covers these aspects together with selection of instruments, needles, sutures and surgical technique for the appropriate surgical procedure.

Tubal surgery is no longer a surgical procedure for every gynaecologist; it requires dedication, training and time, and is best concentrated in selected centres where a consultant with a special interest in tubal surgery is available to maintain an adequate service.

Anatomy and physiology

The fallopian tube is 8–10 cm in length and can be divided into distinct segments by virtue of its structure. Figure 16.1 illustrates schematically a fallopian tube and its muscular wall. At the medial end of each fallopian tube the circular muscle coat is thick and continuous with the uterine myometrium (Fig. 16.1c),

the internal diameter is narrow (0.5 mm), and the portion of the tubal lumen within the myometrium (intramural) is subject to closure due to uterine contraction; this can easily be seen at hysteroscopy.

The medial portion of the tube is called the isthmus and also has a thick circular muscular wall (Fig. 16.1b); the endothelium lining the lumen is arranged in primary folds, often five in number. The tube then expands in diameter—the ampullary–isthmic junction—and becomes the ampullary portion of the tube with numerous folds of endothelium and a weak circular muscle coat (Fig. 16.1a). The tube then opens at the outer end into numerous delicate folds, the fimbriae.

The blood supply to the tube is via a double-arcade system anastomosing with the uterine and ovarian arteries. Numerous smaller arteries supply the tube but major branches of significance in tubal surgery enter the inferior aspect of the tube at the cornu of the uterus, the ampullary–isthmic junction and the inferior aspect of the ampulla just adjacent to the fimbriae (see Fig. 16.1).

The tube has two main functions:
1 The transport of sperm and the fertilized eggs.
2 The pick-up of the egg.
The normal tube is lined with ciliated epithelium and these cilia with the ampulla beat towards the ampullary–isthmic junction.

The egg pick-up mechanisms are complex, but depend mainly upon the intimate relationship between the fimbriae and the surface of the ovary, and the peristaltic movements of the fimbriae and the ciliated epithelium. At the time of ovulation the egg is captured by these mechanisms from the surface of the ruptured ovarian follicle and rapidly propelled into the ampulla.

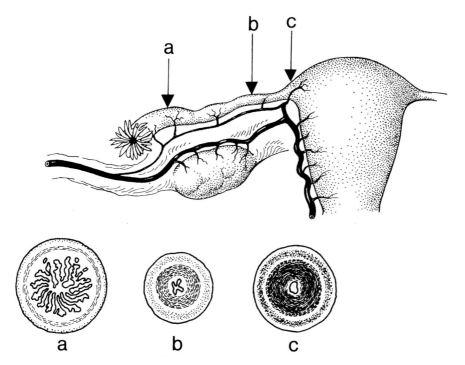

Fig. 16.1 Anatomy of the fallopian tube and its blood supply.

Pathology of tubal disease

Ascending infection of the genital tract leading to an endometritis or salpingitis or both remains the main cause of distal tubal disease and tubal blockage. However, in some countries there is still a high incidence of pelvic tuberculosis leading to tubal blockage. Gonococcal salpingitis now may affect 1 in 5 women in the large metropolitan areas of the Western world, and up to 17% of women will develop tubal occlusion following an attack of acute salpingitis and will therefore be infertile.

The use of intrauterine contraceptive devices has also been implicated in the development of pelvic sepsis, though these patients may in many situations be an 'at risk' group, having multiple sexual partners, and be exposed to ascending infection more often.

Up to 15% of women undergoing laparoscopy for infertility investigation have been found to have asymptomatic endometriosis.

The diagnosis of pelvic inflammatory disease (PID) is often difficult and poorly investigated. To confirm the diagnosis, laparoscopy is needed and the following minimum criteria should be present:
1 A sticky tubal exudate (also seen at the fimbria if patent).
2 Hyperaemia of the tubal surface.
3 Oedema of the tubal wall.

Adequate and prompt antibiotic therapy after correct diagnosis (including laparoscopic assessment) is the key to success; failure to act may lead to blocked tubes and adhesion formation.

For endometriosis, a full suppressive progestogen or danazol treatment regimen is needed for a minimum of 6–9 months with alleviation of all symptoms and menstruation. Laparoscopic assessment should be carried out to confirm clearance of the disease, as suboptimal treatment often leads to recurrence, tubal damage or occlusion.

The rise in the number of female sterilizations, and the increase in the divorce and remarriage rates have both contributed to a rise in requests for reversal of sterilization. Unfortunately, some methods cannot be reversed—those where total salpingectomy, tubal ligation plus fimbrectomy, or removal of the major part of the tube have taken place. Other methods, e.g. unipolar diathermy, often lead to necrosis of large parts of the tube and are not amenable to reconstructive surgery. Tubal sterilization using Falope rings destroys up to 3 cm of tube while clips only destroy 2–4 mm.

Consequent upon the rise in the incidence of pelvic sepsis, there has also been an increase in the incidence of ectopic pregnancy. All too often, total salpingectomy is carried out whereas conservative surgery with local excision of the ectopic mass will leave the patient with a chance of reconstructive surgery at a later date (see Chapter 18).

Assessment prior to definitive surgery

It is essential to have an accurate and up-to-date assessment of tubal and pelvic pathology before embarking on surgery. A full discussion with the couple at the time of referral will enable the gynaecologist to decide on an appropriate course of action. The minimum work-up should include:
1 History and examination of both partners.
2 A full seminal fluid analysis.
3 Confirmation of ovulation.
4 Assessment of tubal status.

With answers to the above examinations and tests, a full discussion can then take place on the risks and success rates of tubal surgery. At this stage some couples will opt for no further treatment.

Assessment of tubal status

Given the error rates of tubal patency testing due to tubal spasm, and the difficulty of defining pelvic adhesion on X-ray salpingography, the test of choice is laparoscopy with tubal hydrotubation using methylene blue. Some gynaecologists combine this test with hysteroscopy to assess the uterine cavity and tubal ostia. Laparoscopy by direct vision allows accurate description of pelvic pathology, adhesions and tubal status, and an assessment of the feasibility of tubal surgery. It may be necessary to repeat this test if previous laparoscopy has occurred some years earlier or all information is not available. It should not immediately precede tubal surgery, i.e. it should not take place under the same anaesthetic.

Counselling and contraindications

While preliminary discussion will take place at the initial referral and should include all alternatives to tubal surgery, i.e. remaining childless, adoption, fostering, tubal surgery and in vitro fertilization. Full discussion, including a prognosis and selection of the treatment most likely to succeed, cannot take place until all preoperative tests are complete. The most important factors to be considered are:
1 Age—those over 35 have to balance lowered fertility and an increased fetal abnormality risk during pregnancy against possible success.
2 The previous sterilization procedure may not be compatible with reversal.
3 Previous pelvic sepsis may have led to severe damage not amenable to surgery.
4 Unexpected male infertility may be present and may not be amenable to treatment. Here surgery is not usually indicated.
5 Some couples find the prospect of major surgery and long hospitalization unacceptable and too risky for their own circumstances.
6 The low pregnancy rates associated with distal tubal disease may not be acceptable.
7 Risks of surgery—the risks include failure of surgery, postoperative complications, postoperative adhesion formations and ectopic pregnancy (more common after tubal surgery).

Strong motivation, coupled with a complete understanding of the chances of success and the risks of tubal surgery, will enable a couple to reach a decision with their counsellor. Time is important but hasty decision-making is not sensible. At this stage some couples will opt for no further treatment.

Contraindications to tubal surgery are both relative and absolute. Surgery is contraindicated if there exists:
1 A serious psychological or medical disease which contraindicates pregnancy.
2 Pelvic tuberculosis.
3 Congenital or acquired absence of the fallopian tubes.
4 A frozen pelvis.
5 Active PID.
6 A normal pelvis.

Other situations which require careful consideration before proceeding with surgery are:
1 Tubal destruction following sterilization—if this

leaves less than 5 cm of viable tube, then surgery is best avoided.

2 Age—as indicated above, fertility declines after 35 years; the 'grey area' is 35–38 years and a balance must be achieved between benefit and risk.

3 Previous surgery—a reasonable attempt, using microsurgery, usually contraindicates a second tubal procedure. However, in certain cases it may be useful to try microsurgery, e.g. after failed macrosurgery if tubal assessment gives a realistic prognosis.

There are many patients who use an attempt at tubal surgery to bolster up a failing marriage or psychologically inadequate personality. Psychological assessment is valuable in many cases to avoid this trap.

Surgery

For many years, conventional macrosurgery was used for fallopian tube surgery; no magnification aids were used and fine sutures were not available. Given the internal diameter of the tube, it is remarkable that any of these operations were successful.

In recent years, microsurgery has shown a definite improvement in tubal patency rates and pregnancy rates following surgery. The word 'microsurgery' embraces not only the use of optical aids, but also a discipline of surgery and therapy that has been responsible for this increased success rate.

Laser surgery is still in its infancy. It is a precise surgical tool for excision and vaporization of tissue. It is claimed that healing following laser surgery is better and postoperative adhesions are less likely to form. Time will tell whether this new method is useful in all cases of tubal surgery.

Principles of microsurgery

The aim of microsurgery is to produce reconstruction of the anatomical relationships of the tubes and ovary with minimal damage to pelvic structures and peritoneum, to achieve healing without postoperative adhesion formation, and to leave the patient with a functional tube. To this end, adequate exposure with the correct size incision is essential to prevent unnecessary retraction and bruising of tissues.

In addition, the following points are essential for microsurgery:

1 *Tissue wetting or irrigation.* When viewed through the operating microscope, tissues dry rapidly and an exudate, which is clearly visible after a few minutes forms. This interferes with healing. To overcome this, constant irrigation with an isotonic solution, e.g. Ringer's lactate solution, prevents tissue drying and improves healing.

2 *Careful haemostasis.* Intraperitoneal blood promotes postoperative adhesion formation; meticulous attention to haemostasis is essential. The use of an operating microscope plus bipolar diathermy or the CO_2 laser enables atraumatic division of adhesions with complete haemostasis. When combined with irrigation, the identification of small blood vessels is easy and allows accurate and discrete sealing of these vessels without damage to surrounding tissues.

3 *Avoidance of peritoneal damage.* It is now clear that even small areas of peritoneal damage will lead to postoperative adhesion formation. For this reason, adequate instrumentation is used to prevent raw areas occurring, i.e. glass rods, a dental mirror and the uterine elevator. When a raw area is caused and cannot be adequately closed, then peritoneal grafting using a small area of peritoneum taken from the anterior aspect of the incision will cover the area adequately.

4 *Suture material.* Tissue reaction from certain absorbable suture materials can give inferior results. By using non-absorbable sutures, e.g. fine nylon, results can be improved.

Instruments

Operating loupes and microscopes

Since the early 1950s, operating microscopes have been used in several branches of medicine for microsurgery. Often, the gynaecologist will have to share a microscope with another discipline, e.g. neurosurgery, but the basic operating microscope produced by Zeiss is ideal for tubal microsurgery, provided the correct focal length lens (250–300 mm) is used.

Operating loupes—low-power magnification units attached to spectacles—can be used for microsurgery. The magnification is ×2 to ×8, but the field of view is restricted, being 20–100 mm. This restriction, together with movement of the field in the opposite direction to head movement, limits their use and many people find them irritating to use.

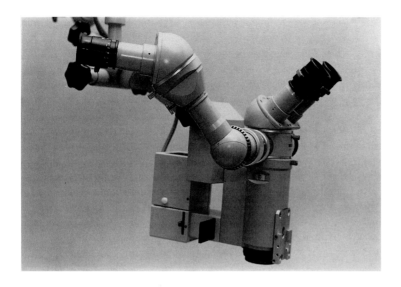

Fig. 16.2 The Zeiss operating microscope.

Microscopes (Fig. 16.2), either single- or double-headed, are much easier to use for tubal and pelvic microsurgery. The basic unit consists of an objective lens with a focal length of 250–300 mm with a foot-operated motor driven 300 mm system giving magnification changes of ×2 to ×30. This covers the complete range needed for dissection, identification of structure, and suturing. Above this is attached the beam splitter and then the binocular units with angled adjustable eye pieces. These eye pieces also have variable magnification of ×10, ×12.5, ×15 or ×20, depending upon the operator's choice. The beam splitter allows a variety of accessories to be attached—additional eye piece (monocular tube) for an observer, still or ciné photography or TV single tube or 3-chip, or light-weight cameras. With the dual-head microscopes two identical binocular heads are attached opposite one another for the surgeon and assistant.

Illumination is critical for good microsurgery and most modern microscopes have two cold-light cables from tungsten halogen light sources. These light sources are housed in the microscope stand.

The stand is a critical part of the microscope as the old-fashioned multiple-jointed operating stand wastes operating time (up to 40%) due to the large number of joints and difficulty experienced in adjusting the microscope position. The modern stand is counterbalanced, easy to set and adjust, and does not get in the way of the surgeon.

To use the microscope effectively, the surgeon should be comfortable, either standing with the arms resting on supports or sitting. If the surgeon sits, then the standard gynaecological central pillar operating table will cause great discomfort and an extension to the foot piece will be needed. This allows the operating area to be moved down beyond the central pillar and then the surgeon can sit with his legs comfortably positioned under the table.

Diathermy units

A modern solid-state multipurpose machine is essential giving both unipolar and bipolar diathermy, with variable intensity. The unipolar machine should have blended cutting and coagulation modes in addition. For ease of use, bearing in mind the foot-pedal control of the microscope, the unipolar unit should be controlled by a hand piece incorporating a rocker switch. It will also need an insulated pelvic extension piece and a selection of plug-in tips. The bipolar unit can be controlled by a foot switch, but it is advisable to have this mounted on the front of the microscope foot switch to save moving one's foot. The bipolar forceps should be angled titanium neurosurgical fine-pointed forceps. They are angled to keep the operator's hand out of the field of view.

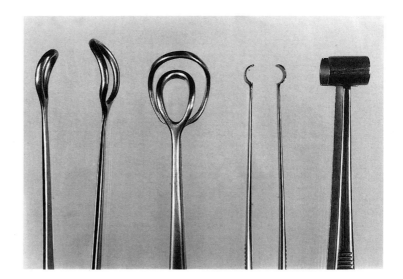

Fig. 16.3 Ovarian and tube-holding forceps.

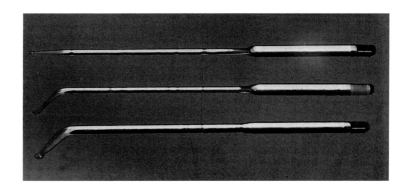

Fig. 16.4 Glass probes.

General surgical instruments

In addition to a routine abdominal set of the surgeon's preference, other instruments will be necessary for tubal surgery. These are:

1 An *intermediate set* of needle holder, scissors and fine non-toothed forceps similar to those used for plastic surgery. Atraumatic tube-holding forceps and ovarian forceps are also useful (Fig. 16.3).

2 *Retractors*. A square-frame Kirschner retractor with four adjustable blades is essential for adequate exposure. A circular-frame retractor can also be used but the blades usually supplied are too small for routine use.

3 *Glass probes* (quartz). These are essential for easy dissection of adhesions, opening of the tube, diathermy and laser use. They consist of a set of four probes — one straight, two angled and one flat-plate. The first three have olive ends and all are fitted with a standard cold-light cable collar (Fig. 16.4). This allows an ordinary laparoscopy light lead to be attached, so transillumination of the adhesion and tube can be accomplished easily (Fig. 16.5). Diathermy division or laser vaporization of tissue overlying these probes is easily dealt with, without damage to adjacent tissues (Fig. 16.6).

4 *HUMI cervical adaptor*. There are many methods of intrauterine instillation of methylene blue dye to test tubal patency during the operation. All can fail and leak, but the HUMI transcervical adaptor is the easiest and most reliable (Fig. 16.7); connected to this is a three-way tap and syringe. It has the additional advantage of providing uterine manipulation as well as instillation of dye. This is applied prior to the start of the operation after catheterization.

173

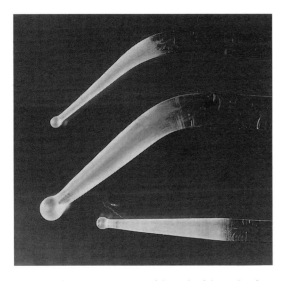

Fig. 16.5 Close-up appearance of the ends of the probes for transmitting light.

5 *The microsurgical set* These are very delicate instruments and, when not in use, should be kept inside their own steel box (Fig. 16.8). The basic set (Fig. 16.9) consists of:

2 pairs fine-pointed jeweller's forceps;
1 pair swan's necked forceps;
1 pair needle holders;
1 pair scissors.

Additional instruments, e.g. fine-toothed forceps, probe, combined scissors and needle holders, can be added, together with a set of atraumatic tubal clamps.

There are many types on the market; what is essential is that the instruments should be light, long enough to fit comfortably into the surgeon's hand and have rounded handles to allow 'pill rolling' movements of the fingers. Otherwise, rotation of an instrument with flatsided handles requires movement of the wrist, and this will lead to unnecessary hand movement.

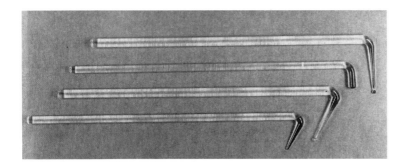

Fig. 16.6 Glass rods.

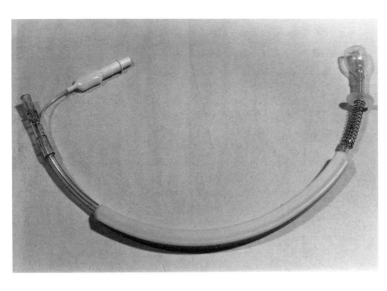

Fig. 16.7 HUMI cervical adaptor.

6 *Combined irrigator and sucker* (Fig. 16.10). Disposable units, which are efficient and cheap, are now available. They consist of a hand unit incorporating a switch; attached to this basic unit, a series of micro-double tubes are available in different sizes. Suction tubes are placed through the bottom tube; when the switch is depressed, suction ceases and irrigation fluid is dispensed. To provide enough pressure we use a 1 L bag of Hartmann's solution in a Fenlow pressure bag.

Suture materials and needles

For microsurgery it is important to choose materials that have the least or no tissue reaction and have not been shown to produce postsurgical fibrosis. Needles made out of fine stainless steel wire and swaged onto the suture material should be nearly the same diameter as the suture to avoid tearing of tissues. The points can either be tapercut or needle point. Tapercut are easier to use for muscle suturing and needle point for peritoneum. Either 3/8 circle or 1/2 circle needles are made but, for most microsurgical muscle wall sutures, 3/8 circle allows easy manipulation of the suture, needle and tissue.

For suture material the choice at first sight seems difficult but Table 16.1 will be of assistance.

For routine microsurgical work I therefore prefer either Vicryl or monofilament nylon, Vicryl being easier to handle and less difficult to tie. For reanastomosis a 6.0 or 8.0 suture is adequate, but on a 1/3 or 1/2

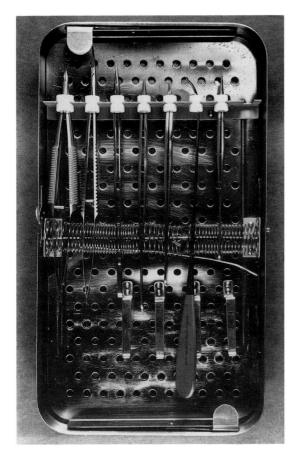

Fig. 16.8 Instruments in their steel box ready for autoclaving.

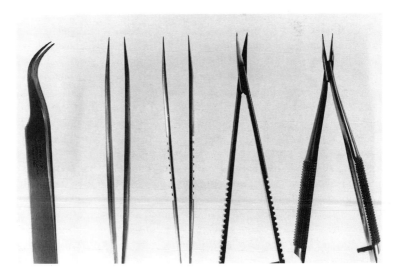

Fig. 16.9 Basic microsurgery set.

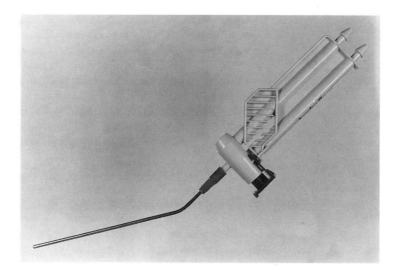

Fig. 16.10 Irrigator and sucker.

Table 16.1 Suture materials

Suture material	Tissue reaction	Suture size
Plain catgut	Marked reactions plus fibrosis	4.0 to 8.0
Polyglycolic acid (Dexon)	Moderate reaction	Up to 10.0
Polyglactin (Vicryl)	Minimal	Up to 10.0
Monofilament nylon	Non-absorbable, no reactions	Up to 10.0

length, to avoid difficulties in pulling through the suture and in tying the knot. Prepacked atraumatic needles of 3/8 circle, 3.7 mm radius and 130 μm diameter are usually used for anastomosis. Similar needles and sutures can be used for salpingostomy. However, for approximating the broad ligament more support is needed and Vicryl or nylon of 4.0 can be used on either a 3/8 or 1/2 circle needle.

CO$_2$ laser instruments

There are many companies that currently produce lasers suitable for abdominal surgery. Power outputs required are higher than those needed for some outpatient work; power of 30–90 W at the tissue may be needed, together with the ability to pulse the laser beam.

The articulated arm should be light, easy to move through 360° and capable of attachment to a micromanipulator and hand pieces.

Abdominal use

The CO$_2$ laser beam can be used as a very discrete surgical knife for removing adhesions, opening tubes, coagulating small vessels and vaporizing endometriosis deposits. It is vital to protect tissue behind the laser beam. This is done by the use of quartz glass rods and stainless steel or aluminium instruments with matt black surfaces. As the beam is absorbed by water, fluid in the pouch of Douglas and fluid-soaked swabs will protect other tissues.

Setting up the theatre and preparation of the patient

With microsurgical procedures, two large pieces of additional equipment are used in addition to the usual surgical team plus surgical instrument tables. Positioning these pieces of equipment correctly is essential if easy, comfortable surgery is to be carried out.

The ideal situation is to have the microscope ceiling-mounted with the lights so that the floor space is not cluttered. However, this is expensive and not the usual situation. If a laser is used, then the cabinet and laser optical bench will need to be adjacent to the microscope with the ability to couple the articulated arm to the microscope or to use this 'free hand' when required.

Prior to surgery the microscope is checked, the eye pieces set to the operator's own eye correction, and the lights checked. The arm is then positioned over the projected abdominal position and set up for middle magnification. Once the patient is in position this can be checked and then the microscope has only to be lowered 5 cm to be in focus so saving time in surgery. The use of video equipment attached to the microscope is invaluable when used together with a monitor in theatre. This allows all staff to see what is happening without disturbing the surgeon.

Surgical scrub-up is the same as for any major surgical procedure, but orthopaedic sterile gowns (with sterile backs) are recommended, and, to avoid talc contamination, gloves without powder should be used and hands rinsed prior to surgery.

Initially, it is necessary to catheterize the patient and then insert a uterine cannula (transcervically).

Following insertion of the cannula the patient is positioned on the table with a foot extension to allow the surgeon to sit comfortably with his legs under the table away from the pedestal. After preparation of the abdomen and upper legs the patient is draped with surgical towels, leaving an area suitable for a lower abdominal transverse incision.

Salpingolysis/ovariolysis

The operation

The surgeon's approach to adhesions has changed dramatically since the use of microsurgery and operating microscopy. The vascular supply and extent of adhesions are clearly revealed, together with the correct tissue plane for incision and excision. In the past, dissection across the middle of an adhesion band or sheet was considered enough; however, the adhesion then often coiled up upon itself leaving the ideal nidus for postoperative adhesion formation.

The aetiology of adhesions is complex but includes

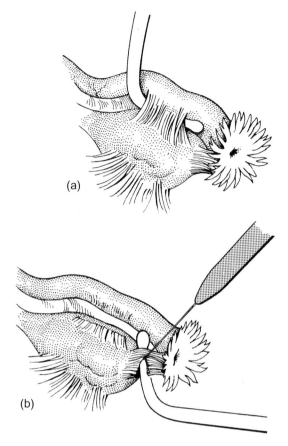

Fig. 16.11 (a) Glass rod elevating tubal adhesions; (b) micro-electrode dividing adhesions.

previous pelvic sepsis, endometriosis and operative trauma. Also implicated are drying of the serosa, contact with blood, infection and foreign-body contamination (e.g. talc granules). To combat these, routine microsurgical principles are used: constant irrigation, absolute haemostasis, antibiotic therapy when needed, and the use of surgical gloves with no added talc.

Incising the adhesions

Microsurgery, combined with clear visualization and removal of each layer of adhesions, is the key to this surgical procedure. Adhesion bands or sheets are stretched over quartz glass rods (Fig. 16.11a) and removed with low-power blended cutting and coagulation current (Fig. 16.11b), using a micro-electrode (Fig. 16.12) or a CO_2 laser, cutting through the adhesions on to the glass rod which protects deeper tissues.

177

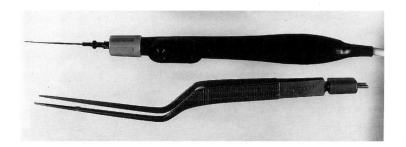

Fig. 16.12 Bipolar forceps and hand operated unipolar probe.

Clearing the pelvis

The adhesions are carefully removed, systematically clearing the pelvis, freeing both fallopian tubes and ovaries and clearing the fimbriae. It may be necessary for the assistant to hold the adhesions stretched with fine-toothed forceps to clear all adhesions. Finally, the surface of the ovary is carefully checked and the capsule cleaned either with diathermy or more easily using low-power CO_2 laser light. Any spots of endometriosis will need to be vaporized as well. Should ovarian endometriosis be present, then these are dealt with in a routine manner. However, to prevent adhesion formation postoperatively, laser vaporization of the inside of the endometrioma plus ovarian microsuturing of the capsule using 6.0 nylon will prevent recurrence. Routine postoperative medical suppressive therapy should also be used in these cases.

Removing ovarian adhesions

Common sites of adhesions are from the inferior part of the ovary to the broad ligament. In this situation, inspection of the adhesions using the dental mirror is essential prior to removal; otherwise, unnecessary bleeding will occur. Ovarian and fimbrial adhesions often occur in pelvic sepsis and may completely cover the fimbriae. In the mid-tubal portion, adhesions often distort and fix the tube to the ovary; or, adhesions between the bowel and tubes may occur more commonly on the left side.

Postoperative management

The essential feature of this operation is to restore normal anatomy and normal mobility of the tubes, fimbriae and ovaries without promoting post-operative adhesion formation. After removal of adhe-sions, tubal patency is tested and routine postoperative care instituted.

Results of salpingolysis/ovariolysis

These will depend on the underlying disease, coincident endometriosis or tubal damage from pelvic sepsis, all of which will reduce the pregnancy rate. Simple lysis of adhesion should leave the patient with patent tubes, and pregnancy rates up to 67% have been reported.

Fimbrioplasty

The operation

This operation is used when there has been distortion of the fimbriae by adhesions or partial closure of the fimbriated end of the tube. In some cases this may present as a phimosis or a constriction band around the fimbriated end. In the past this has been called salpingoplasty.

Releasing the fimbriae

In early stages, two or three folds of fimbriae are agglutinated and all that is required is dissection down the line of the fused fold using diathermy or laser with a glass rod placed inside the tube to stretch the fimbriae and protect other tissues. Microhaemostasis, if necessary, is with bipolar or laser coagulation.

End result

If a phimotic band is present (Fig. 16.13a), with a glass rod inside the band, the tissue is incised with diathermy or laser (Fig. 16.13b); usually, the fimbriae then open up and no stay-suturing is required. Occasionally, one or two stay-sutures are needed with 8.0 or 10.0 nylon (Fig. 16.13c). Magnification, using the operating

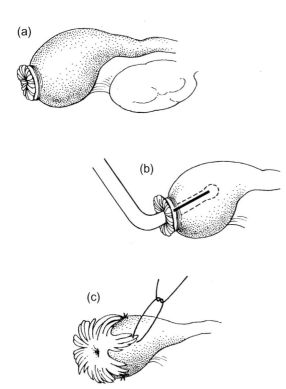

Fig. 16.13 (a) Preoperative appearance of the fimbrial phimosis; (b) incision of the adhesive band; (c) end result of the procedure with stay-sutures in position.

microscope, is invaluable for determining the correct line of incision and depth of cut; low-power magnification only is needed. Staining the fimbrial folds with dilute 1/1000 methylene blue (a vital stain) often aids the surgeon in identifying normal fimbrial tissues and the direction of the fimbrial folds.

Salpingostomy/salpingoneostomy

Much has been written about the surgery of distal tubal disease and many variations of macrosurgery were used in attempts to increase the pregnancy rate. More recent experimental work, combined with microsurgical techniques, has identified the need to assess the degree of distension of the closed ampulla, the wall thickness, and, when opened, the extent of tubal epithelial destruction and replacement by fibrosis. In general, the thicker the wall and the greater the loss of fimbrial folds, the lower the pregnancy rate.

Salpingostomy, or the creation of a new tubal stoma, must take into account the direction of fimbrial folds and restore anatomy to the original situation as much as possible.

The operation

Surgery should concentrate on the following points:
1 *Removal of periampullary and pelvic adhesions.* The objective here is to free the tube and restore its mobility, in the hope that ovum pick-up will be increased.
2 *Freeing the tube from the ovary.* Often, the distal portion of the tube, the site of the fimbriae, is turned down on itself and adherent to the ovary. The correct plane of cleavage needs to be found and the tube carefully freed from the ovary — magnification is essential if this is to be a bloodless procedure.

To assist in these first two steps, distension of the fallopian tube with methylene blue via the cervical cannula helps to define the tubal margins, especially the terminal portion of tube (see Fig. 16.14a). Dissection against a rigidly distended tube is also much easier.

During dissection, as much tubal tissue as possible, especially at the distal end, should be conserved; excess fibrosis can be removed at a later stage.
3 *Creation of the new stoma* (Fig. 16.14a). Having freed the outer portion of the tube, under magnification a small dimple will be found together, in some cases, with small white lines of fibrosis, indicating the old ostium and site of fusion of the fimbriae. With the tube distended, an opening is made into the hydrosalpinx at the site of the dimple with low-power cutting diathermy or laser beam. Using the glass rods and retraction, the white lines can then be incised to enlarge the opening, care being taken to follow the line of the fimbrial folds and not to cut across them (Fig. 16.14b). Cutting across these folds will reduce egg and sperm transport and encourages adhesion formation.

At this time, it is useful to assess the degree of intratubal fibrosis and the extent of remaining tubal folds. This will help to determine the prognosis. Staining of the tissue with methylene blue will help to identify fibrotic and normal areas.
4 *Eversion of the fimbriae.* After control of bleeding either with bipolar or laser coagulation, the edges of the stoma are everted (Fig. 16.14c). Traditionally, this is carried out by a few fine nylon stay-sutures to maintain this eversion. Too much eversion and impaired blood supply may result. However, a simpler way is to defocus

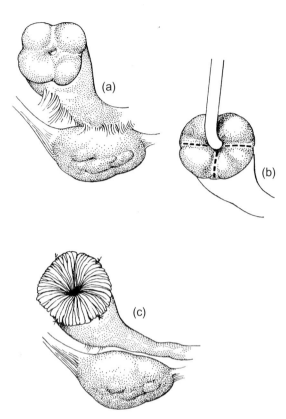

Fig. 16.14 (a) Preoperative appearance; (b) incision of the dimple and widening of the ostium; (c) the end result of a salpingostomy.

the laser beam and run this longitudinally from the ostium down the outer surface of the tube. This precipitates protein, shortening the molecules and everting the edges without the need to suture.

It is essential during the surgical creation of the stoma to restore the normal relationship of fimbriae to ovary to assist in egg pick-up.

Variations in technique
Linear salpingostomy When the distal portion of the tube has been excised, e.g. after an ectopic pregnancy or distal tubal disease has so damaged the terminal ampullary portion that excision is necessary, then the diameter of the tubal lumen is reduced and there are no fimbriae. To try and create a 'spoon' to collect the egg, the tube is opened laterally for 5–8 mm in order to create a linear or lateral salpingostomy.

Using a glass rod to protect the tube, the incision is made with either the CO_2 laser or a knife. Haemostasis is achieved and then a few stay-sutures with 8.0 or 10.0 nylon are used to evert the edges of the tube to create a spoon end. This needs to be adjacent to the ovary and all intervening adhesions need to be removed.

The prognosis following this operation is poor and patients will often need to be referred for IVF as secondary closure of the linear salpingostomy is a common complication.

Prosthetic devices Studies with tubal splints left in for several weeks postoperatively or with prosthetic devices to hold open the salpingostomy stoma (Mulligan Rock Hoods) have been shown to damage the lining of the tube. They are also associated with a reduced pregnancy rate. Intraoperative splints can be used for anastomosis, but the use of other devices for longer periods postoperatively is not recommended.

Tubo–tubal anastomosis

The type of anastomosis is usually described by its site and the diameter of the tube, i.e.:
1 Ampullary–ampullary (same size).
2 Ampullary–isthmic (different sizes).
3 Isthmic–isthmic (same size).
4 Isthmic–cornual.

Operations that leave the end result with a tubal length of less than 5 cm have such a significantly lower pregnancy rate that they are not worthwhile.

The operation

Resecting the obstruction
The basic anastomotic operation is the same for all types: the fibrous tissue or pathology is excised under magnification ($\times10$ to $\times20$), care being taken to maintain haemostasis. This initial excision can be carried out by low-power cutting diathermy or laser. The peritoneum is then removed for 2 mm from the tubal muscle to allow easy suturing of the muscle layer. This is done with either laser or scissors. The tube is then cut vertically until patency is easily recognized; the anatomy of the isthmus is helpful as it has a thick muscle wall with the mucosa thrown into four or five primary folds (see Fig. 16.1b), whereas the ampulla has a thinner muscle wall and many complex folds of the mucosa.

The proximal portion of the tube can be distended with methylene blue via the uterine cannula which aids identification of the lumen. The distal portion can then be distended with either methylene blue via the fimbriae or with a fine silver probe. Once patency of both ends is achieved with high power magnification (×30), a further slice of tube is taken (1 mm) to ensure removal of all fibrous material. The mucosal lining is then stained with concentrated methylene blue and excess dye washed away. This is to aid positioning of the sutures.

Primary suturing

The defect in the broad ligament is then repaired with nylon sutures to bring the ends of the tube together and remove tension on tubal sutures. This also makes the placing and tying of the two-layer anastomotic sutures much easier.

The muscle layer is then approximated using four or five cardinal sutures only, of 8.0 or 10.0 nylon or Vicryl. The lumen needs to be correctly aligned and the sutures should be placed at the same depth in the muscle and not involve the mucosa (Fig. 16.15); the sutures are placed at 12, 3, 6 and 9 o'clock. The posterior suture should always be placed first; then, the tube can be rotated by the assistant using glass rods. The anastomosis must not be under tension.

The second layer of sutures

A second layer is then placed in the peritoneum, usually five or six sutures of either 4.0 or 6.0 nylon or Vicryl. Then the tube is checked for patency and the anastomosis site checked for leakage. Additional sutures can be placed if there is leakage, which is unusual (Fig. 16.16).

If the defect in the broad ligament has not been completely closed, then additional sutures can be added.

With ampullary–isthmic anastomosis there is a difference in size. Here the two unequal diameter portions of tube are prepared as before, and then cut diagonally. The ampullary portion is then partially closed from the antemesenteric border until the open portion has the same diameter as the isthmus. A routine two-layer repair then is completed (see Figs 16.15 and 16.16).

For sterilization reversal following diathermy, Falope rings and Pomeroy-type procedures, tubal blockage may involve the isthmus or the ampullary–isthmic junction; so the two methods described above will be needed. For sterilization using Hulka or Filshie

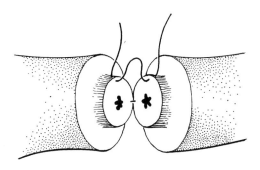

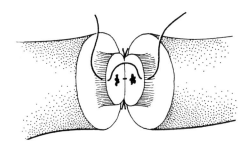

Fig. 16.15 Preparation of the tube, excision of the fibrosis and insertion of the first layer of sutures.

clips, the isthmus only has been involved and therefore an isthmic–isthmic anastomosis is used.

Tubo–cornual anastomosis

Until the pathology of cornual blockage was reevaluated, reimplantation of the tube was considered the only option. However, detailed observations of the radiographic site of the cornual block, and hysteroscopic observation, confirmed the usual site for the block to be at the outer end of the intramural portion of the tube. This enables a tubo–cornual anastomosis to be performed, in many cases with, as we shall see, a better prognosis.

The operation

Identifying the blockage The intrauterine HUMI catheter is used to distend the uterine cavity with methylene blue and to identify the site of the blockage — often seen as a distended knob (Fig. 16.17). Using the microscope, fine slices of tissue are carefully removed

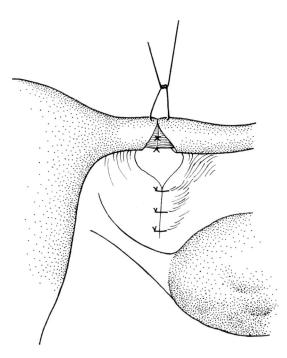

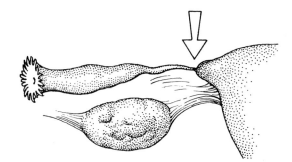

Fig. 16.17 Tubocorneal obstruction before operation.

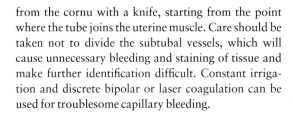

Fig. 16.16 Suturing the peritoneum with the second layer of sutures.

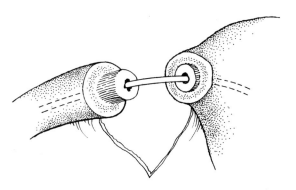

Fig. 16.18 Distal and proximal prepared ends of the tube.

from the cornu with a knife, starting from the point where the tube joins the uterine muscle. Care should be taken not to divide the subtubal vessels, which will cause unnecessary bleeding and staining of tissue and make further identification difficult. Constant irrigation and discrete bipolar or laser coagulation can be used for troublesome capillary bleeding.

Preparing the fallopian tubes Dissection is continued, care being taken not to remove too large an area of uterine peritoneum and muscle, as this will leave a raw area later. Magnification (×20 or ×25) aids the identification of tubal mucosa and dissection is continued until patency (a fine blue jet) and normal tubal mucosa are seen.

The distal portion of the tube is prepared for anastomosis as for tubo–tubal anastomosis.

The anastomosis Broad ligament stay-sutures are then inserted to approximate the two prepared areas—the tube and the uterine cornu. This avoids tension on the anastomotic sutures and makes the anastomosis easier to perform. A fine polythene splint or nylon suture (1.0

or 2.0) can be used as an intraoperative tubal splint to assist in correct alignment of the tubal lumen (Fig. 16.18). This is inserted either down the tube from the fimbriae, through the two prepared ends and into the uterus, or into the uterus first and then placed in a fine hollow probe and threaded carefully up the distal portion of the tube to the fimbriae. The important point here is to avoid tubal damage and to use the method that has least resistance. At the end of the anastomosis, the splint is removed from the fimbrial end and not left in place.

The anastomosis is then carried out using a standard two-layer approach, the first layer (muscle only) using 8.0 or 10.0 sutures of nylon or Vicryl. A 1/2 circle needle is often easier to use, especially on the cornu. Four cardinal sutures are placed through the muscle of both prepared ends (Fig. 16.19) and then the distal portion of the tube is 'railroaded' down onto the cornu over the intraoperative splint. The first layer of sutures is then tied and the peritoneum is closed using five or six sutures as for tubo–tubal anastomosis (Fig. 16.20). If

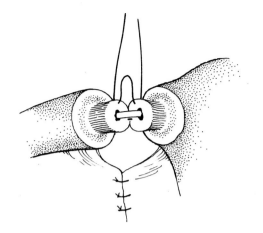

Fig. 16.19 First layer of muscle sutures.

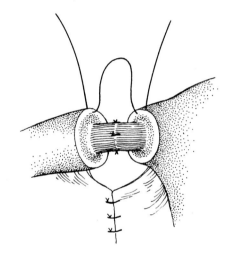

Fig. 16.20 Second layer of sutures.

there is a raw area of muscle on the cornu, a peritoneal graft should be used to cover this.

'Railroading' the tubes together It is usually easy to prepare the distal portion of the tube for anastomosis as shown in Fig. 16.18 with a combination of laser or scissors, knife and low-power diathermy. However, if the cornual block is deep in the myometrium, it may be necessary to open up the cornu. This should be done towards the fundus of the uterus and not inferiorly as this is where a main branch of the uterine–tubal artery arcade enters the myometrium. Once tubal patency has

been demonstrated, a routine anastomosis is carried out; however, it may be necessary to strip the distal tube peritoneum for up to 4mm to allow for the greater depth of the anastomosis. After the first layer of sutures, the uterine myometrium can then be closed above the anastomosis with interrupted nylon sutures.

Haemostasis Haemostasis can also be a problem with tubo–cornual anastomosis, but constant irrigation with Hartmann's solution or the use locally of a dilute solution (1/100 000) of phenylephrine on a small pledget or intravenous Syntocinon (oxytocin) 20 units as a bolus injection at the start of the dissection will help to contain unnecessary bleeding. Alternatively, CO_2 laser coagulation or fine bipolar diathermy can be used. In practice, one uses a combination of these aids to achieve a bloodless field.

Once the intratubal splint has been removed, tubal patency should be checked with methylene blue via the HUMI cannula.

Reimplantation

It is preferable to perform tubo–cornual anastomosis whenever this is feasible. But if during an operation, or after preoperative assessment, it is clear that the intramural portion of the tube is completely blocked, then implantation is the only hope of success. There are two methods—closed and open. The closed method is shown in Figs 16.21–16.23.

The operation

Preparation of the cornua
Under magnification, the distal portion of the tube is prepared as for anastomosis. The cornual preparation is different. Using ×20 magnification the intramural tube site is identified, the uterus is distended with dye and then, using a CO_2 laser, a core of tissue is vaporized (Fig. 16.21), producing a hole through the uterine muscle into the cavity. Its diameter should be the same as the diameter of the prepared muscle of the distal tube. Alternatively, for those surgeons who do not have a laser, a circular stainless steel borer can be used to 'core out' a portion of the myometrium to take the tube. Entry into the cavity of the uterus is marked by a jet of methylene blue dye.

Haemostasis is achieved as for anastomosis.

183

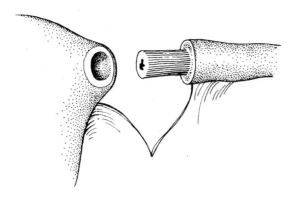

Fig. 16.21 Reimplantation, preparation appearance.

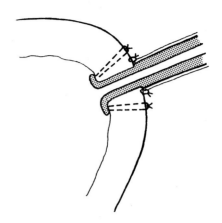

Fig. 16.23 Cross-sectional view of the reimplanted tube.

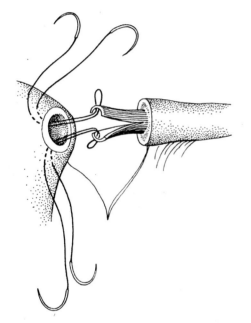

Fig. 16.22 Suturing the tube into the cornua.

Preparation of the tube
The distal portion of the tube is then split into two halves (Fig. 16.22) and double-ended 4.0 nylon arterial sutures (needle on both ends) are then inserted and tied halfway down the suture on the anterior and posterior lips of the tubal muscle.

Fixing the tube
The needles are inserted into the cavity and brought out through the myometrium so as to lock the tube in place

with the ends open and against the uterine cavity wall (Fig. 16.23).

A layer of peritoneal sutures is then inserted to attach the tubal peritoneum to the uterine peritoneal coat.

Variation in technique
The alternative, open, method involves opening the uterine fundus completely down to the cavity, laying the prepared tubes into the defect, suturing open the end of the tube as described above, and then closing the fundus of the uterus in two layers over the tubes. This method causes more bleeding, haemostasis is difficult, and a tubal splint is necessary to keep the tubes patent. There is no evidence that this method is any better than the closed method and it is not recommended.

Results of reversal of sterilization

Ectopic pregnancy still remains a problem with all types of surgery; however, microsurgery has shown an improvement in pregnancy rates. When coupled with a sterilization method that destroys little of the tube, e.g. Filshie clips, then pregnancy rates as high as 80% have been recorded.

Other operations

These are described for completeness, but the results in terms of pregnancy are so low that alternatives such as IVF are preferable.

Double operations of the same tube

Here a combination of pathology requires the surgeon to carry out some type of tubal or tubo–uterine anastomosis plus a salpingostomy. This is not recommended.

However, if the only disease process affecting the distal portion of the tube is adhesion formation with intact fimbriae then adhesiolysis plus anastomosis is a reasonable choice.

Ovarian implantation into the uterus (Estes operation)

Here the intact ovary on its pedicle is implanted into the uterine cavity. A posterolateral incision in the uterus allows access to the cavity. After mobilization of the ovary and division of the ovario–uterine ligament, the ovary is introduced into the uterine cavity and held in place by stay-sutures. The myometrium is closed over the ovary. This operation, carried out in the early part of the 20th century, achieved some success, but it has now been replaced by IVF.

Transplantation of portions of the tube

When, due to disease or previous surgery, all that is left of the fallopian tubes is an isthmus on one side and an ampulla on the other, some surgeons recommend transplantation. The ampulla, together with its intact blood supply, is moved to the isthmus and a complex microvascular anastomosis of artery and veins is then followed by an ampullary–isthmic anastomosis. While some have been successful, i.e. a satisfactory blood supply maintained and tubal patency achieved, IVF is a more logical alternative.

Postoperative management and follow-up

Steroid therapy

Many surgeons use steroids in the belief that postoperative adhesion formation is reduced, and this regimen has been shown to give improved pregnancy rates. The regimens vary but all produce a sense of well-being and euphoria in the patient postoperatively which can be of help. Two examples are given in Table 16.2.

Most surgeons restrict the use of steroids to those patients with distal tubal disease and adhesions, and do

Table 16.2 Steroid regimens

Regimen A
20 mg dexamethasone IM 2–3 h preoperatively
20 mg dexamethasone into peritoneal cavity at end of surgery

Starting 4 h postoperatively 20 mg dexamethasone; 12 doses at 4-hourly intervals (i.l. +52 h after surgery at end of course)

Regimen B
8 mg IM dexamethasone evening prior to surgery
20 mg IM dexamethasone 1 h prior to surgery
8 mg IM dexamethasone the evening after surgery
8 mg IM dexamethasone twice a day on day 1
1 mg oral dexamethasone four times a day on day 2
0.5 mg oral dexamethasone four times a day on day 3
0.5 mg oral dexamethasone once on day 4

not give them for reversal of sterilization. Others recommend their use for all cases regardless of pathology.

Antibiotics

Especially if steroids are to be used, routine antibiotic therapy is helpful to prevent any unnecessary postoperative infection. A combination of a broad-spectrum antibiotic plus Flagyl (metronidazole) is used to cover all possibilities.

Intraperitoneal solutions

At the end of the operation, peritoneal lavage with Ringer's lactate solution is useful to remove any small blood clot or debris. Instillation of dextran 70 into the peritoneal cavity (100–200 ml) has been shown to reduce peritoneal adhesion by causing a peritoneal transudate; it also appears to have a siliconizing effect upon raw surfaces and to alter fibrin structure.

Other agents to decrease postoperative adhesion formation

Anticoagulants
These are of no value and the complications reported do not make their use worthwhile.

Chymotrypsin
This appears to be of little value.

Postoperative hydrotubation

Controlled studies have not been carried out and there is little evidence to suggest this procedure is worthwhile. With conventional microsurgery, postoperative hydrotubation is not needed.

Prostaglandin synthetase inhibitors

These also have little effect on postoperative results.

Postoperative mobilization

Patients should be mobilized early and worked up from oral fluids to a normal diet within a few days. Abdominal sutures should be removed on the fifth day and the patient allowed home. Many patients may be ready for earlier discharge and if home circumstances permit it, then this should be encouraged.

Follow-up

All patients should be seen 6–8 weeks after surgery for a routine check. Continuation of regular ovulatory cycles and postoperative abdominal healing are both assessed.

The patient is encouraged to try for a pregnancy after one normal period and regular fertility follow-up is continued.

If pregnancy has not occurred after 6 months, then repeat laparoscopy to check tubal patency and adhesion formation is desirable, and preferable to hysterosalpingography.

Further reading

Textbooks

As well as John Newton the author of this chapter, Mr R.M.L. Winston is the leading authority on microsurgical technique in Britain; the editor feels that the student's attention should be drawn to three of his review articles, 'Progress in Tubal Surgery' (Chapter 7 in *Clinics in Obstetrics and Gynaecology*, vol. 8, no. 3, December 1981), 'Developments in Infertility Practice', Michael G.R. Hull (ed.), published by W.B. Saunders, London, and Chapter 22 'Tubal Microsurgery' in *Progress in Obstetrics and Gynaecology*, vol. 1, 1981, John Studd (ed.), published by Churchill Livingstone.

References

Two of the historical references related to tubal surgery are the classics of Jeffcoate and Shirodkar:

Jeffcoate TNA. Salpingectomy or salpingo-oophorectomy? *J Obstet Gynaecol Br Empire* 1955.

Shirodkar VN. Plastic surgery of the fallopian tubes. *West J Surg* 1961;69:253.

Other significant references include:

Gomel V. Reconstructive surgery of the oviduct. *J Reprod Med* 1977;18:181–90.

Gomel V. Microsurgical reversal of female sterilisation: a re-appraisal. *Fertil Steril* 1980;33:587.

Siegler AM. Surgical treatment for tuboperitoneal causes of infertility since 1967. *Fertil Steril* 1977;28:1019–32.

17 Laparoscopy and other minimal access surgery

Laparoscopy

Since the mid 1960s laparoscopy has grown from very simplistic beginnings to become one of the most commonly performed and most valuable of gynaecological procedures. The procedure is used extensively in the assessment of infertility, in the diagnosis of pelvic infection and endometriosis, and for sterilization procedures.

During the late 1980s and 1990s, laparoscopic surgery began to develop into what is now generally called 'minimal access surgery' (MAS), being applied to a wide variety of conditions and gynaecological problems, changing from a mere observational process into one which has become the mainstay of effective management and treatment of a wide variety of conditions including a number of cancers. MAS is now widely established throughout gynaecological surgery, particularly in gynaecological oncology, and has developed to a significant extent initially from the efforts made by general surgeons who, although taking up laparoscopy late, realized its major value as an operative technique, rapidly developing MAS techniques for gall bladder disease, and in urology. The technique is now widely used throughout the body, including the thorax, and in any place in the body where a space can be developed to generate access. The major changes which have allowed this development have been the massive improvements in instrumentation, particularly the generation of high-quality video cameras which now allow the surgery to be performed remotely with the surgeon and assistants observing the procedure on video monitors. Indeed in some circumstances surgery can be carried out even more remotely at a distance with a single surgeon leading other surgeons in their activities.

The laparoscopic equipment has also improved markedly and it is now normal to use very small diameter instruments (5 mm) and even smaller diagnostic instrumentation down to 2 mm has been developed. Most of these give superb views of the intra-abdominal and pelvic structures.

In recent times, the development of MAS has meant that patients with significant pelvic inflammatory disease, endometriosis and oncological problems, can be diagnosed and effectively treated using techniques which allow for rapid recovery and return to normal activity.

Instrumentation

Modern instrumentation for MAS is complex and should include high-quality laparoscopes of the smallest diameter available to give the maximum access and vision of intra-abdominal and pelvic structures. Access to the abdomen is via a series of trocars, virtually all of which should be disposable in order to produce high-quality consistent sharpness of access and the most advanced safety devices to reduce the risk of trauma.

Verres needle
This narrow needle continues to be used as the main method of introducing gas into the abdominal cavity, although some clinicians will use other trocar systems. The Verres needle remains the mainstay of our technique.

Abdominal insufflation equipment

These have become increasingly sophisticated and allow the surgeon to make accurate measurements of volume of gas pressure; they also have a number of safety devices set within them.

The gas used for insufflation is carbon dioxide because of its ability to be rapidly absorbed into the patient's bloodstream and excreted through the lungs and kidneys. The instrumentation has both high and low flow rates allowing initial safe low-pressure insufflation which can then be accelerated during the subsequent phases of the procedure. In most circumstances, the intra-abdominal cavity pressure should run at approximately 14 mm of mercury, although some clinicians utilize much higher pressures at the time of the placement of the trocars to reduce risk of injury to intra-abdominal structures.

Other instrumentation

There are a variety of instruments for manipulation of the uterus during the procedure, and a wide range of graspers, scissors and cutting devices have been developed.

Diathermy

Whilst monopolar diathermy remains a mainstay of most MAS procedures, some clinicians prefer bipolar and the use of the 'harmonic scalpel', which is a form of ultrasound initiated by vibration in an instrument.

The use of a variety of lasers, particularly the Nd:YAG laser, has been popular, but is used only in a minority of circumstances.

Light source

Modern fibre optic light sources provide tremendous intra-abdominal illumination as long as their fibres remain intact. Cables should be checked regularly to make sure that there is no loss of fibres and a consequent reduction in light availability.

Preparation

Patients do not require special preparation for these procedures. Many of the simple diagnostic tests are performed as day cases and even a number of small MAS procedures will be performed as day cases.

Anaesthesia

Laparoscopic surgery should be performed under general anaesthesia with the patient intubated and fully relaxed. The use of laryngeal masks has become popular and for short procedures can be used. The use of local anaesthetic techniques is difficult and renders operations more complex and potentially dangerous.

Diagnostic laparoscopy

Operation

Positioning and preparation

The patient should be positioned on the operating table in the lithotomy position with the legs tilted slightly forward so that the operator has easy access to the lower abdomen. This position is most accurately achieved by using multijoint supports such as the Lloyd-Davis stirrups. Simple lithotomy poles may be used, tilted slightly forwards. The vulva and the vagina are swabbed and the bladder meticulously emptied using a disposable catheter. At the same time, the lower abdomen is swabbed and the patient draped.

Grasping the uterus

The pelvis must be examined prior to the procedure to determine the size, position and mobility of the uterus. The cervix is visualized by inserting a Sims' speculum into the vagina and grasped by placing a single-toothed tenaculum transversely across the anterior lip of the cervix and attaching it to a simple intrauterine device, such as that used for injecting methylene blue into the uterus, or the Hulka tenaculum which combines a tenaculum and a sound. These devices allow the assistant to manipulate the uterus to different positions to improve access and visibility for the surgeon.

Producing the pneumoperitoneum

The surgeon now makes a small transverse or vertical cut in the fold of skin at the lower part of the umbilicus. (Some operators prefer to insert the Verres needle directly through the centre of the umbilicus, although this is not the authors' choice.) The surgeon then grasps the skin of the relaxed lower abdomen with his left hand and elevates the abdominal wall. The right hand now firmly introduces the Verres needle through the abdominal wall via the small cut (Fig. 17.1). Resistance is felt at the level of the rectus sheath causing the blunt obtu-

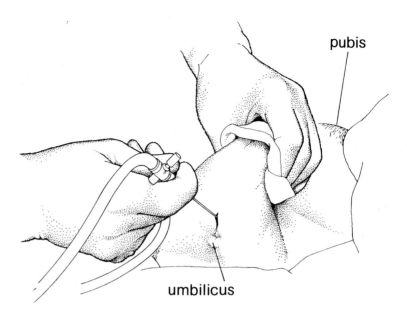

pubis

umbilicus

Fig. 17.1 Verres needle inserted through the abdominal wall into the abdominal cavity and producing a pneumoperitoneum.

rator in the needle to be forced back, allowing the needle's cutting edge to pass through the sheath into the abdomen. At this point the spring-loaded obturator moves forward protecting the abdominal contents from the sharp cutting edge. Utilizing modern disposable Verres needles, a double click may be heard as the needle passes through the layers of the abdominal wall.

Variations in technique
Although the umbilical site is the commonest one used for straightforward laparoscopic procedures, in patients where there has been any evidence of previous surgery or intra-abdominal or pelvic infection, it is prudent to utilize an alternative site of entry. Statistically, the left hypochondrium is the site in the abdomen where the surgeon is at least risk of hitting an intra-abdominal structure. The site usually chosen is the point roughly in the line of the left nipple, some two fingers below the lower margin of the rib cage. This technique of placing the gas insufflation in the left hypochondrium is that described by Palmer and the point chosen is that of Palmer's point. At this point a small incision some 3 mm wide is made in the skin. The Verres needle is now inserted vertically through the abdominal wall. It is prudent to grasp the needle in the right hand with the fingers of the right hand lying along the shaft of the needle to act as a buffer as the needle is inserted through the skin. Once more the abdominal

wall is elevated with the left hand and the needle is passed through the wall, once more hearing the two clicks of the disposable needle as it passes through the rectus sheath and then through the peritoneum into the abdominal cavity. The gas may be running as the needle is inserted. However, many clinicians do not utilize this technique and adopt a series of small tests including the water test, which consists of attaching a syringe full of sterile water to the Verres needle, opening and observing the gentle change in pressure associated with respiration.

Initially the gas is allowed to flow in at a low pressure, less than 10 mm of mercury. Once flowing freely with clear signs of wide distribution throughout the abdominal cavity, as can be demonstrated by percussion of the expanding abdomen, the pace of insufflation can be raised to a high flow. It is important in the operation notes to record the flow rates and the volume of gas put in during the procedure. It is remarkable that even quite high intra-abdominal pressures do not seem to cause concern to the anaesthetic process.

Insertion of the laparoscope
Once gas flow is proceeding smoothly and evenly, the operation table can be tipped to a very slight head-down position so that the bowel may fall away from the pelvis. The surgeon should check that the intra-abdominal pressure has reached at least 14 mm; usual-

189

ly more than 3 L of gas will have been insufflated at this time. At this point, if the Verres needle has been inserted in the periumbilical region it can be removed and the gas tube is attached to the laparoscopic trocar. For most diagnostic procedures a 5 mm trocar and a 5 mm laparoscope will be used to minimize trauma. For insertion of the disposable trocar, the trocar is grasped in the surgeon's right hand with the index finger passing along the length of the trocar. Once more the index finger will act as a buffer so that the trocar is not inserted any further than the depth of the abdominal wall. At this point the abdominal wall will be firm from the insufflating gas, but it is prudent to once more hold the abdominal wall with the left hand and to insert the trocar boldly with the right hand directing the trocar down towards the pelvis. The modern disposable trocars are very sharp and safety devices built into them immediately spring to cover the sharp blade as soon as the trocar passes through the abdominal wall. The trocar can be felt passing through the various layers of the abdominal wall and as soon as this is achieved the laparoscope can be inserted, the gas attached to the trocar and observation of the intra-abdominal structures begun (Fig. 17.2). It is often useful to apply demisting solutions to the laparoscope tip prior to insertion, or in some centres gas can be warmed prior to being put into the abdomen as it is merely the gas cooling the laparoscope which causes misting. A fibre optic light is attached to the laparoscope, and the pelvis and abdomen can then be visualized. If the laparoscope mists while inside the abdomen (this often occurs in the initial phases of a laparoscopy) it is usually not necessary to remove it from the abdomen. All that is needed is to touch the laparoscope gently on to a nearby piece of bowel.

Insertion of other devices into the pneumoperitoneum
In modern practice the video camera is attached to the laparoscope inserted in the first trocar so that a full inspection of the abdomen can be made and all further instrumentation can be inserted under direct vision.

In most procedures other instruments are inserted into the abdominal cavity. This is facilitated by illuminating the abdominal wall if it is thin using the laparoscope or choosing a spot where large vessels such as the inferior epigastric artery can be avoided. Once more the same technique of inserting trocars can be applied, this time under direct vision via the video camera which has now been attached to the laparoscope.

Diagnostic laparoscopy consists simply of recording appearances within the abdomen and pelvis. These can be recorded either in the operation notes or using more

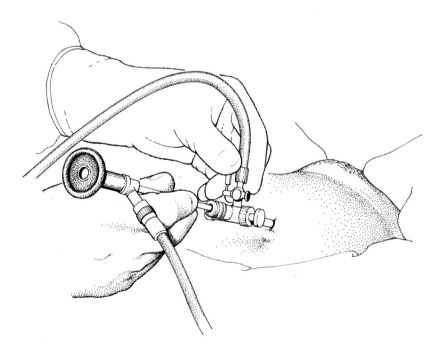

Fig. 17.2 Insertion of the laparoscope via the trocar.

modern techniques with individual photographic records of elements which are of importance. Modern digital cameras can generate a number of images which can be stored or printed out and put into the patient's clinical record. These are of particular value in the recording of sterilization procedures and when wishing to discuss further more complex management which may be necessary following the diagnostic procedure.

Completing the procedure

Once the diagnostic laparoscopic procedure is complete the laparoscope can be removed and gas released from the abdomen. When a number of ports have been used, it is prudent to observe individual trocars being taken out to make sure that no untoward bleeding occurs. Finally, having released all the gas from the abdomen, the final trocar can be removed and the various incisions closed, usually with a single stitch for 5 mm laparoscopic procedures.

Problems and complications associated with laparoscopy

Although the basic procedure is simple in concept there are a number of traps and pitfalls which must be avoided:

1 Failure to examine the patient prior to the procedure may result in missing uterine enlargement or masses in the pelvis which can be put in significant danger when the various instrumentation is being inserted into the abdomen.

2 Failure to catheterize the bladder increases the risk of damage to that organ.

3 A tentative approach to the production of the pneumoperitoneum may result in gas being inserted in the fatty layer of the anterior abdominal wall. The Verres needle must be inserted through the abdominal wall at almost a vertical angle down towards the pelvis and not at a shallow angle as this will generate problems. The double click of the disposable Verres needle is reassuring. The use of Palmer's point will markedly reduce the risk of failure to develop a pneumoperitoneum.

4 Failure to produce an adequate pneumoperitoneum either because of problems mentioned above, or because of failure to put in an adequate volume of gas, jeopardizes the bowel when the laparoscopic trocar is being inserted.

5 Many complications of laparoscopy have been reported including bowel damage and arterial damage. These can all be avoided by using a careful technique,

producing an adequate pneumoperitoneum and assiduous practice.

Traumatic complications have been categorized as follows:

Type I. These are complications which occur to fixed structures such as the arteries and veins of the posterior abdominal wall and the pelvic rim, or of the small and large bowel mesentery.

Type II. These complications occur where structures have become fixed, usually due to adhesions. This applies particularly to the bowel. Such structures are inadvertently damaged as the Verres needle or trocars are passed through the abdominal wall. The risk of such trauma is low (approximately 1 in 1500 cases), but it is important that all patients should understand these small risks prior to the procedure. Risks should be carefully explained and in the consenting process all patients should be warned of the possible need for an open procedure, i.e. a laparotomy, if significant trauma or difficulties occur during the laparoscopic process.

Laparoscopic surgery for endometriosis

Endometriosis continues to be a major problem of modern Western society. Its management was hoped to become almost entirely medical. However, it has become clear in recent years that surgical management will remain the cornerstone of the care of the patient with both small volume painful endometriosis as well as those with advanced and recurrent endometriotic disease. The scope of this subject is enormous and the authors would refer the interested clinician to a text such as that of Sutton and Diamond's *Endoscopic Surgery for Gynaecologists*, published in 1998 by W. B. Saunders (pp. 349–98).

MAS in gynaecological oncology

For many years after the introduction of laparoscopy, the technique was almost entirely utilized in the management of minor gynaecological problems. However, in more recent times MAS has expanded its role, particularly in gynaecological oncology, and predominantly in the area of lymphadenectomy.

A significant number of advances have been made, mainly by the French school of gynaecological surgery, that have been taken up by many other centres around the world. It became clear that MAS would meet the modern requirements of both gynaecology and gynaecological oncology in terms of ease of access, reduction of impact of surgery on patients, rapid recovery and, in many Western countries most importantly, an early discharge from hospital thus reducing overall costs of surgery.

This pressure to speed up the process of care had to be tempered by the need to be effective and ensure that new technologies were at least equal in efficacy to previous open surgical techniques. There is little doubt that the major proponents of MAS have been able to demonstrate the ease with which major and at times extremely radical procedures can be performed using MAS techniques. However, it is also clear that such techniques require a considerable experience of standard surgery. They require a prolonged period of training and the equipment which is necessary has to be of the highest order. All the services associated with surgical care, including anaesthetics, nursing and operating theatre skills, have to be comparable, and it is vital that surgeons accept that the same prolonged period of training will be required for MAS as is accepted for open surgery.

The major areas of practice have been in the use of MAS in the performance of lymphadenectomy. Pelvic lymphadenectomy is now widely accepted as a standard procedure in MAS, and periaortic lymphadenectomy of varying levels of radicality can also be satisfactorily performed using these techniques.

By definition the acceptance of MAS in lymphadenectomy has meant that it is mainly used in the management of early stage cervical cancer and early stage corpus cancer. At the present time, except in the very exceptional circumstances of early (stage Ia) ovarian cancer, MAS is not used as a treatment technique in ovarian carcinoma. Although the techniques have been used for lymphadenectomy in the groin in the management of vulval cancer, these have met with problems and have not been accepted into the mainstream of management of this disease.

We will therefore concentrate on the use of MAS in pelvic and periaortic lymphadenectomy in the management of early cervical cancer and corpus cancer.

Equipment

The equipment required is as for other MAS. It is vital that not only the surgeon but also the assistants are trained in MAS as there is an enormous reliance on the assistants being entirely in tune with the needs of the surgeon. The use of high-quality cameras and monitors is paramount, and the surgeon must spend a considerable period of time developing the hand skills required to dissect out the tissues of the pelvic side wall. In essence, MAS should simply translate the techniques of open surgery.

The operation

Preparation
No special preparation is required for the patient. The position generally adopted is that of the patient supine or with the legs slightly elevated in Lloyd-Davis stirrups. The abdominal wall is prepared and gas insufflation completed utilizing either the standard periumbilical insertion or Palmer's point.

Equipment
As material will be removed from the abdominal cavity it is generally accepted that larger diameter trocars will be required and usually 10–12 mm trocars are utilized.

Stage 1
After gas insufflation a 10 mm trocar is placed centrally and periumbilically and the laparoscope inserted. Under direct vision, the author's preference is to place trocars alongside but slightly caudal to the central trocars. A fourth trocar is placed suprapubically. This fourth trocar is usually 5 mm and is to be utilized solely for grasping the upper part of the uterus to produce tissue tension during the dissection. Once the trocars are in place, the laparoscope is transferred to the right-sided trocar with the surgeon standing on the left side of the patient. In his left hand he should have a pair of diathermy scissors and in the right hand dissecting forceps, ideally those with a flick off ratchet which will allow rapid and easy grasping and manipulation of tissues (Figs 17.3 and 17.4).

Stage 2
The uterus is grasped close to the insertion of the round ligament into the fundus by a ratcheted forceps passed through the fourth trocar which has been inserted some 7 cm above the pubis in the mid-line. A second assistant will move the grasping forcep to put the triangle of tissue which has developed between the round ligament, the infundibulopelvic ligament and the pelvic

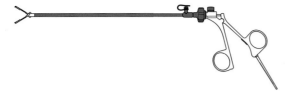

Fig. 17.3 Tissue grasping forceps.

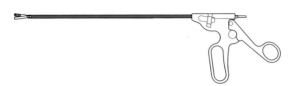

Fig. 17.4 Laparoscope dissecting scissors.

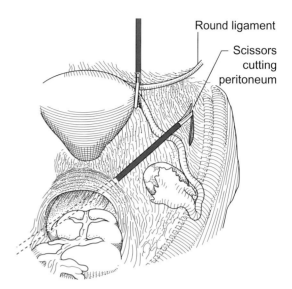

Round ligament

Scissors cutting peritoneum

Fig. 17.5 Incision in the stretched peritoneum over the external iliac vessels on the right side.

side wall on tension. As the fundus of the uterus is moved across to the left side of the abdomen, the triangle of tissues tighten and it is then possible to visualize the external iliac artery passing just beneath the peritoneum on the right side of the triangle.

Opening the peritoneum

With the forceps in the left hand, the peritoneum just lateral to the external iliac artery is picked up and incised with the scissors held in the surgeon's right hand. It is usually possible to see tiny blood vessels running across the peritoneum and these can be individually diathermied if necessary. The incision in the peritoneum is then carried forwards and backwards opening up a line of peritoneum between the round ligament anteriorly over the external iliac artery and posteriorly to the infundibulopelvic ligament which is now on tension (Fig. 17.5).

Opening the pelvic side wall

The incision which has been made along the line lateral to the external iliac artery can now be extended medially across the stretched peritoneum of the middle part of the triangle. This then allows the forceps in the left hand and scissors in the right hand to be used as gentle blunt dissectors to open up the space around the external iliac artery.

Pelvic lymphadenectomy

If a pelvic lymphadenectomy alone is to be performed

and the procedure is not to be part of a Coelio-Schauta procedure, it is the author's preference to remove the lymph nodes beginning from the lateral part of the external iliac chain. However, if the procedure is part of a Coelio-Schauta procedure, it is the authors' preference at this early stage to identify the ureter, the uterine artery and to divide the uterine artery prior to the performance of the lymphadenectomy.

Once the peritoneum has been opened and the external iliac vessels and their surrounding tissues displaced, the fascia covering over the tissues to the lateral side of the external iliac artery can be picked up and divided. Occasional small vessels will require diathermy, but in general terms diathermy is little used in this procedure. Working anteriorly, the lateral part of the external iliac artery is cleaned and then, moving posteriorly, the dissection is continued down to the identification of the common iliac node which is clearly seen lying slightly lateral to the external iliac artery. Pelvic lymphadenectomy is unlike the open lymphadenectomy which is generally performed as an *en bloc* procedure. The nodal tissue is removed in small volumes and can be 'stored' anterior to the round ligament which is kept on tension by the fourth suprapubic trocar.

193

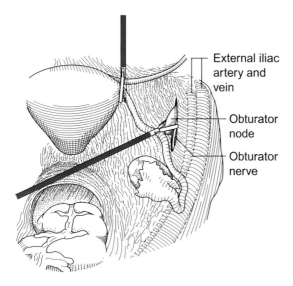

External iliac artery and vein

Obturator node

Obturator nerve

Fig. 17.6 Opening of the right obturator fossa and removing the node.

Cleaning lymphatic tissue from the vessels
The dissection of the external iliac artery continues and, as it is cleaned, the external iliac vein becomes apparent and this also can be cleaned of lymphatic tissue from anterior to posterior. On the right side and with the laparoscope in the right port, vision behind the lateral part of the external iliac artery is very straightforward and this area can be cleaned down into the obturator fossa.

Removing nodes from the obturator fossa
Once the external iliac vessels have been cleaned, it is possible using the scissors in the right hand to retract the vessels laterally and the grasping forceps in the left hand can then be used to dissect gently and bluntly down into the obturator fossa, identifying the lateral wall of the obturator fossa and obturator internus muscle (Fig. 17.6). On the medial side of the obturator fossa the obliterated hypogastric artery is visible and will function as the medial limit of the obturator fossa. Lying centrally within the fossa is the long, thin obturator node which is now defined on both its sides and, as it is drawn medially away from the obturator internus muscle, the obturator nerve can be seen running through the lower part of the tissue under the node. The nerve is cleaned from its most anterior part to the posterior part of the fossa, and the node then lies free.

Carrying the dissection of the node forwards above the obturator foramen it will be found to narrow, and at this point it is prudent to place two small clips (surgiclips) across the node and divide it. The nodal tissue at this point may also be divided utilizing the diathermy scissors. Sometimes an abnormal obturator vein will cross this area and this can be dissected clear, and clipped and divided. The obturator node is then stripped posteriorly from the nerve and once more 'stored' anterior to the round ligament. At this point it is straightforward to remove any internal iliac nodes which may be lying close to the internal iliac vein and artery, and moving the external iliac artery and vein medially it is possible to dissect the pelvic side wall clear down to the point at which the obturator nerve exits the muscles of the posterior part of the pelvis. At this point, the interiliac node dissection is virtually complete. The internal iliac artery is defined on the medial side of the obturator fossa and if necessary the uterine artery can be divided at this point. The ureter is now lying slightly lateral to the internal iliac artery running across the face of the peritoneum and should be identified.

Removal of the nodes
It is important to reduce the risk of contamination of the port sites wherever possible and we have for some years used a simple system of removing nodes by drawing them into a non-disposable 10 mm port which fits down the 12 mm ports. The nodes are grasped from the storage place anterior to the round ligament and are individually drawn into the 10 mm trocar which is then brought out with the node inside it through the 12 mm port. This means that the risk of contamination of the port sites with nodal material is reduced markedly.

It is occasionally necessary to clean the area of the dissection with suction but suction is rarely necessary during a standard lymphadenectomy.

Dissection of the left side
It has been the authors' experience that moving from one side of the operating table to the other to dissect the opposite side of the pelvis is not without its difficulties. It has therefore been our practice for the surgeon and camera assistant to remain in the same position, and for the surgeon to move further across the table to dissect the left side of the pelvis. Clearly with the laparoscope in the right-sided port, the view of the left side of the pelvis is rather different from the view given for the right side of the pelvis. This does not, however, present

major difficulties except that the dissection of the uterine artery sometimes is a little more obscure and requires a wider opening of the triangle of tissue between the round ligament and the infundibulopelvic ligaments.

Completion of the procedure

Once the lymphadenectomy is complete and haemostasis is seen to be secure, all that is required is serial removal of the ports observing each as it is removed from the abdomen. If the procedure is part of another procedure, such as a laparoscopic assisted vaginal hysterectomy for corpus cancer or a Coelio-Schauta procedure for carcinoma of the cervix, then the remaining part of the procedure is completed and at the end of all the procedures the pelvis is inspected, haemostasis checked and the ports are closed. It has not been the author's constant practice to close the internal part of the port although some authors would recommend closure of all ports where a trocar of greater than 5 mm in diameter is used.

Complications

Risk of port site metastases

There has been a small but important series of individual case reports and comments concerning the risks of port site recurrences associated with MAS in gynaecological oncology. There is no doubt that when laparoscopic techniques are used in association with ovarian cancer the risk of port site recurrence is significant, particularly when there is a long gap between the surgical procedure and the inception of chemotherapy. However, there have also been reports of port site recurrences following the treatment of both cervical and corpus cancers, even when very early cancers have been treated. The mechanism of development is uncertain, but it is likely that the major problem is contamination of the port with material containing cancer cells, the so-called implantation theory. However, this theory seems to fall down when it is noted how rarely the vaginal vault is involved in recurrences, particularly in the case of cancer of the cervix. Various gas pressure theories have also been promulgated but to date there is no certain aetiology.

Port site hernia

Port site hernia continue to be a debilitating but rare problem for a small number of patients. The result of extensive study has shown the higher risk of hernia associated with the use of larger ports. The result of these studies is that many experts now consider that closure of the large ports (larger than 5 mm), is of value. It has been the authors' experience that the most likely sites are lateral 12 mm ports.

Port site haematoma

Port site haematomata can be extremely debilitating slowing recovery and causing considerable pain and distress. Avoidance of large vessels such as the inferior epigastric is mandatory. However, when the lateral ports are inserted through a muscular abdomen, particularly through the rectus muscle, damage to contained vessels may be unavoidable. Damage to these vessels may result in a haematoma developing or may manifest itself as continuing pain after the procedure or even in extreme cases a significant drop in haemoglobin in the days following surgery.

Recovery from laparoscopic surgery

In general terms, the most significant characteristic of the postsurgical period following MAS is the rapid and progressive recovery of the patient. Any patient who does not do so or suddenly develops new pain or symptomatology must be carefully examined for complications. Early discharge of such a patient is a formula for progressive and sometimes long-term problems including litigation.

Further reading

Textbooks

The confidential report by the Royal College of Obstetricians and Gynaecologists on Gynaecological Laparoscopy is hardly a textbook but is well worth studying as it is a masterpiece of sound advice. The report is entitled 'Gynaecological Laparoscopy: The Report of the Working Party of the Confidential Enquiry into Gynaecological Laparoscopy, Chamberlain G and Brown JC (eds) (1978) Royal College of Obstetricians and Gynaecologists, London.

Hulka, in *Textbook of Laparoscopy* (1985) published by Grune and Stratton, New York, is an authoritative monograph.

18 Management of extrauterine gestation and sterilization procedures

Extrauterine gestation

Extrauterine gestation or ectopic pregnancy remains a serious pregnancy-related cause of morbidity and mortality, being the most common cause of deaths in early pregnancy and the fourth leading cause of direct deaths, during the 1997–99 triennia. Many deaths still occur as a result of misdiagnosis or an inability to appreciate the severity of the condition. The management of the collapsed patient exsanguinating from a ruptured ectopic pregnancy must be immediate, and relies on an experienced team of gynaecologist, anaesthetist and haematologist with an early recourse to laparotomy. However, for the majority of cases, sensitive urinary and serum β-human chorionic gonadotropin tests and transvaginal ultrasound scanning have improved the possibility of early identification and, for these women, laparoscopy remains the cornerstone of diagnosis.

Aetiology

Ectopic pregnancy is a condition which has no single aetiological factor. Women at higher risk are those who have:
1 A previous history of ectopic pregnancy.
2 A previous history of pelvic infection.
3 An intrauterine contraceptive device (IUD) *in situ*.
4 Congenital malformations of the fallopian tubes or uterus.
5 Endometriosis.
6 Previous surgery to the fallopian tubes, particularly sterilization procedures and reconstructive surgery.
7 IVF pregnancy.

Suggested factors such as altered physiology of the tubes, including slowing of the transmission times for the ovum, are more difficult to demonstrate.

Ectopic sites

Most (95%) ectopic pregnancies occur in the fallopian tube, 55% being in the ampulla. Ovarian ectopic pregnancy represents 2% of the total and abdominal pregnancy 1%. The condition is almost always unilateral.

Symptoms and signs

It should always be remembered that this condition is a form of pregnancy, of which the patient will show signs and symptoms.

Amenorrhoea will have occurred; usually, at least one menstrual period will have been missed.

Pain in the lower abdomen will occur at a varying time after missing a period depending on the site of implantation of the ectopic pregnancy. (If the site is a distensible part of the tube then the pregnancy may reach a more advanced stage than at constrictive sites).

Bleeding, often slight, will occur vaginally in the majority of patients but is not a constant feature. Rarely, the endometrium is expelled as a 'cast' upon the death of the pregnancy.

Clinical pattern

Acute rupture
This may produce a disastrous, life-threatening situation; the patient experiences extreme lower abdominal

196

pain, occasionally being felt in the shoulder due to irritation of the diaphragm by the blood tracking from the pelvis, after she has been lying down. The patient becomes shocked, the pulse rises, blood pressure falls, peripheral vascular shutdown produces pallor and eventually 'air hunger' develops. If the heavy bleeding is not stopped the patient eventually succumbs. The management is immediate laparotomy, coupled with large transfusions of blood expanders until whole blood for transfusion is available. There is no place for delay; resuscitation should occur simultaneously with laparotomy. Indeed, the patient usually cannot be resuscitated without laparotomy and ligation of the bleeding vessels.

Subacute syndrome

This condition will arise if the pregnancy continues to develop. Intermittent pain associated with intraabdominal bleeding will occur. There is a pattern of more chronic symptoms with vague bowel and urinary symptoms being produced by peritoneal irritation and the development of a pelvic haematocele.

The proper diagnosis may be confused with a threatened miscarriage, appendicitis, salpingitis, complications of ovarian cysts and pelvic malignancies.

It is important to make a certain diagnosis. The most useful investigation is laparoscopy. This should be carried out with the patient prepared and consent obtained for a laparotomy.

Management

It is vitally important in the acute state for the patient to be rapidly transported to the nearest available operating theatre. Intravenous transfusions are erected at the same time and an emergency laparotomy is performed.

Opening the abdomen

The patient is anaesthetized quickly, ideally in the theatre; the abdomen is cleansed and draped and a mid-line subumbilical incision is made. The peritoneum usually has a bluish tinge due to the blood in the peritoneal cavity. As soon as the peritoneum is incised, blood and clots may pour out. Do not waste time mopping them away.

Stopping the bleeding

The surgeon should immediately reach into the abdomen and grasp the uterus with the left hand, bringing it up into the wound. If the uterine artery on the affected side is firmly grasped, the blood pressure monitor on the anaesthetic machine will often show an immediate favourable response.

Identifying the source of bleeding

As the uterus is elevated it is usually immediately apparent where the bleeding is emanating from. If the isthmus of the tube has ruptured it may not be necessary to remove the entire tube: the central portion can be taken and the fimbrial end and the uterine portion retained for future repair. If the whole tube is involved and damaged by the extravasated blood, a total salpingectomy will be necessary. Rarely will a tubal abortion produce a massive bleed but if it has, when the contents of the tube have been milked out, it may be possible to preserve the entire tube. If the bleeding is due to rupture close to the uterine part of the tube it will be necessary to run a mattress suture into the substance of the uterine muscle in order to stem the flow.

Surgical procedure

The different surgical procedures are described below.

Peritoneal toilet

After the tubal operation has been performed it is important to remove all blood from the peritoneal cavity, especially that which has tracked up into the paracolic gutters.

Closure of the abdomen

The abdomen is closed as described in Chapter 6, without drainage.

The subacute state

When the condition of ectopic pregnancy has been diagnosed by laparoscopy, there is not quite the same urgency as in the acute state. The patient should be operated on immediately after the diagnosis has been made. Therefore, all the possible surgical procedures should have been explained to the patient prior to anaesthesia. The abdomen may be opened using a low transverse incision as there is not the same need for speed and the surgery can err more towards the conservative if that is the patient's wish.

Whenever possible, attempts should be made to manage the entire procedure laparoscopically, whether the tube is to be preserved or not. With experience, it is possible to surgically manage the majority of ectopic pregnancies in this manner.

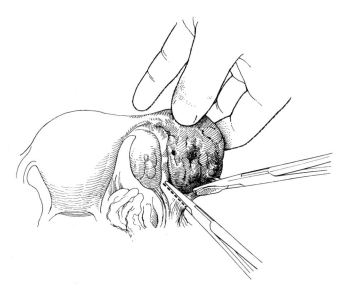

Fig. 18.1 Total salpingectomy for a tubal pregnancy.

Partial and total salpingectomy
The operation Having identified the source of the bleeding, the tube and its contents are elevated and separated from the ovary. If the tube contains a large haematosalpinx it may be necessary to disengage this from the pouch of Douglas. Tissue forceps should now be applied serially along the tube as shown in Fig. 18.1. The tube is progressively removed using Monaghan's scissors as each forceps is applied. Each forceps is stitch ligatured and complete haemostasis achieved.

Partial salpingectomy may be carried out if only a short section of the tube is involved. This procedure allows the chance of later tubal surgery to achieve function in the future; the forceps are placed as shown in Fig. 18.2.

Conservation of the fallopian tube
Gentle tissue handling, copious irrigation, meticulous haemostasis and the use of fine, non-reactive suture material are important.

The operation When the fallopian tube has been fully mobilized, a 'linear salpingostomy' may be performed. The surgeon steadies the tube in the left hand and incises the tube in a longitudinal manner on the antimesenteric border over the length of the swelling (Fig. 18.3). The material contained within the tube is then extruded or gently scraped out with the scalpel handle. All bleeding points are carefully ligated and the tube is reconstituted using a fine (3.0) absorbable suture. Alternatively, the

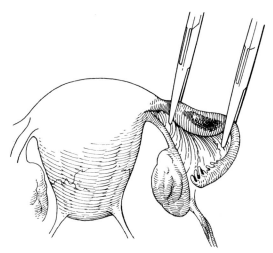

Fig. 18.2 Partial salpingectomy for a tubal pregnancy.

opening can be left to close by secondary intention. Meticulous peritoneal toilet is then performed and the abdomen closed.

Operative management of an intra-abdominal extrauterine pregnancy

In the very rare circumstances of this diagnosis being made, it is important to perform a laparotomy as soon as possible after the patient and the operating theatre

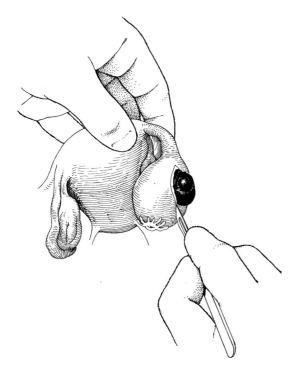

Fig. 18.3 Removing an ampullary tubal pregnancy with conservation of the tube.

have been fully prepared. Blood should be readily available, the anaesthesia should be of the highest quality, and if there is any prospect of extracting a viable child, full paediatric staffing is mandatory.

The operation
The abdomen must be opened with great care as the placenta may be attached to any intra-abdominal structure. Omental adhesions are also very common. A large incision to give good access is essential; the subumbilical mid-line incision is recommended. If the placenta is attached to the anterior abdominal wall it is important to undersew large vessels and to try and choose a relatively avascular area to gain access to the abdominal cavity.

The fetus is delivered and the cord clamped and cut close to the placenta. It is important to resist the temptation to try to separate the placenta from surrounding structures as this can be disastrous. The placenta and the membranes will be absorbed once the fetus is delivered.

Operations on the fallopian tubes for female sterilization

In many parts of the world it has become commonplace for both men and women to choose some permanent form of contraception once they have achieved their optimal size of family.

Preoperative counselling is of utmost importance and evidence of the discussions held with the patient highlighting relevant points should be clearly documented within the medical case notes. Also, it is imperative that specially designed consent forms are used in relation to all forms of sterilization, detailing the principles and pitfalls of the procedure. The author also recommends obtaining an intraoperative photographic record of the appliances accurately placed on each fallopian tube for storage within the case notes and potential future use. Despite these recommendations, sterilization procedures remain a major cause of medical litigation.

In women, techniques to obstruct the fallopian tubes are the most popular. Methods available include:
1 Total salpingectomy.
2 Ligation of the tube.
3 Laparoscopic controlled diathermy and cutting of the tube.
4 Laparoscopic controlled application of metal or Silastic clips and Silastic rings to the tubes.
5 Resection of a portion of the tube and tying or burial of the ends.

Resection of the fallopian tubes

This procedure is rarely performed except where there is evidence of unilateral tubal infection or ectopic pregnancy. It is not recommended as a sterilization technique.

Ligation of the fallopian tube

This simple procedure consists of grasping the tube close to its mid pont, elevating it and tying a ligature around the tube and the mesosalpinx (Fig. 18.4). A variation of the technique is to resect that part of the tube contained within the ligature, taking care not to cut too close to the ligature. This technique, which forms the basis of the Pomeroy operation, has the major disadvantage that it carries an unacceptably high failure risk, as the tubes have a tendency to recanalize after the ligature has been absorbed.

199

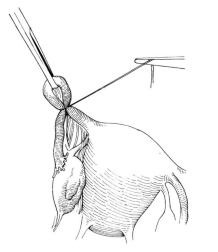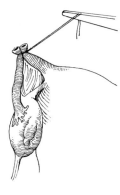

Fig. 18.4 Ligation and resection of the fallopian tube.

Laparoscopic methods

The technique of laparoscopy is described in Chapter 17. The ease with which the tubes can be visualized and manipulated has virtually eliminated the need to perform open tubal ligation procedures.

After introduction of the laparoscope and an additional trocar/introducer into the abdominal cavity, various appliances can be used to perform the tubal occlusion procedure.

Shortly after the first use of laparoscopy, there developed a great vogue for diathermy of the tubes and resection of the diathermied area. Although this technique has been successfully used to sterilize many thousands of women, it is potentially dangerous and has been superseded by the application of tubal occlusion devices to the tubes using applicators specially designed for this purpose.

The devices include the Falope rings, small Silastic rings which are applied by drawing the fallopian tubes up into a hollow applicator and then releasing the ring from the end of the applicator so that the ring lies firmly around the loop of tube. These techniques carry the same disadvantages as the Pomeroy operation.

The Hulka and Filshie clips are small locking devices, which are applied to the tubes using special applicators, and if applied appropriately will seal the tubes completely. Despite common practice, it is not recommended that the clips be applied in pairs to each tube because of the potential risk of a symptomatic hydrosalpinx developing between the two clips.

The material of which all these devices are constructed is inert and remains with the patient for the rest of her life, although on occasions following fibrosis of the surrounding tissues they can dislodge from the fallopian tubes and can be seen lying within the pouch of Douglas.

It is said that the advantage of these mechanical obstructive devices is that they damage only a small portion of the tube so that it is relatively straightforward to reconstruct the tubes in the future, giving a realistic prospect of pregnancy. The authors would stress that it should not be the policy of any doctor to recommend sterilization techniques on the basis that they may be reversed; all patients embarking on a sterilization operation must do so in the knowledge that the procedure is permanent.

Further reading

Why Women Die 1997–1999: The fifth report of the confidential enquiries into maternal deaths in the United Kingdom. London: RCOG, 2001.

References

Ectopic pregnancy is multifactorial in its aetiology. Breen JL (1970) A 21-year survey of 654 ectopic pregnancies (*Am J Obstet Gynecol* 106:1004–19) reviews the disease process, particularly predisposing factors and site of ectopic.

Bronson RA (1977) Tubal pregnancy and infertility (*Fertil*

Steril 28:221–8) demonstrates the high risk of ectopic pregnancy arising in those women who have undergone surgery on the fallopian tubes with a view to correcting infertility.

Nicholas Kadar has reappraised the aetiology, diagnosis and treatment of ectopic pregnancy in a chapter in the *Progress in Obstetrics and Gynaecology* series (vol. 3, 1983) John Studd (ed.), published by Churchill Livingstone.

One of the original references to silicone rubber ring sterilization (Falope ring) is Yoon IB, Wheeless CR and King TMA (1974) Preliminary report on a new laparoscopic sterilization approach. The silicone rubber band technique. *Am J Obstet Gynecol* 120: 132–6.

Details of the technique of clip sterilization is contained in the original articles by Hulka *et al* and Filshie *et al*.

Hulka JF, Omran KF, Lieberman BA and Gordon AG. Laparoscopic sterilization with the spring clip: instrumentation, development and current clinical experience. *Am J Obstet Gynecol* 1979;135: 1016–20.

Filshie GM, Casey D, Pogmore JR, Dutton AG, Symmonds EM and Peake AB. The titanium/silicone rubber clip for female sterilisation. *Br J Obstet Gynaecol* 1981;88:655–62.

19 Operations for benign ovarian disease

Ovarian cysts are said to be the fourth most common gynaecological cause for hospital admissions. They are classified as non-neoplastic functional cysts such as follicular or corpus luteum cysts, or neoplastic cysts. Their ratios vary with age but approximately:

1 25% are functional cysts.
2 40% are benign cystadenomas.
3 15% are dermoid cysts (benign).
4 10% are endometriotic cysts.
5 10% are malignant cystadenocarcinomas.

The rapid development of ultrasound technology and its increasing use in routine gynaecological practice has led to an increased diagnosis of ovarian cysts in women of all age groups. In premenopausal women the majority of lesions are benign functional cysts which usually disappear with menstruation or can be managed conservatively by suppression of ovulation with the combined oral contraceptive pill. Persistent cysts or those suspicious of malignancy require surgical removal. In recent years there has been an increasing use of the laparoscope for assessment and removal of adnexal cysts thought to be benign in nature.

Diagnosis of an ovarian mass

The normal ovary is usually palpable in the premenopausal woman but barely palpable in the postmenopausal. Consequently, almost any enlargement should be looked upon with suspicion and warrants further investigation. Transvaginal sonography is the investigation of choice not only in the detection of the ovarian cyst, but also in the assessment of potential malignancy. Features such as multiple cysts, solid areas, papillae, thickened septae, bilateral lesions and ascites are suggestive of malignancy, as is an increased blood flow on doppler studies. In these cases an abdominal ultrasound scan should also be performed to assess the upper abdomen (liver, omentum and para-aortic lymph nodes) for evidence of malignant spread.

The determination of serum levels of the tumour marker CA125 is also useful in differentiating benign from malignant cysts, especially in the postmenopausal woman. The authors currently use the ultrasound findings combined with a serum CA125 level and menopausal status to calculate the risk of malignancy index (RMI) to differentiate benign from malignant lesions. Those with a RMI of >200 are at increased risk of malignancy and are managed by gynaecological oncologists, whilst those with RMI <200 are managed by the gynaecologist.

Surgery

The role of surgery for an ovarian cyst is its removal and histological diagnosis. In women under 40 years of age, benign cysts should be managed using ovarian-preserving procedures, but above that age an oophorectomy may be more appropriate. If there is doubt about the nature of the cyst, frozen section of the cyst should be undertaken.

Since the last edition of this textbook, laparoscopic surgery has become the gold standard in the treatment of benign ovarian masses in many centres, with laparotomy being reserved for the treatment of malignant tumours. However, the laparoscopic management of ovarian cysts has been controversial because of the concern of accelerating intraperitoneal dissemination of an unsuspected ovarian cancer. Although the evidence for this is not overwhelming, definitive surgery in this situation should be undertaken within 2–3 weeks and the trocar sites should be excised as part of the procedure. With careful preoperative assessment and appropriate selection of cases the situation should arise infrequently.

The principles of laparoscopic surgery for ovarian cysts are similar to that at open surgery, but the approach and technique differ and have been described in Chapter 17.

Ovarian cystectomy

Victor Bonney gave this name to the procedure whereby the cyst is removed without compromising the function of the ovary. The same technique is used for the enucleation of a small solid ovarian tumour such as a fibroma.

For ovarian cystectomy to be successfully carried out, the mass to be enucleated must have a capsule (a characteristic of most benign tumours), the most common exception being endometriotic cysts, which rarely have a recognizable capsule and can usually only be separated from the ovary by sharp dissection.

The benign tumours of the ovary which are amenable to the technique include:
1 Benign teratomas (dermoids).
2 Serous cystadenomas.
3 Corpus luteum cysts.
4 Fibromas.

The procedure should always be considered in young women where ovarian preservation is to be desired, particularly where the cysts are bilateral and total loss of the ovaries would produce a premature climacteric.

The operation (laparotomy)

Opening the abdominal cavity
This is described in Chapter 6. The decision to use either the transverse or the longitudinal incision will obviously depend on the size of the ovarian cyst and whether there is any possibility of the tumour being malignant. If there is any likelihood that the mass is malignant, a vertical incision must be carried out.

Exploration of the abdomen
The examination of the entire abdominal cavity is meticulously performed as described in Chapter 6, together with the collection of washings from the peritoneal cavity. If there is any free fluid in the abdomen its presence should be recorded and it should be removed before washings are taken and sent separately for cytology. Washings are best carried out by instilling 100–200 ml of normal saline into the pelvis and along the paracolic gutters and then collecting the fluid using a large syringe. *NB*: it is not unusual to find a small quantity (20–50 ml) of fluid in the peritoneal cavity in association with benign lesions.

Extraction of the enlarged ovary
If the cyst is large, it is easily delivered from the wound; if the cyst is relatively small, or the tubes and infundibulopelvic ligaments are resistant, the procedure can be performed within the abdomen, using a self-retaining retractor to give adequate access.

Incising the capsule of the cyst
It is often possible to identify the edge of the normal ovarian tissue running along the lower part of the ovary. If this is so, the knife should be lightly run along this line (Fig. 19.1); the plane of cleavage will readily

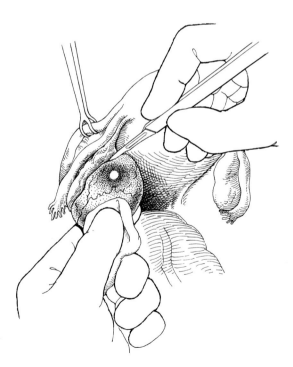

Fig. 19.1 Incising the capsule of an ovarian cyst.

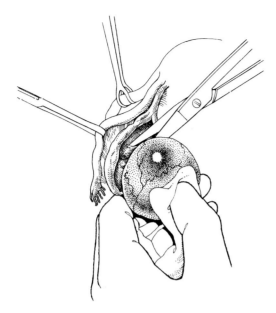

Fig. 19.2 Removing the ovarian cyst intact.

become apparent and should now be developed using blunt dissection either with the handle of the scalpel, or, as the authors prefer, with Monaghan's scissors, using the blunt points to separate and develop the plane.

The incision is now carried further around the cyst
The cyst is gently peeled back from the normal ovarian tissue (Fig. 19.2) until all that is left is a thin strip of normal ovary which is cut with the scissors.

Repair of the remaining ovarian tissue
Usually, there is a thin rim of redundant capsule which should be resected back to the thicker normal ovarian stroma. The edges of the ovarian tissue are brought together using fine interrupted sutures.

Abdominal closure
The ovary is returned to the abdomen and the wound closed as described in Chapter 6.

The operation (laparoscopy)

Insertion of trocars
Unless contraindicated, a 12 mm trocar is inserted into the umbilicus either by an open technique or following insufflation followed by the laparoscope. Two further

5 mm trocars are inserted either side of the lower abdomen for instrumentation and occasionally a further suprapubic port may be necessary. Using a 5 mm laparoscope increases the flexibility as it can be inserted into any port.

Exploration of the abdomen
This is identical to the open approach and washings should also be taken for cytology. If there is any suspicion of malignancy, a biopsy should be performed and the operation abandoned with referral to a gynaecological oncologist, or if appropriate converted to a laparotomy.

Incising the capsule of the cyst
Using laparoscopic scissors and forceps an attempt is made to find a plane of cleavage to remove the cyst intact. For large cysts and where there is difficulty finding a plane, the cyst may be punctured and the fluid aspirated. This should be performed in an endobag inserted through the umbilical port to avoid leakage into the peritoneal cavity. The cyst lining is examined for any areas suspicious of malignancy and if not the cyst wall is excised. Haemostasis is obtained and there is no need to repair the ovary.

Removal of the ovarian cyst
The ovarian cyst is placed in an endobag and removed through the umbilical port which may need to be extended or the cyst is aspirated in the bag before removal. It is frequently simple to insert the Verres needle through the entrance to the endobag which has been brought out of the port and then by applying countertraction the needle can be inserted cleanly into the cyst and the fluid content extracted. This procedure eliminates contamination of the port by the cyst or its contents.

Port closure
The umbilical port site is closed in layers.

Removal of a retroperitoneal cyst

The majority of retroperitoneal (or broad ligament) cysts are ovarian cysts which have grown retroperitoneally. This is more likely to occur after hysterectomy with ovarian conservation when the ovaries frequently become retroperitoneal structures.

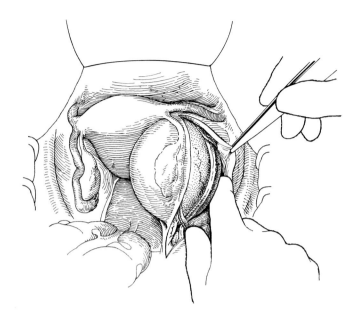

Fig. 19.3 Opening the peritoneum and identifying the ureter.

The exact position of the ureter will vary depending on the size and extent of the retroperitoneal extension of the cyst, stressing the vital importance of identifying the ureter at an early stage in the procedure and following it for the full length of its course across the cyst. Clear identification and separation of the ureter will remove the most important danger in this procedure.

The operation

Identification of the cyst
Having opened the abdomen as described in Chapter 6, the cyst is palpated and its limits defined.

Opening the peritoneum and identifying the ureter
The safest area to open the peritoneum is between the fallopian tube and the round ligament. The peritoneum is incised and the edges picked up (Fig. 19.3). The incision is now curved posteriorly so that by separating between the cyst and the lateral pelvic side wall, using the fingers, the ureter can be isolated as it courses in the peritoneum over the cyst. Usually, the plane of cleavage is easily found and the cyst is rapidly circumnavigated.

Enucleation
If the cyst is not ovarian in origin it usually shells out without great difficulty, but if it has burrowed below the uterine artery this can be sacrificed together with small veins which lie in the same position. If oozing does occur, tissue must not be blindly clamped; the best technique is to insert a swab into the bleeding space, applying a little pressure and wait for 2 min, taking care to inform the scrub nurse that a swab has been inserted and is marked up. When the swab is removed the whole field is dry and the small bleeding points can be identified and ligated. If the cyst is ovarian in origin one can either perform a cystectomy or oophorectomy.

Dealing with the peritoneum
After the cyst or ovary has been removed and haemostasis secured, no attempt is made to repair the pelvic peritoneum.

Abdominal closure
The abdomen is closed in the manner described in Chapter 6.

Difficulties and dangers
If the safeguards mentioned above are taken with respect to the ureters and to the uterine vessels, then this procedure should not produce any problems. Haemorrhage may be troublesome and the anatomy distorted and discoloured, making identification of structures problematic.

Proper identification of all structures will make this a simple procedure, 'short cuts tend to make long operations'.

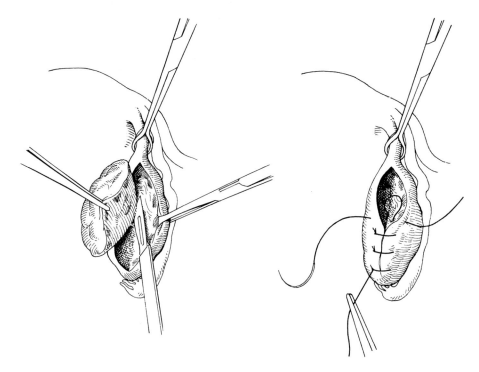

Fig. 19.4 Wedge resection of the ovary.

Variations

It is possible for an ovarian cyst to grow downwards and forwards into the broad ligament so that it mimics a true broad ligament cyst. The management is as described above except that the cyst will have a pedicle which must be identified, clamped and cut.

Wedge resection of the ovary

This procedure had a much greater vogue in the past, possibly out of misdiagnosis and a failure to understand that an ovary with multiple small follicular cysts is in no way abnormal. Unfortunately, small cysts on the ovary are often all that is found when laparotomies are performed for unattributable pelvic pain. It is very doubtful whether these small cysts can ever be blamed for the pain which has provoked the laparotomy. Puncturing of the cysts or wedge resection of the ovary was often performed.

The procedure was also popularized in the management of Stein–Leventhal syndrome but has now been superseded as first-line management by the use of clomiphene and the human gonadotropins.

The operation consists of delivering the ovary and taking out a longitudinal 'orange segment' of the ovarian tissue. The two halves of the ovary are then reapposed using interrupted Vicryl or nylon sutures (Fig. 19.4).

Further reading

M Canis from Clermont Ferrand, France has one of the largest experiences in laparoscopic surgery for adnexal masses having managed over 1 600 cases and published widely on the subject. Recent articles include:

Canis M, Botchorishvili R, Manhes H, Wattiez A, Mage G, Pouly JL and Bruhat MA. Management of adnexal masses: role and risk of laparoscopy. *Semin Surg Oncol* 2000; 19:28–35.

Canis M, Rabischong B, Houlle C, Botchorishvili R, Jardon K. Safi A, Wattiez A, Mage G, Pouly JL and Bruhat MA. Laparoscopic management of adnexal masses: a gold standard? *Curr Opin Obstet Gynecol* 2002;14:423–8.

20 Operations for malignant ovarian disease

Surgery for malignant ovarian disease can be the most challenging of surgical procedures in gynaecological practice. The disease invariably presents late in its course, at which point there is widespread peritoneal dissemination of tumour. Currently, the standard treatment consists of a combination of primary surgical debulking in an attempt to achieve complete or optimal cytoreduction, followed by a course of chemotherapy. Recent evidence has also confirmed the significant value of surgical cytoreduction as an interval procedure during the course of chemotherapy if optimal debulking was either not performed or not achievable in the primary setting. In addition, surgical cytoreduction of recurrent disease would appear to be of significant benefit not only in relieving symptoms, but also in improving outcome survival.

These operations are best performed under the auspices of a gynaecological oncology centre by highly trained, accredited gynaecological oncologists who are more able to achieve maximum cytoreduction, and are better placed to provide the multidisciplinary care that is required to allow the greatest likelihood of cure.

Ovariotomy

Ovariotomy was first performed successfully in 1809 by McDowell in the USA, replacing the procedure of tapping of ovarian cysts with a potentially curative operation. The term ovariotomy or ovariectomy is limited to the removal of a diseased ovary, whether benign or malignant.

Preparation of the patient

The patient should be prepared as for any laparotomy, but with certain special considerations:

1 All patients with a suspected ovarian mass should have a preoperative risk of malignancy index (RMI) calculated to determine the likelihood of the mass being of malignant origin. The RMI is calculated using a simple and useable formula that incorporates a combination of ultrasound scan features of the ovarian mass, the serum CA125 tumour marker result and the menopausal status.

2 If the RMI result is suggestive of malignancy, then the patient is best referred to a gynaecological oncology centre for treatment.

3 Various other tumour markers including carcinoembryonic antigen (CEA), CA199 and CA153 should also be considered to determine the possibility of the ovarian mass being due to metastatic spread from another site. In young patients, the clinician should be alerted to the possibility that the ovarian mass is of germ cell type, and include α-fetoprotein, human chorionic gonadotropin (HCG) and lactate dehydrogenase (LDH) serum estimations as part of their tumour marker screen.

4 The bowel should be prepared prior to surgery for possible resection by use of a low-residue diet together with large bowel clearance and a non-absorbable antibiotic for 2 days prior to surgery. Stoma siting is advisable as the patient will not be thankful for a troublesome stoma, which might have been better placed.

5 A chest X-ray is necessary to exclude obvious chest metastases and pleural effusions, which may require drainage prior to surgery.

6 Preoperative drainage of ascites should be avoided as much as possible, as port site tumour implantations can be particularly symptomatic to the patient and will require excision during the cytoreductive surgical procedure.

7 When there is little doubt about the diagnosis, there is virtually no need for preoperative assessment by intravenous urogram (IVU), CT scan, MRI, barium enema or colonoscopy/sigmoidoscopy.

8 A full blood count is mandatory as many women are anaemic at presentation, and if not adequately dealt with this can exacerbate the problems associated with the significant blood loss that often accompanies the complex and prolonged procedures required during the cytoreductive surgical intervention.

9 A biochemical profile is also required as many patients show considerable fluid, electrolyte and protein derangement at presentation. An experienced anaesthetist is invaluable during the perioperative period as management of fluid balance often requires a cocktail of ingredients first to optimize the patient, and secondly to maintain optimization during this crucial period.

10 Nutritional status is often neglected in these patients. Assesment by dietitians can usually identify those most at risk, thereby allowing intervention during the perioperative period by the use of various forms of supplementation.

11 An indwelling transurethral urinary catheter should be inserted to allow adequate monitoring of fluid balance during surgery and the early postoperative period.

Anaesthesia

As so many patients who come to ovariotomy have late-stage carcinoma of the ovary with associated embarrassment of their cardiopulmonary function due to ascites and pleural effusions, it is important to use careful anaesthetic techniques. The authors prefer light general anaesthesia combined with epidural or spinal analgesia; this allows complete relaxation without the toxic effects of full muscle relaxant general anaesthesia.

Instruments

The instruments in the gynaecological general set outlined in Chapter 2 will be required together with appropriate bowel stapling devices, a pair of Babcock's tissue forceps, some iodine solution and a surgiclip device.

The operation

The incision

This must be of an adequate size to remove the ovarian mass intact. It must be possible to lengthen the wound easily and quickly, and allow a full visual inspection of the entire abdomen. These requirements indicate that there is no place for the low transverse or Pfannenstiel incision.

Exploration of the abdomen

This is carried out in a meticulous manner, paying particular attention to the leaves of the diaphragm, the liver, the para-aortic lymph nodes and the omentum as well as a complete pelvic assessment. Ideally, these findings should be recorded on a 'tick sheet' in theatre.

Peritoneal washings

If present, a small amount of ascitic fluid should be sent for cytological assessment. In addition, the amount of ascitic fluid removed should be recorded. In the absence of ascites, peritoneal washings should be performed from within the pelvis, both paracolic gutters and the upper abdomen, in association with the performance of smears obtained from both diaphragmatic leaves.

Tapping of the cyst

This section is only retained to reaffirm that there is no place for the tapping of ovarian cysts; every effort should be made to remove the cyst intact and the wound lengthened to accommodate this removal.

Delivery of the ovarian mass

As many ovarian tumours reach an enormous size before the patient presents for treatment, it is not infrequently found that there are adhesions to bowel and other peritoneal surfaces (Fig. 20.1). Where the mass is carcinomatous, there may be direct extension of the tumour into surrounding structures. At the time of the preliminary examination, the extent of these adhesions must be noted. The cyst must be released from its adhesive attachments before delivery from the abdomen. This process often involves considerable manoeuvring of the mass and extension of the wound will often ren-

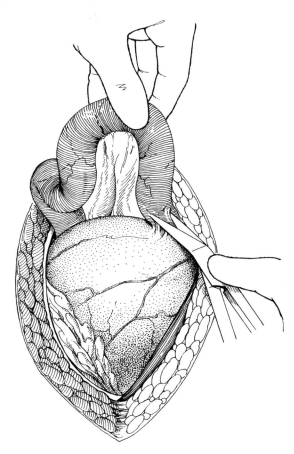

Fig. 20.1 Separation of adhesions from an ovarian carcinoma.

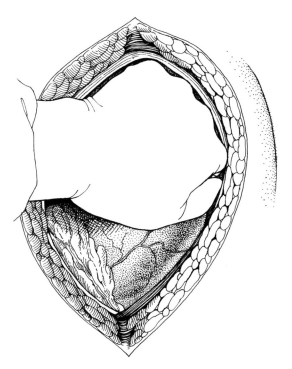

Fig. 20.2 Delivery of the ovarian cyst from the wound.

der a difficult task simple. Once adhesions are clear, the surgeon should elevate the cyst with the left hand; at the same time, the assistant can gently depress the sides of the wound so that the mass delivers through the wound (Fig. 20.2). Great care should be taken not to tear the pedicle, which, although large, contains many delicate veins.

Often, very large tumours are multicystic with large bosselated projections; it is easier to deliver these tumours by rotating the cyst so that one projection at a time is delivered from the wound.

There is no merit in attempting to force a large mass through a small wound and rupturing the capsule; if the tumour is malignant, the prospects for the patient will be significantly reduced.

Examination of the opposite ovary

If the patient is young and there is no suspicion of malignancy, the opposite ovary should be preserved and an ovarian cystectomy performed on the diseased side. However, if the ovarian mass shows any suggestions of malignancy, the authors advocate removal of the entire diseased ovary, which should be sent for immediate frozen section analysis, a technique that has been shown to be extremely accurate and useful under these circumstances. If the mass is confirmed to be malignant, it is mandatory that a full staging procedure is carried out. This would include removal of any suspicious intraperitoneal tissues, systematic bilateral pelvic and para-aortic lymphadenectomy, complete omentectomy and multiple random peritoneal biopsies from various sites within the abdominal and pelvic cavity. If subsequent fertility is not a relevant issue, the staging procedure should be combined with a total abdominal hysterectomy and removal of the remaining ovary and both fallopian tubes. If immediate frozen section analysis is not available, an alternative approach would be to close the abdomen after removal of the diseased ovary

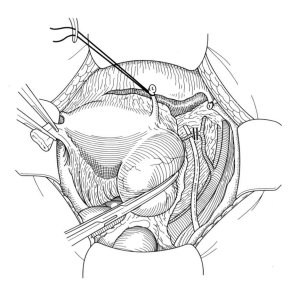

Fig. 20.3 Entry into the retroperitoneum, and identification of the ureter and ovarian vessels.

and to await formal sectioning and pathological assessment with a view to performing a second staging/completion procedure if primary ovarian malignancy is confirmed.

Removal of the diseased ovary

Ovariotomy may be the entire procedure or it may form part of the total management of ovarian carcinoma. Once the cystic mass has been delivered, the pedicle is easily identified. The pedicle is often extremely wide and careful thought must be given to the placing of clamps. The cyst may have elevated and altered the position of the ureter; it is important to identify the ureter before clamping the pedicles. This is best performed by incising a loose fold of peritoneum on the pelvic side wall lateral to the ovarian vessels allowing entry into the retroperitoneal space. Once adequate exposure is achieved, the ureter can be identified and the ovarian vessels can be clamped safely under direct vision (Fig. 20.3). Frequently the tumour mass has a long pedicle and tissue clamps can be placed in pairs beginning at each edge of the pedicle (Fig. 20.4); rarely, it may be necessary to use more than two pairs of clamps. The pedicle should be divided between clamps so that there is no spillage of the contents of the pedicle or the blood vessels. Do not be too ambitious; small bites and multiple clamps are better than one large pedicle which slips.

Suturing the pedicle

The individual pedicles can be ligature tied or dealt with using transfixion stitches, taking each clamp separately. If transfixion stitches are used, the surgeon should carefully inspect the pedicle and try to avoid piercing the veins, which are always present. It is not necessary to double-tie or double-stitch the pedicles.

Closing the abdominal cavity

Once a large ovarian mass has been removed, closure of the abdomen is simple and as described in Chapter 6. Drainage of the cavity is not necessary even when the cystic mass has inadvertently ruptured during removal.

Difficulties and complications

When delivering the cyst, adhesions to bowel may be found; if they require sharp dissection, the wall of the bowel may be damaged. If there is a possibility of damage, it is a wise precaution to oversew that part of the bowel with a fine suture.

The retroperitoneal operation for carcinoma of the ovary

The basic operation for the primary surgical management of carcinoma of the ovary should consist of bilateral salpingo-oophorectomy, total hysterectomy, omentectomy and retroperitoneal lymphadenectomy. It is now felt that this procedure should be performed so as to remove all visible tumour, including those areas that affect bowel, and all accessible peritoneal surfaces and retroperitoneal structures. Obviously this instruction must be tempered with judgement—often it is impossible to set about removing every tiny mass studded on peritoneal surfaces, especially when the whole underside of the diaphragm or much of the bowel surface may be involved. The surgeon must also decide how extensive a removal of involved bowel he will carry out, as the performance of an exenterative-type procedure for ovarian carcinoma was shown by Brunschwig to have little impact on long-term survival and greatly increased the morbidity and mortality of management.

There is, however, a variation in technique which the authors have used for a number of years, which if used more frequently would render more patients operable and reduce the amount of tumour left behind.

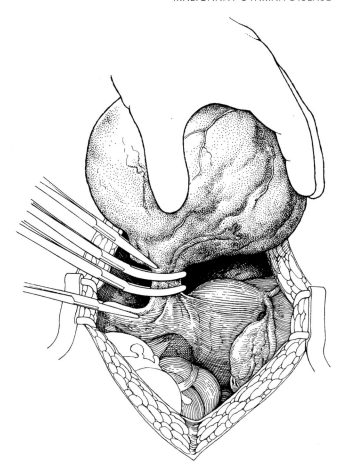

Fig. 20.4 Resection of the pedicle of the ovarian cyst.

It is frequently found that ovarian carcinoma grows in the pelvis so that it becomes adherent to and then invades the peritoneum, especially that over the back of the uterus, round ligament, pelvic side wall and the anterior surface of the bowel. It is very tempting to attempt to separate the tumour from these structures, normally by blunt dissection. The usual end result is that a considerable quantity of tumour is left behind adherent to and invading these surfaces.

Using a retroperitoneal approach, the ovary, together with the peritoneum to which it is adherent, is completely removed. The retroperitoneal dissection allows complete visualization of the ureters and the external and internal iliac vessels, and it is possible to separate the rectum from its peritoneal covering without jeopardizing the integrity of the bowel. Also, if necessary the rectum and sigmoid colon can be removed with the other pelvic structures as an *en-bloc* specimen.

The operation

The abdomen is opened via a vertical mid-line sub-umbilical incision of appropriate length for the size of tumour mass envisaged. The abdomen is explored and documented as described under 'ovariotomy' (p. 207).

Removing mobile structures
If one ovary is impacted and adherent in the pelvis, it is useful to deliver the other and remove it as described under 'Ovariotomy' (p. 207). This produces easier access to the remaining pelvic structures.

Identifying structures in the pelvis and separating the bladder
It is often very difficult to see exactly where one organ begins and the next one ends in a pelvis filled with carcinoma; it is in these circumstances that the retroperi-

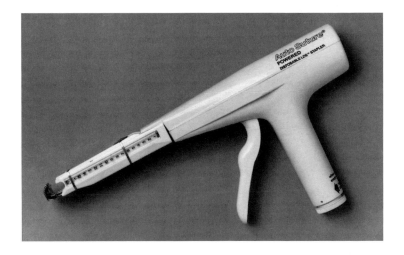

Fig. 20.5 The powered ligating and dividing stapler (PLDS) (by kind permission of Autosuture UK Ltd; this artwork was originally prepared for the United States Surgical Corporation's General Atlas and for publications by Professors Mark Ravitch MD and Felicien Steichen MD, ©USSC 1981).

toneal approach has major advantages. The round ligament should be picked up on either side and divided. If the round ligaments are not identifiable at the onset of the operation, a loose fold of peritoneum on the pelvic side wall is incised and the incision continued inferiorly and medially until the round ligaments are approached, at which point they can be divided. The incision is now carried across the uterovesical sulcus, making sure that any nodules of tumour on the peritoneum are skirted and included in the uterine specimen.

Opening of the lateral retroperitoneal space
The incised round ligament is now drawn laterally on its clip and the peritoneum incised in a posterior direction along the line of the pelvic brim. This serves to identify the infundibulopelvic ligaments which are often much more easily seen from behind the peritoneum. The vessels contained within the ligament are cut and ligated. Using the fingers, it is now a simple task to open the fascial space down the side of the pelvis.

Deepening the pelvic side wall dissection
The ureter is readily identified on the peritoneum and the uterine artery crossing over the ureter is picked up and divided.

Separating the bladder
The anterior incision in the peritoneum allows the bladder to be pushed down away from the cervix and upper vagina. At this point there are many variations in this operation:

1 The ureters can be dissected as in a radical hysterectomy, allowing full access to the upper vagina.
2 The vagina can be entered anteriorly and separated on its lateral and posterior part, not disturbing the paracolpos or the ureters.
3 Having transected the vagina, the tissue plane below the pouch of Douglas is entered and the peritoneum separated from the anterior surface of the rectum. The separation continues upwards and laterally to meet the dissection on the pelvic side wall. The uterosacral ligaments are clamped in the course of this manoeuvre.

Removing the tumour mass
On completion of these dissections, the central tumour mass, consisting of the uterus, ovary or ovaries together with the peritoneal surfaces to which they are attached, will be lying freely within the pelvis and are removed.

Omentectomy
This is rapidly and easily performed using the powered ligating and dividing stapler (LDS) (Fig. 20.5). This is shown in use in Fig. 20.6.

If the omentum is heavily involved in tumour, forming the 'omental cake', surgeons may be worried about breaching the transverse colon when removing the mass. It is surprising how often there is a relatively avascular plane running along the surface of the colon which allows the mass of omentum and tumour to be removed without danger. If stapling devices are not available, then the omentum must be removed by

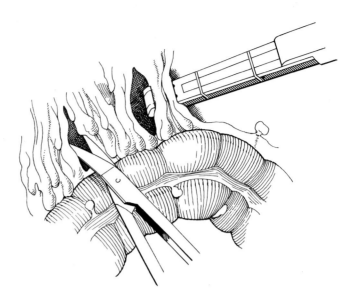

Fig. 20.6 Using the powered LDS to remove the omentum.

painstaking clipping, cutting and tying along the full length of the transverse colon. If the assistant holds up the omentum, it is surprisingly easy to identify the vessels and rapidly clip and cut them. Following mobilization of the transverse colon from the leaves of the greater omentum, it is also possible to continue the omental dissection in close proximity to the inferior aspects of the stomach via the lesser sac, thereby allowing removal of the supracolic omentum, which all too often is part of the 'omental cake' or is studded with separate tumour masses.

Bowel resection

If isolated areas of bowel are involved in carcinoma and in particular when obstruction is present, it is in the patient's best interest for a resection to be performed. The advent of stapling devices has made this part of the procedure much less time-consuming than it used to be and also made the quality of the anastomoses so much better. The techniques involved are shown in Chapter 26.

Pelvic lymphadenectomy

This is performed either as part of a staging procedure in the absence of obvious metastatic disease, or as part of the cytoreductive attempt when bulky nodal disease is present. The technique is previously described in Chapter 11.

Para-aortic lymphadenectomy

Access to the para-aortic area is easily achieved by incising the peritoneum lateral to the caecum and ascending colon in association with a second adjoining incision, which passes medial to the caecum and the mesentery of the small bowel. Care is required to keep the previously identified ureters in full view to prevent unnecessary mishap. This dissection allows complete mobilization of the intestine, which can then be lifted out of the abdominal cavity allowing access to the retroperitoneum and the para-aortic areas (Fig. 20.7). The bowel can either be protected with a warm, moist pack or alternatively placed into a 'bowel bag'. The assistants are then instructed to place two large Morris retractors cranially on either side of the great vessels allowing adequate exposure up to the point where the great vessels are crossed by the duodenum, above the point of entry by the ovarian vessels. A delicate approach showing considerable respect to the vessels, the inferior vena cava in particular, and judicious use of the liga clip should then result in a systematic dissection of the nodal and fatty surrounds commencing at the bifurcation and progressing superiorly up to the renal vessels (Fig. 20.8). The procedure is relatively straightforward if the correct plane lying in close proximity to the surface of the vessels is identified. A rolling technique as described for the pelvic node dissection will allow a complete dissection of the nodal and fatty

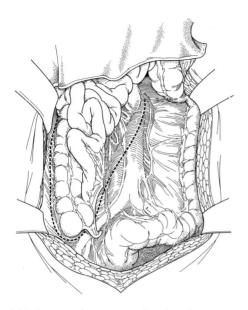

Fig. 20.7 Access to the para-aortic lymph nodes.

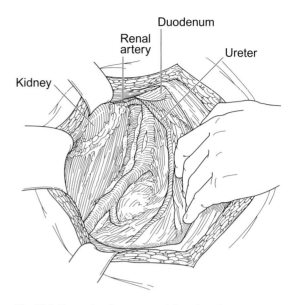

Fig. 20.8 Removing the para-aortic lymph nodes.

tissue. The occasional vessels perforating from the inferior vena cava if breached can be associated with considerable bleeding. Immediate pressure either digitally or by use of a small swab can control such bleeding instantly without difficulty. This manoeuvre will then allow sufficient time to place the suction point appropriately and allow a satisfactory view of the breached vessel for application of liga clips if appropriate or, alternatively, carefully placed sutures into the wall of the inferior vena cava encompassing the breached area and the point of bleeding.

Upper abdominal disease
A splenectomy may occasionally be required during the attempt to achieve complete cytoreduction. The procedure is easily achieved by extending the incision up to the xiphisternum allowing adequate exposure and access to the upper abdomen. The peritoneal attachments to the spleen are then tackled by incising the gastrosplenic ligament and the leinorenal ligament, allowing mobilization of the spleen medially and inferiorly. A Zeppelin clamp is then placed medial to the splenic hilum to incorporate the splenic vessels, which are then divided. A ligature tie is then applied to the vessels using a strong Vicryl or Dexon suture material. Attention should be given to the tail of the pancreas, which lies in

close proximity and can be damaged during the procedure especially when the spleen is surrounded by a mass of vascular tumour. When a splenectomy is performed, the patient should be vaccinated with a polyvalent pneumococcal vaccine during the postoperative period.

Disease involving the undersurfaces of the diaphagmatic leaves, the liver or other areas of the upper abdomen including the porta hepatis can be particularly challenging and require a conjunctive approach with an experienced upper gastrointestinal surgeon or liver surgeon. Further comments will not be made here.

Surgery to the bladder and ureter
Ovarian cancer very rarely invades the bladder or ureter, and with a patient and cautious approach, a plane of cleavage is virtually always identified obviating any need to resect ureter or bladder, even in the presence of a hydroureter. Occasionally, however, the integrity of the ureter is so weakened by the dissection that it may be sensible to insert a ureteric stent. This is easily performed by use of a double pig-tail catheter and a small longitudinal incision into a relatively healthy area of the ureter. The incision is repaired using fine monocryl and performed in a transverse manner to avoid causing subsequent ureteric constriction.

Small volume residual disease

After completing the above steps, there are often small volume deposits of peritoneal disease (less than 1 cm size) remaining scattered throughout the abdominal and pelvic peritoneal cavity. Attempts can be made to remove or destroy each of these deposits individually in an attempt to convert the final operative result from one of optimal cytoreduction to complete cytoreduction. A decision must be made on an individual basis, based on severity and extent of residual disease. A combination of surgical excision (peritoneal stripping) in association with surgical destruction by use of the Argon beam coagulator is a technique that is currently being used by the authors.

Further reading

Textbooks

Ovarian carcinoma has become such a major scourge that every gynaecological text has significant sections on the subject. JS Shepherd, in Chapter 11 of *Clinical Gynaecological Oncology*, Shepherd and Monaghan (eds), published by Blackwell Scientific, Oxford (1985), has made a comprehensive review of the present state. He has emphasized the role of surgery in the accurate assessment of the disease and in its primary management.

'Ovarian Malignancy', the monograph by S. Piver in the current reviews in *Obstetrics and Gynaecology*, published by Churchill Livingstone, is well worth reading.

Barber HRK *Ovarian carcinoma: Etiology, Diagnosis and Treatment* (1978) Masson, New York.

References

Notable references include:

Scully RE. Ovarian tumours. *Am J Pathol* 1977;87: 686–720.

Rutledge F, Boronow RC, Wharton JT. 'Treatment of Epithelial Cancer of the Ovary' in *Gynecologic Oncology* (1976), published by Wiley, New York. The MD Anderson hospital have made many notable contributions towards cancer knowledge over the years, ably led by Professor Felix Rutledge. 1976.

Dembo AJ, Bush RS, Beale FA, Bean HA, Pringle JF, Sturgeon JFG. The Princess Margaret Hospital study of ovarian cancer: stages I, II, and asymptomatic III presentations. *Cancer Treat Rep* 1979;63: 249–254.

The same group also produced startling results with a combination of surgery and postoperative whole abdominal irradiation; Dembo AJ, Bush RS and Beale FA *et al.* Ovarian carcinoma: improved survival following abdomino-pelvic irradiation in patients with complete pelvic operation. *Am J Obstet Gynecol* 1979;134: 793–800.

21 Operations for urinary incontinence

Stuart L. Stanton

Gynaecological urology surgery includes operations for the control of incontinence, whether due to urethral sphincter incompetence (USI) (also known as genuine stress incontinence, GSI) or fistula and voiding difficulties. There are over 100 operations to correct USI and the author will review here those that are currently used and of proven value. Anterior colporrhaphy will not be described in detail as it is covered in Chapter 22. Similarly, fistulae will not be discussed as these are covered in Chapter 15.

There is still controversy about the most effective procedure to correct primary stress incontinence due to USI. Many gynaecologists, including the author, favour a suprapubic rather than a vaginal approach. The principle 'do the best operation first' is fundamental. The choice of which of the many suprapubic operations depends on clinical and urodynamic factors such as mobility and capacity of the vagina, and surgical training and expertise (Fig. 21.1). Additional factors include the patient's physical health, her weight and her age. Conditions such as detrusor instability and voiding disorder are frequently aggravated by a suprapubic procedure and need separate consideration. Finally, additional gynaecological surgery may be required, e.g. hysterectomy for menorrhagia or posterior colporrhaphy for rectocele.

Role of urodynamic assessment

The need to confirm the cause of incontinence before proceeding with surgery for its correction is becoming increasingly evident. Failure to demonstrate stress incontinence by clinical means should be followed by one of several urodynamic procedures to confirm incontinence before surgery is attempted.

Where the patient's sole symptom is stress incontinence, there is a 90% chance that this is due to uncomplicated USI (GSI).

Urodynamic assessment is indicated where:
1 There are symptoms of urgency, urge incontinence, frequency, nocturnal enuresis (suggesting detrusor instability or symptoms of poor stream, incomplete emptying or straining to a void) which may indicate a voiding difficulty.
2 There has been a previous attempt to correct stress incontinence.
3 Overt or occult neuropathy is present or suspect.

Urodynamic studies include midstream specimen of urine (MSU) for culture and drug sensitivity, two-channel subtracted cystometry (CMG) (Fig. 21.2), or videocystourethrography, and uroflowmetry. Ultrasound is preferable to catheterization (unless in the course of cystometry) to detect residual urine.

Cystoscopy is relevant:
1 To investigate urgency and frequency.
2 Under general anaesthesia, to confirm or refute a small capacity bladder already found on cystometry.
3 To detect intravesical pathology such as an unabsorbable suture after previous continent surgery.

It is of little use to determine urethral sphincteric function.

The author finds no use for Q-tip testing. Dynamic urethral pressure measurement is subject to wide variation, and significant artefacts due to catheter stiffness have been found, especially when there has been previous bladder neck surgery. It has clinical and research

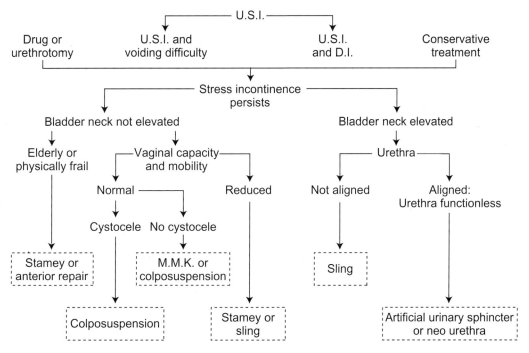

Fig. 21.1 Choice of surgery. Urodynamic studies will be required to detect voiding difficulty and detrusor instability (DI) in a patient who presents with urethral sphincter incompetence (USI). Then, it is necessary to determine bladder neck elevation. If this is inadequate, the vaginal capacity and mobility, and the presence or absence of a cystocele, should be determined by clinical examination.

If there is adequate bladder neck elevation, the alignment of the proximal urethra to the symphysis pubis should be checked using a lateral straining chain cystogram. If the proximal urethra is well aligned or the urethra is scarred and functionless, one of the two procedures designed to raise urethral resistance will be required.

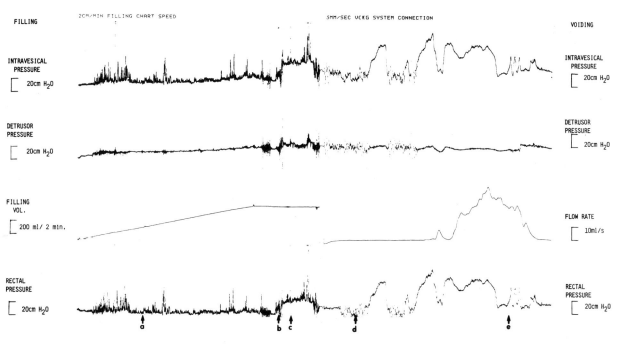

Fig. 21.2 Two-channel subtracted cystometry, showing normal filling (left) and normal voiding (right).

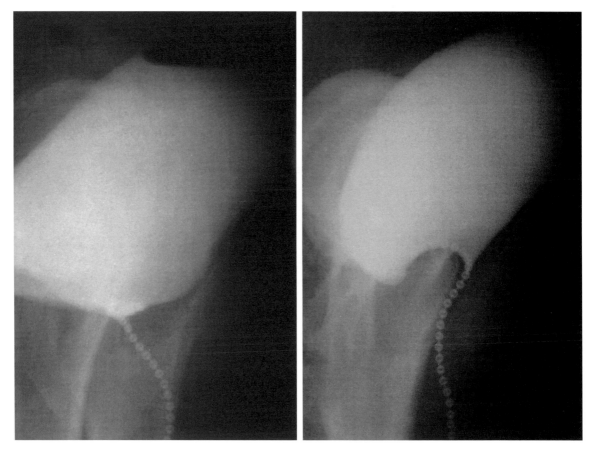

Fig. 21.3 Erect straining lateral chain cystogram before (left) and after (right) successful colposuspension for urethral sphincter incompetence.

applications, e.g. to study the effects of drugs on the sphincteric mechanism.

Strain chain urethrocystography will determine the precise elevation and alignment of the bladder neck and proximal urethra to the symphysis pubis at the moment of physical effort (Fig. 21.3).

Bladder drainage

It is advisable to drain the bladder after most operations for incontinence. A suprapubic rather than a urethral catheter is preferred, as with the former it is easier to initiate voiding and the patient is more comfortable and less prone to urinary tract infection. Either a

Bonanno (Fig. 21.4a) or a Stamey (Fig. 21.4b) catheter may be used. The regimen is as follows. A fluid intake of 2–2.5 L/day is encouraged and a strict fluid chart maintained. The catheter is clamped at about 08.00 hours on the second postoperative day and it is released about 8–10 h later, or earlier if the patient is in pain or has failed to void. A residual urine is measured by allowing the suprapubic catheter to drain for half an hour; once the patient is voiding more than 200 ml of urine at a time, the evening residual urine is likely to be below 150 ml. When this occurs, the catheter is clamped overnight and the patient woken once or twice in the night to void. The morning residual urine is measured: if the patient has voided at least 200 ml at a time during the night and the morning residual is less than 200 ml,

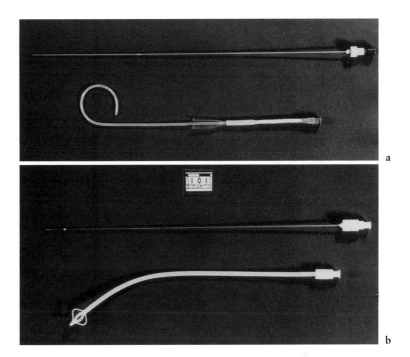

a

b

Fig. 21.4 Suprapubic catheters: (a) Bonanno and (b) Stamey.

the catheter can be removed. Antimicrobial therapy is not routinely used but regular specimens of urine are sent for culture and drug sensitivity.

Classification of operations

The route of access can be used to classify the various surgical procedures—either vaginal, or vaginal and suprapubic, or suprapubic alone. Each procedure has its clinical and urodynamic indications.

Vaginal (anterior colporrhaphy)

The use of the anterior colporrhaphy, or repair to correct stress incontinence and anterior vaginal wall prolapse, is well established. Special emphasis is placed on elevating and supporting the bladder neck by deep sutures placed and tied either side of it. The sutures are either inserted as Kelly has described, into bladder muscle, or placed in paraurethral tissues and in the anterior portion of pubococcygeus, or pubourethral ligament plication or levator ani (pubococcygeus) approximation.

Indications
The author does not feel that an anterior repair is the first operation of choice for primary correction of stress incontinence due to USI for the reasons given above. He also found that comparison with a colposuspension indicated the latter to have a significantly higher cure rate. However, the anterior repair may be more appropriate where a shorter operating time with less blood loss, postoperative pain and postoperative morbidity are desirable, e.g. in the elderly or physically frail.

Instruments
The gynaecological general set described in Chapter 2 is required.

Preoperative preparation
Metronidazole (1 g) is given *per rectum* 1 h before surgery at the same time as the premedication, to inactivate *Bacteroides* organisms in the vagina.

Anaesthesia
A general anaesthetic is required, but if the patient is frail or elderly an epidural or spinal anaesthetic has advantages.

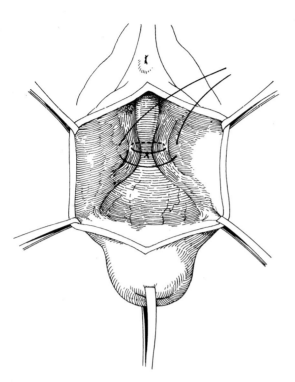

Fig. 21.5 Anterior colporrhaphy: a vertical anterior vaginal wall incision has exposed the proximal urethra, bladder neck and bladder base. The first suture has already been inserted into paraurethral tissues and tied. The second suture is inserted lateral to this and about to be tied.

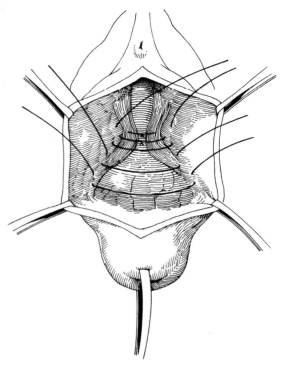

Fig. 21.6 Anterior colporrhaphy: bladder neck suture is tied and three sutures inserted into the pubocervical fascia (on the underside of the anterior vaginal wall flap).

The operation

A 3–4 cm vertical incision is made on the anterior vaginal wall, starting about 0.5 cm below the external urethral meatus. The precise length will depend on the extent of anterior vaginal wall prolapse. The proximal urethra, bladder neck and bladder base are exposed. The dissection is carried out such that the pubocervical fascia is left behind on the anterior vaginal wallflaps. Two absorbable sutures (no. 1 Vicryl or Dexon) are inserted at the bladder neck region: the first is placed deep and lateral to each side of the bladder neck and tied. The next suture is inserted lateral to this and tied (Fig. 21.5). Then, three or four sutures are inserted into the pubocervical fascia on the medial side of the vaginal skin flap (and not on the surface of the bladder) alongside the length of the urethra and bladder, and are then tied (Fig. 21.6) to form a shelf of pubocervical fascia which supports the structures of the anterior vaginal

wall. Excess vaginal skin is trimmed and the vaginal wall is closed by a continuous locking suture (no. 0 Vicryl or Dexon) which is haemostatic and also avoids vaginal shortening. A suprapubic catheter is inserted.

Variations in techniques Some gynaecologists believe that pubocervical fascia is found adherent to the bladder, and consequently their sutures are placed on the bladder surface as opposed to the lateral vaginal skin flap.

The anterior vaginal wall can of course be closed with interrupted sutures if a locking stitch is not satisfactory.

Major complications

Occasionally, a urethral diverticulum is found and the urethra may be entered during the course of dissection. The urethra should be closed with interrupted sutures of 3.0 Dexon without tension and the bladder drained for 7 days before clamping the suprapubic catheter.

Both venous and arterial haemorrhage can occur. Using diathermy and oversewing, haemostasis should be achieved during the operation, and a vaginal pack can be left in place for 24h, though this is not the author's practice.

Postoperative care
Mobilization of the patient starts on the first postoperative day and is gradually increased until the patient is fit to be discharged home on the sixth or seventh day. Intercourse should be avoided until after the follow-up appointment at six weeks. Heavy lifting is preferably eschewed forever; if this is not possible, it should certainly be avoided in the immediate six weeks following surgery.

Vaginal and suprapubic (Stamey procedure)

Indications
This procedure is brief and relatively free of postoperative pain and is therefore ideal for the physically frail, the obese and the elderly. It can be performed where there is some vaginal contraction.

Instruments
The gynaecological general set described in Chapter 2 with the addition of the Stamey needles are required. Three types of Stamey needles are available (Fig. 21.7).

The author finds the 15° to be the most acceptable. At present, a 30° needle (Stundey needle) is available from Rocket of London Ltd (Watford). Two lengths of no. 2 monofilament nylon with two 0.5 cm long 'buffers' of Dacron tubing are required.

Preoperative preparation
A 1g suppository of metronidazole is inserted *per rectum* at the time of premedication.

Anaesthesia
A general anaesthetic is required.

The operation
Positioning of the patient The patient is placed in the horizontal lithotomy position with the legs on Lloyd-Davies stirrups. The abdomen and perineum are prepared with Betadine and draped so that access is possible to both the abdomen and vulval areas. A 14 gauge Foley catheter is inserted into the urethra.

The incision Both vaginal and suprapubic incisions are used.

Either a 3 cm transverse incision is made in the anterior vaginal wall, just below the external urethral meatus (Fig. 21.8) or a 3 cm vertical incision is made over the bladder neck (the author's preference); the bladder neck is dissected free on either side.

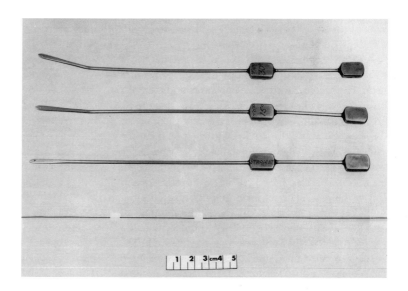

Fig. 21.7 Three Stamey needles and, below, a length of 2 nylon suture and 2 Dacron buffers.

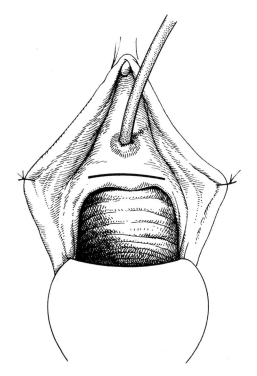

Fig. 21.8 Stamey procedure: transverse anterior vaginal wall incision just distal to the bladder neck.

Insertion of the Stamey needles Stamey needles are used to place nylon sutures either side of the bladder neck. The author prefers to insert the needle from the vaginal aspect, although Stamey's description shows the needle being inserted from above.

A 15° or 30° Stamey needle is loaded with the nylon suture and the point placed just lateral to the bladder neck. The needle is then passed upwards and laterally, behind the symphysis pubis into the retropubic area and then through the rectus fascia; it is felt under the skin, just above the inguinal ligament on the same side. The abdominal surgeon cuts down onto the needle with a 3–4 cm long incision parallel to the inguinal ligament (Fig. 21.9). The needle is now retrieved and Dacron buffers are placed on both ends of the nylon suture. The lower end of the suture is now re-threaded onto the needle, which is reinserted about 1 cm lateral to the original on the same side of the bladder neck. The needle is again passed upwards and laterally, behind the symphysis pubis, to emerge at the same abdominal

incision. The needle is removed from the nylon and retrieved. There is now a loop of nylon lateral to the bladder neck on one side, passing between periurethral tissue and rectus fascia with both ends extruded at the abdominal incision; a buffer is in place on the vaginal aspect and another on the suprapubic aspect to prevent the nylon tearing through at either site (Fig. 21.10).

The procedure is now repeated on the other side.

Assessment of the bladder The Foley catheter is removed and the patient cystoscoped. This is a vital step to ensure that a suture has not entered the bladder or urethra. If it has, it is removed and the procedure is repeated; then, the patient is recystoscoped. When the sutures are elevated, the bladder neck will be seen to rise and close.

Closure of the vaginal incision After ensuring haemostasis, the vaginal incision is the first to be closed, with interrupted sutures of no. 0 Vicryl or Dexon.

Tying the nylon suture and closure of the abdominal wound The vaginal surgeon elevates one lateral fornix so as to allow the abdominal surgeon to tie the appropriate nylon suture with sufficient tension to maintain that elevation. This must be tied cautiously to avoid tearing through. This is repeated on the other side. The abdominal wounds are now closed and a suprapubic catheter inserted.

Variations in technique As mentioned already, the author inserts the needle from a suprapubic aspect. The sutures can then be placed with greater accuracy in relation to the bladder neck by inserting them upwards from the vaginal aspect.

Complications
Intraoperative insertion of a suture into the bladder or urethra is a known hazard; therefore, the patient must be cystoscoped at the end of the operation. Occasionally, the suture tears through the paraurethral tissue as it is being tightened and care needs to be exercised to avoid this. Late complications include voiding difficulties, fracture of the nylon, and infection around the nylon suture.

Postoperative care
This is as with the other urological procedures.

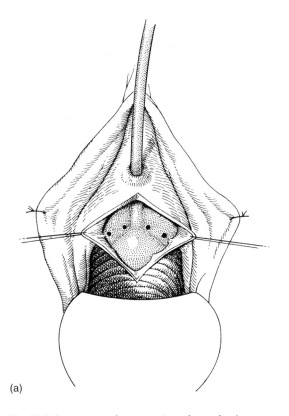

(a)

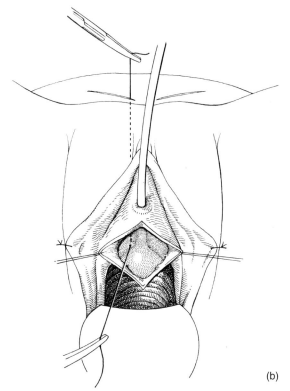

(b)

Fig. 21.9 Stamey procedure: (a) points of entry for the Stamey needle shown either side of the bladder neck;

(b) suture passing through the right side at its first insertion. The next passage of the suture on this side will be lateral to this.

Suprapubic

Marshall–Marchetti–Krantz operation
This was first described in 1949 and remains one of the most important procedures for the control of urinary incontinence.

Indications This technique is indicated for primary or secondary procedures without significant anterior vaginal wall descent.

Instruments The gynaecological general set shown in Chapter 2 is required with the addition of a Denis Browne four-bladed self-retaining ring retractor, which is recommended for this and all other suprapubic operations (Fig. 21.11).

Preoperative preparation Intramuscular cefradine 500 mg with the premedication and then 6 hourly (in-tramuscularly and then orally) for 48 hours is recommended by the author.

Anaesthesia A general anaesthetic is required.

The operation The patient is placed in the horizontal lithotomy position with the legs abducted and in Lloyd-Davies stirrups. The lower abdomen and perineum are prepared with Betadine solution and draped so that access is provided to both. A transurethral resection (TUR) drape covers the vulva, and the condom is inserted into the vagina to allow the surgeon to work from both the vaginal and abdominal aspects. A 14 gauge Foley urethral catheter is inserted into the urethra and allowed to drain freely.
1 *The incision.* A low Pfannenstiel incision, 1 cm cephalad to the symphysis pubis is made. If there has been a previous lower abdominal incision, a Cherney incision is then made; this incises the tendinous inser-

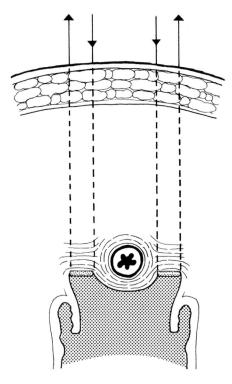

Fig. 21.10 Stamey procedure: showing two sutures in place with their respective buffers.

tion of the recti muscles and allows access to the retropubic space without risk of entering the peritoneal cavity. These incisions give excellent exposure to the retropubic space and bladder neck.

2 *Developing the retropubic space.* The retropubic space is entered in the midline using either blunt or sharp (scissors) dissection to free the bladder from the back of the symphysis (Fig. 21.12). The surgeon dissects with one hand in the abdominal incision and a forefinger of the other hand inserted through the condom of the TUR drape into the vagina to assist the abdominal hand.

3 *Inserting the sutures.* Once the proximal urethra and bladder neck have been adequately freed and mobilized, one or two sutures are placed either side into paraurethral tissue alongside the proximal urethra and also alongside the bladder neck. The most caudal pair of sutures is then inserted at an equivalent point into the periosteum or perichondrium at the back of the symphysis pubis (Fig. 21.13). Next, the more cephalad pair of sutures is inserted similarly. These are tied. Ei-

ther absorbable (Vicryl or Dexon) or non-absorbable (Ethibond) sutures may be used. Catgut is not advised, as it loses its tensile strength within 10 days.

4 *Drainage and skin closure.* Haemostasis is obtained by diathermy or oversewing and a vacuum drain is left in the retropubic space. If a Cherney incision is made, a loop or single-filament no. 1 nylon suture is used to close the sheath and rectus muscle in one layer. No fat stitch is necessary and the skin is closed by sutures or removable clips.

Variations in technique Some clinicians open the bladder to be certain of the exact point of the bladder neck suture. Lengthening of the urethra has been proposed as an adjunct to this operation, but the author knows of no scientific evidence to suggest that this gives an enhanced cure rate.

Complications Bladder or urethral injury during the course of dissection is managed by prompt recognition and a single- or double-layer repair. The catheter is left on free drainage for about 7 days before being clamped.

Failure of retention of sutures at the back of the symphysis is a known difficulty and the Burch colposuspension may be used if this occurs.

Haemorrhage from the perivesical plexus of veins can be troublesome; it is managed by diathermy, oversewing or liga clips or, finally, the use of a synthetic clot-promoting agent such as Oxycel (oxidized cellulose).

Osteitis pubis is reported as a late complication in up to 5% of some series and is thought to be due to infection of the periosteum introduced by the suture needle. The patient complains of localized pain and a radiograph may show osteitis or abscess formation (Fig. 21.14). Exploration and curettage may be required.

The retropubic drain is removed after 24 h. The patient is mobilized on the first postoperative day; the catheter management has been described above. Clips or sutures are removed at the standard time.

Burch colposuspension
Burch described this procedure in 1961 and since then it has become the procedure of choice for many gynaecologists and urologists on both sides of the Atlantic.

Indications The colposuspension will cure incontinence and elevate not only the bladder neck but also the bladder base (properties hitherto unique to the anterior colporrhaphy), which makes it a very suitable choice

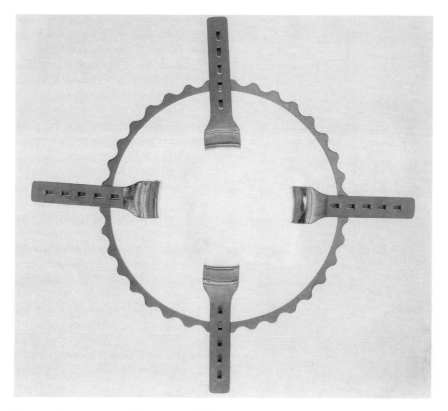

Fig. 21.11 Denis Browne ring retractor with four narrow blades. A larger ring and wider blades are available.

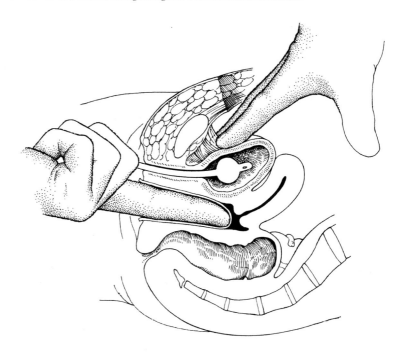

Fig. 21.12 Standard entry to the retropubic space. Note the Foley catheter (5–10 ml balloon) in place.

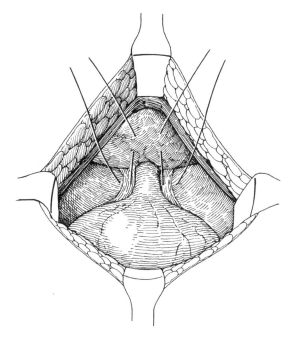

Fig. 21.13 Marshall–Marchetti–Krantz operation: first (most distal or caudal suture) placed on either side of the bladder neck.

when urethral sphincter incompetence and anterior vaginal wall prolapse coexist. It does, however, require normal vaginal capacity and mobility for satisfactory elevation of the lateral vaginal fornices. It is contraindicated if elevation is restricted by scarring due to previous surgery or menopausal atrophy.

Instruments As well as the gynaecological set described in Chapter 2, the following are required. An 8″ Finochetti needle holder, with the jaws angled at about 15° to the shaft, is ideal for insertion of sutures into paravaginal fascia and ileopectineal ligaments (Fig. 21.15). The author prefers to use a non-absorbable suture no. 1 Ethibond (braided polyester coated with polybutylate) inserted on a heavy, round-bodied J needle size 30 mm. A Lahey swab mounted on a curved Roberts forceps is ideal for blunt dissection. The four-bladed Denis Browne ring retractor is standard.

Preoperative preparation This is as for the Marshall–Marchetti–Krantz operation.

Anaesthesia A general anaesthetic is required.

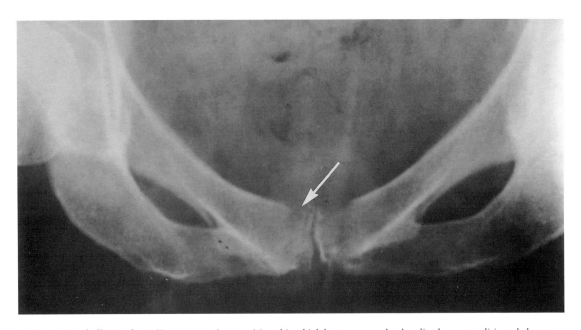

Fig. 21.14 Marshall–Marchetti–Krantz operation: osteitis pubis which has progressed to localized osteomyelitis and abscess cavity.

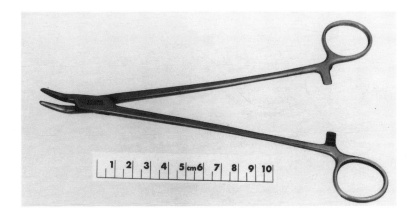

Fig. 21.15 Finochetti needle holder.

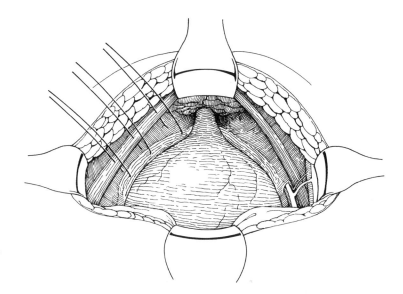

Fig. 21.16 Colposuspension operation: diagrammatic representation of anatomy via a Pfannenstiel incision.

The operation The position, draping and incision are the same as for the Marshall–Marchetti–Krantz procedure.

1 *Opening the retropubic space.* A plan of the anatomy is shown in Fig. 21.16. The bladder and urethra are separated gently from the symphysis and the retropubic space is exposed. With the finger of the surgeon's left hand in the condom portion of the TUR drape inside the vagina, pressure is exerted upwards in one or other lateral vaginal fornix (Fig. 21.17).

2 *Identifying the paravaginal fascia.* The lateral edge of the bladder base is dissected medially off the paravaginal fascia (Fig. 21.18), which shows as a whitened sheet. Large veins are either cautiously avoided or over-sewn: diathermy may exacerbate bleeding. When there is adequate exposure of the fascia, two or three sutures of no. 1 Ethibond are inserted from the highest (most cephalad) point of the lateral fornix, parallel to the bladder base. Subsequent sutures are inserted caudally but *not* below the bladder neck, as these will lead to delay in spontaneous micturition and possibly to post-operative voiding difficulties.

3 *Tying the sutures.* Each suture is tied on the fascia (to aid haemostasis and prevent movement of the suture through the fascia) and then anchored to the corresponding part (by approximation) of the ipsilateral ileopectineal ligament (Fig. 21.19). This is repeated on the other side. When all the sutures are in place, they are

227

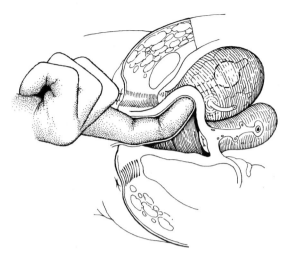

Fig. 21.17 Colposuspension operation: surgeon's 'vaginal' finger elevates one or other of the lateral vaginal fornices prior to dissection of the bladder base from the paravaginal fascia.

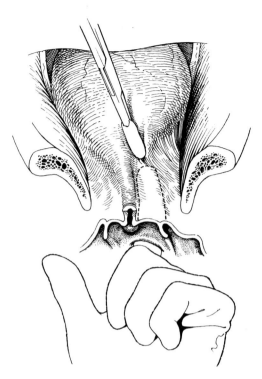

Fig. 21.18 Colposuspension operation: start of dissection of the bladder base off the paravaginal fascia in a medial direction.

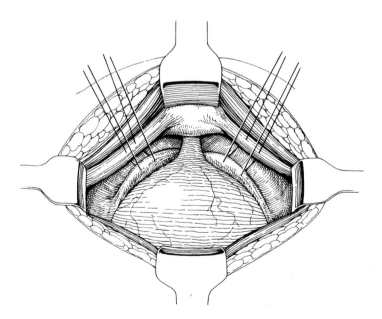

Fig. 21.19 Colposuspension operation: two sutures inserted into the paravaginal fascia and ipsilateral ileopectineal ligament. Note the most distal (caudal) suture is never lower than the bladder neck. The sutures are tied initially on the vaginal fascia prior to passage through the ileopectineal ligament.

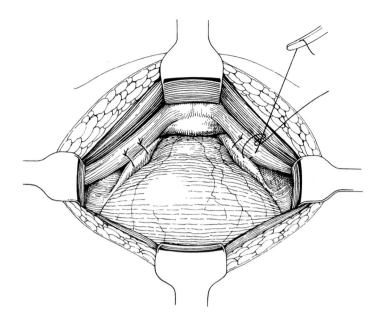

Fig. 21.20 Colposuspension operation: tying of sutures. Note the technique: the limb of a suture passing through the ileopectineal ligament is pulled taut, so elevating the paravaginal fascia; then the other limb is tied on to this, obviating the need for an assistant to elevate the lateral fornix and allowing the operator himself to judge tension in a suture.

tied alternately, starting from the most caudal suture and moving proximally. There is no need for the assistant to elevate the lateral vaginal fornix, as this is achieved by holding taut the limb of the suture which passes through the ileopectineal ligament and knotting the remaining limb around this (Fig. 21.20). Often, there is incomplete approximation of the fascia to the ileopectineal ligament at the most caudal suture, leaving some 'bow-string'. This looks surgically inept, but does not seem to mar the cure rate. Failure of all sutures to approximate the fascia to the ligament or pelvic side wall indicates that the vagina is significantly contracted and the colposuspension should not have been chosen. Passage of an unabsorbable suture completely through the vaginal skin does not seem to be disadvantageous. If, however, a suture is placed in the bladder, this should be removed because of the risk of calculus formation.

4 *Haemostasis and wound drainage.* After haemostasis has been completed, the wound is closed routinely and a vacuum drain placed in the retropubic space. A suprapubic catheter is then inserted.

5 *Final assessment.* Vaginal examination at this stage should show a well-elevated anterior vaginal wall (Fig. 21.21) with some ridging of the posterior vaginal wall, due to elevation of rectovaginal fascia. This is less prominent at the 8-week follow-up examination.

Should a hysterectomy be required, this may be performed first of all as an abdominal procedure. If an en-

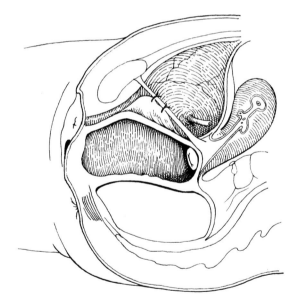

Fig. 21.21 Colposuspension operation: sagittal view illustrating elevation of the bladder neck and the anterior vaginal wall.

terocele is present, this should be corrected irrespective of symptoms, as a colposuspension tends to make it larger. This is carried out prior to the colposuspension using a Moschowitz closure of the pouch of Douglas. A non-absorbable suture material should be used to

229

encircle the peritoneum and close the hiatus between the uterosacral ligaments (Fig. 21.22a and b). Care should be taken to avoid the pelvic ureter at this stage. If a rectocele is present, this again is exacerbated by the colposuspension and needs to be repaired: a posterior repair is performed once all the abdominal procedures have been completed.

Variations in technique Some clinicians find that the amount of elevation required to approximate the lateral vaginal fornices to the ileopectineal ligaments is either unobtainable or excessive, and prefer to attach the paravaginal fascia to the obturator fascia, covering the obturator internus muscle. However, this is not as strong as the ileopectineal ligament and it is doubtful if it is as satisfactory.

Absorbable suture materials such as Dexon or Vicryl or PDS may be used as alternatives, but the author prefers non-absorbable suture materials as he feels they offer a more permanent cure rate.

Complications Bladder and urethral entry and haemorrhage from perivesical veins are the main complications. Methylene blue or milk can be instilled into the bladder to aid its anatomical definition and to disclose where entry has occurred. It is important to recognize trauma to the bladder which is repaired in the routine way with a single- or double-layer closure. Ureteric ligation has been described. Prompt recognition and treatment are necessary and urological referral may be required.

Postoperative complications include failure to void and detrusor instability.

Postoperative care This is similar to the Marshall–Marchetti–Krantz procedure.

Sling operations

There are numerous variations of sling procedure and material to choose from. Probably the most widely used operation is the Aldridge sling. Slings may be constructed from organic tissue (rectus fascia, fascia lata, lyophilized dura, or porcine skin) which, unless it is heterologous, avoids foreign body reaction and is usually readily available. Its tensile strength may not, however, be consistent or permanent. Inorganic materials are stronger and of consistent strength but may enter into indissoluble fibrosis with bladder neck tissues making subsequent removal difficult (e.g. nylon, Mersilene,

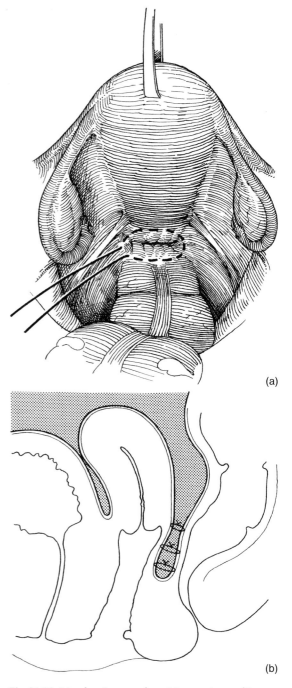

(a)

(b)

Fig. 21.22 Moschowitz procedure: (a) suture inserted into the pouch of Douglas peritoneum including serosa of the colon and both uterosacral ligaments. (b) Sagittal diagram, showing three successive sutures in place to obliterate the pouch of Douglas.

Marlex, Teflon). To overcome this, the author designed a Silastic sling containing woven Dacron (for strength). Apart from provoking a fine sheath reaction, surrounding tissues do not enter into any fibrosis, so the sling is adjustable or readily removable if necessary.

Two methods of sling insertion will be described: the standard Aldridge procedure, which involves a vaginal and abdominal approach, and the suprapubic tunnel approach of Millin.

Indications The sling procedures are usually used:
1 As a secondary procedure after failed previous surgery.
2 Where there is limited vaginal access or significant reduction of vaginal capacity and mobility (rendering a colposuspension technically impossible).
3 Where urodynamic studies indicate adequate bladder neck elevation but absence of posterior support to the proximal urethra and bladder neck.

Preoperative preparation Antibiotic cover, as described for the Marshall–Marchetti–Krantz procedure, is required.

Anaesthesia A general anaesthetic is required.

The Aldridge procedure:
1 *The incision.* Two incisions are made: a low Pfannenstiel and a midline anterior vaginal wall incision.

2 *Exposure of the rectus abdomnis and preparation of the 'sling strips'.* Through the Pfannenstiel incision, the rectus sheath is exposed; two limbs of the sling are cut transversely from the aponeurosis, each about 7–8 cm in length and 1.5 cm wide, starting from the lateral edge and ending 2 cm from the midline where the sling is left attached (Fig. 21.23). If an adequate sling cannot be taken from the rectus fascia, due to previous scarring, a fascia lata graft, 1 cm wide and 17 cm long, is cut. It is optional at this stage, but probably safer, to carry out a retropubic dissection and display the bladder neck.
3 *Exposing the bladder neck from the vaginal incision.* Next, the anterior vaginal wall is infiltrated in the midline with 0.5% lidocaine and 1 in 200 000 adrenaline for haemostasis and definition of anatomical layers. An anterior vaginal wall incision is made from about 1 cm proximal to the external urethral meatus and continuing for about 3 cm proximally to expose the bladder neck area. This is deepened and a plane of dissection is developed laterally between the vaginal side wall and the bladder neck. A finger is passed into this plane in an upwards direction towards the pubic crest, on either side of the bladder neck (Fig. 21.24).
4 *Passing the fascial sling.* A curved clamp is now passed from the vaginal aspect upwards alongside the bladder neck to grasp one of the fascial slings and pull it down to the vaginal dissection; this is repeated on the other side (Fig. 21.25). The slings are then sutured together across the bladder neck with just sufficient tension to slightly elevate it. Excess sling may be

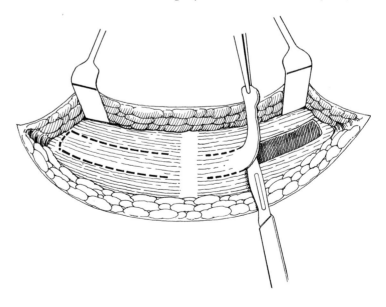

Fig. 21.23 The Aldridge procedure: sling flaps being cut from the rectus sheath.

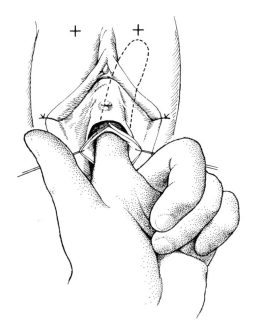

Fig. 21.24 The Aldridge procedure: finger being passed via the vaginal dissection, lateral to the bladder and up behind the symphysis pubis.

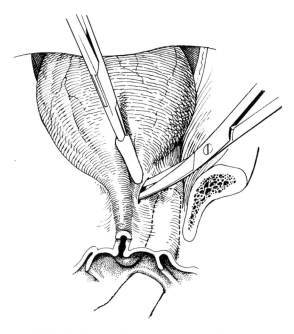

Fig. 21.26 The Silastic sling procedure: dissection commences with an incision between the bladder neck and paravaginal tissue.

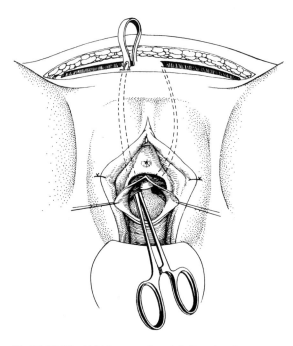

Fig. 21.25 The Aldridge procedure: left sling already brought down and attached to the bladder neck, right sling being brought down.

sutured together to the base of the bladder to provide extra support.

5 *Closure of the incisions.* Excess vaginal skin is trimmed and the vaginal wall closed with interrupted or continuous locking no. 0 Dexon or Vicryl sutures.

The rectus sheath is closed with Dexon or Vicryl sutures and then the abdominal skin is closed. A suprapubic catheter is inserted and managed in the standard way.

The Silastic sling procedure A low Pfannenstiel incision with a Cherney incision, if necessary, is performed and the retropubic space dissected to expose the bladder neck. Gentle traction of the urethral catheter by the operator's 'vaginal' hand will display the bladder neck. On one side of the bladder neck, a 0.5 cm incision is made with scissors and the underlining paravaginal fascia is exposed (Fig. 21.26). Gentle dissection in a medial direction using a Lahey swab mounted on a Roberts forceps is used to commence the suburethral tunnel. Diathermy may be needed for haemostasis. The tunnel is extended using curved scissors (Metzenbaum or Nelson) guided by the surgeon's vaginal forefinger in the TUR vaginal drape. The dissection is repeated on

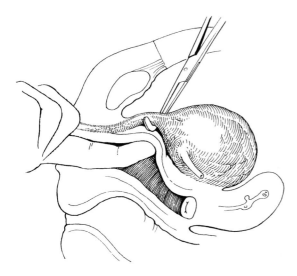

Fig. 21.27 The Silastic sling procedure: a suburethral tunnel has been created using scissor dissection and a Negus forceps introduced to insert the sling under the bladder neck prior to anchoring it to both ileopectineal ligaments.

the other side of the bladder neck and eventually a continuous suburethral tunnel is formed. A pair of Moynihan forceps may be helpful in the dissection. Next, a curved Negus forceps is introduced into the tunnel to grasp the sling and retrieve it (Fig. 21.27).

Each end of the sling is sutured with no. 1 Ethibond suture to the ipsilateral ileopectineal ligament, ensuring that only minimal tension is present in the sling, i.e. just enough to elevate the bladder neck off the underlying vaginal skin, but without leaving the sling taut.

Haemostasis is secured and the abdominal wound closed in the routine way. A vacuum retropubic drain and a suprapubic catheter are inserted.

Variations in technique Other authors have used inorganic materials and their original descriptions should be referred to for details of their techniques. In essence, the sling is shaped beforehand and inserted from the vaginal aspect. The middle portion of the sling is sutured to the bladder neck area and each limb is retrieved in the retropubic area and sutured laterally either to rectus sheath or ileopectineal ligament.

Complications Injury to the bladder or urethra during the course of dissection is not uncommon and, once recognized, should be repaired in the standard manner

and the operation continued. Venous haemorrhage from the paraurethral dissection can be brisk. Urinary retention is common and frequently results from excess sling tension rather than extensive dissection around the bladder neck. It is here that the benefits of suprapubic catheterization are most obvious.

Postoperative care Postoperative care is similar to previous operations except for the increased incidence of urinary retention. Apart from management by continued suprapubic catheterization, clean intermittent self-catheterization (CISC) may be initiated until the patient voids spontaneously. Resistant cases may require release or removal of the sling. Drug therapy, e.g. bethanechol chloride 25–100 mg four times daily to stimulate the detrusor or an α-adrenergic blocking agent may be used to reduce urethral resistance.

Artificial urinary sphincter

The artificial urinary sphincter (AMS 800) (Fig. 21.28a and b) is the latest in a series of sphincters developed by Brantley Scott and Associates of Houston, USA. It is a fully implantable device, allowing the patient to void per urethram under voluntary control with complete urinary continence. In the female it is used usually for end-stage incontinence, or neuropathic causes of incontinence (e.g. myelomeningocele), or as a preferable alternative to permanent catheterization or urinary diversion. However, the device is expensive, the insertion can be technically difficult, and there are definite complications, so careful selection and meticulous attention to sterility are required.

The sphincter is made of medical grade silicone rubber. It is hydraulically operated and consists of an occlusive cuff (in different sizes) made of silicone elastomer and is placed circumferentially around the bladder neck (Fig. 21.29a and b). It is linked by silicone tubing to a pressure-regulating balloon placed in the retropubic space, which controls the amount of pressure exerted by the cuff. It is also made of silicone elastomer and is available in three commonly used sizes; the surgeon selects the lowest balloon pressure needed to maintain closure of the bladder neck. The third part, the control pump (Fig. 21.30) is implanted into the labium majus, usually the left. It is approximately 1.2 cm wide and 3.3 cm long: the upper part contains resistor valves needed to transfer fluid to and from the cuff, whilst the lower part is a bulb which the patient squeezes to transfer

233

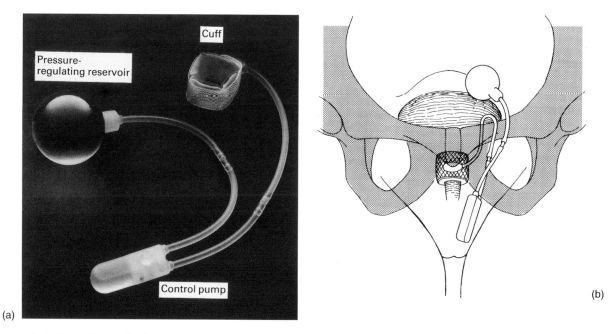

(a)

(b)

Fig. 21.28 (a) The artificial urinary sphincter AMS 800; (b) the sphincter in place.

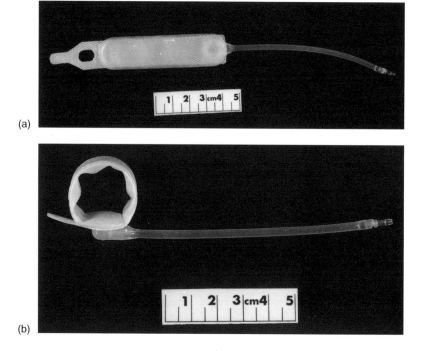

(a)

(b)

Fig. 21.29 Artificial urinary sphincter: occlusive cuff (a) in flat and (b) in circular form.

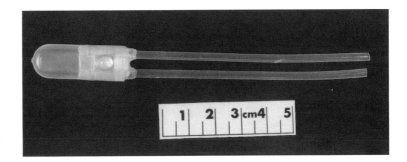

Fig. 21.30 Artificial urinary sphincter: control pump of the AMS 800.

fluid from the cuff to the reservoir; this allows the patient to void. The cuff automatically reinflates after 2–3 min.

Indications The main indications are resistant incontinence due to urethral sphincter incompetence despite at least two appropriate and well-performed conventional incontinence procedures, where the alternative would be continuous incontinence, permanent catheterization or urinary diversion. It is also indicated for neuropathic causes of incontinence; should there be detrusor hyperreflexia, this should be adequately controlled beforehand by drug therapy. Finally, it may be used for congenital causes of incontinence such as epispadias or bladder extropy, where closure has been obtained but the patient is still incontinent.

The patient should be physically fit, have sufficient manual dexterity to work the device, and be mentally aware of the need to be continent.

Prior urodynamic assessment should confirm that:
1 The urine is sterile.
2 The bladder is stable.
3 The bladder has at least 300 ml capacity and is preferably of normal compliance.

Also, there should be no voiding difficulty, upper urinary tract disease or vesicoureteric reflux, and the bladder neck should be well vascularized.

Instruments As well as the general gynaecological set listed in Chapter 2, the following will be required. The cutting diathermy is helpful in the final dissection around the bladder neck. Fine haemostat clamps, used to occlude the tubing, should be shod with silicone rubber. A pair of right-angled scissors may be helpful.

Preoperative preparation Preoperative urodynamic assessment is essential and should include uroflowmetry, videocystourethrography and intravenous urography. Prior to surgery, the MSU must be sterile.

The patient is admitted 2–3 days preoperatively; the night before surgery, the patient showers and uses a Betadine soap preparation. Piperacillin is given as a 2 g dose just prior to surgery and 2 g three times daily for seven days postoperatively. A 1 g suppository of metronidazole is given with the premedication. Once the patient is anaesthetized, the vulva and abdomen are shaved and then scrubbed for 15 min with Betadine.

Anaesthesia A general anaesthetic is required.

The operation
1 *Positioning the patient.* The patient is placed in the lithotomy position with the legs in Lloyd-Davies stirrups. After a careful sterile preparation, the patient's abdomen and perineum are draped; two TUR drapes are used so that one condom may be placed inside the other to allow a double protection for the surgeon's vaginal finger. Some clinicians prefer to pack the vagina instead. Finally, a steridrape sheet is placed on the abdomen.
2 *The incision.* A low Pfannenstiel incision is made, with a Cherney incision if necessary.
3 *Identifying the bladder neck.* The bladder neck is dissected in the manner described above for the Silastic sling, and a 1.5–2 cm wide suburethral tunnel created. If at this stage there is a breach of the vagina, urethra or bladder, it is repaired in the conventional way. If there is doubt about closure or about vascularization of the bladder neck, it is wise to defer cuff placement and to reoperate 6 months later.
4 *Choosing the appropriate cuff size.* Next, a cuff sizer

235

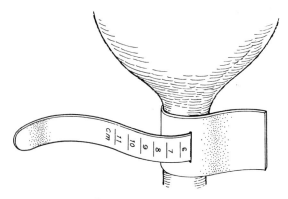

Fig. 21.31 Artificial urinary sphincter: cuff sizer.

(Fig. 21.31) is placed around the bladder neck and the appropriate cuff size is chosen. It is best to err in selecting a larger rather than a smaller size, because cuffs less than 7.5 cm long generally close completely on full inflation.

Once chosen, the snap-on cuff is carefully filled with 12.5% Hypaque (diluted with sterile water and *not* normal saline) and all air bubbles are meticulously excluded. This is vital as air in the system will cause an air lock and lead to malfunction. The cuff is inserted so that the inflatable portion faces the urethra (see Fig. 21.29b).

5 *Placing the tubing in the inguinal canal.* The external inguinal ring is identified, a tubing needle is inserted into the inguinal canal to emerge at the internal inguinal ring, and tubing from the cuff is now withdrawn through the canal.

6 *Choosing and placing the pressure reservoir balloon.* Next, the appropriate pressure reservoir balloon is selected; for female patients whose bladder neck vascularity is not impaired by previous bladder neck surgery, a pressure balloon in the range of 60–70 cm H_2O is appropriate. With previous bladder neck surgery and poor vascularity of the bladder neck, a pressure balloon in the range of 50–60 cm H_2O of water may be more appropriate. When mild detrusor instability exists and bladder neck vascularity is not impaired, a higher pressure of 70–80 cm H_2O may be used, but this is conducive to a greater risk of bladder neck erosion. The appropriate balloon is filled with 18 ml of 12.5% Hypaque and placed in the retropubic space.

7 *Placing the pump control assembly in the labium majus.* Finally, using a no. 12–14 Hegar dilatator, a

space is created in one or other labium majus for the pump control assembly, which has already been carefully filled with 12.5% Hypaque.

8 *Connecting the tubes and testing the device.* All the tubing is checked to exclude air and the final connections are made above the rectus sheath using either 3.0 Prolene ties or the AMS quick-connect sutureless connector. Before wound closure, the device is tested by inflating and deflating the cuff and applying gentle pressure to a full bladder after having withdrawn the urethral catheter.

9 *Drainage of the wound and bladder, and closure of the wound.* The wound is closed in layers. To avoid retropubic infection, neither a drain nor a suprapubic catheter are used. Instead, a no. 14 French Silastic urethral catheter is inserted and left on open drainage for 7 days. The cuff is left in the deactivated mode.

Complications Intraoperative complications include trauma to the urethra, bladder and vagina. Immediate postoperative complications include wound infection and urinary retention. Late complications include erosion of the bladder neck by the cuff and, rarely, of the pump assembly through the labium majus, and mechanical failures. These are commonest with the cuff.

Postoperative care The sphincter is left deactivated for 4–6 weeks. When the patient attends for her first follow-up visit, activation is carried out by giving the lower part of the pump a sharp and forceful squeeze (Fig. 21.32).

Thereafter, follow-up visits are at yearly intervals or earlier should the need arise.

Conclusion

While the procedure for selecting the correct operation is still crude and sometimes deficient, it is appropriate to restate the dicta 'The first operation has the best chance of success' and 'Do the best operation the first time'. A sound knowledge of the pathophysiology and of the indications and limitations of each operation, together with an application of good surgical techniques, are important considerations each time surgery is carried out for incontinence. Urodynamic studies must now be recognized as providing relevant information prior to operations for incontinence and as mandatory if surgery has already been attempted and failed.

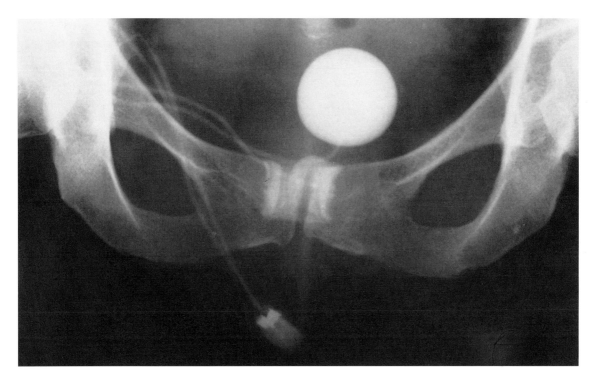

Fig. 21.32 Artificial urinary sphincter: radiograph taken after activation of the AMS 800 at 6 weeks. Contrast is present in all parts of the sphincter.

In recent years TVT has become popular as a technique for treating stress maintenance.

Further reading

Textbooks

Clinical Gynecologic Urology, published by C.V. Mosby, Chicago, in 1985 is a leading text of its type; it comprehensively covers the whole of this rapidly developing subspecialty. Stanton has brought together in this multiauthor text a most stimulating group of writers, each leaders in the field. For the reader who wishes to develop his interest in this field, the editor would recommend this text.

References

For those with an interest in the original articles for the eponymous procedures in gynaecological urology, the editor would recommend the following references:

Aldridge A. Transplantation of fascia for the relief of urinary stress incontinence. *Am J Obstet Gynecol* 1942;44: 398–411.

Kelly H. Incontinence of urine in women. *Urol Cutan Rev* 1913;17:291–3.

Low J. Management of severe anatomic deficiency of urethral sphincter function by a combined procedure with a fascia lata sling. *Am J Obstet Gynecol* 1969;105:149.

Marshall VT, Marchetti AA, Krantz KE. The correction of stress incontinence by simple vesico-urethral suspension. *Surg Gynecol Obstet* 1949;88:509–18.

Millin T. Reported discussion on stress incontinence in micturition. *Proc Roy Soc Med* 1917;40:361–70.

Pacey K. Pathology and repair of genital prolapse. *J Obstet Gynaecol Br Empire* 1949;56:1–15.

Stamey TA. Endoscopic suspension of the vesical neck for urinary incontinence. *Surg Gynecol Obstet* 1973;136:547–54.

Stanton SL, Brindley G, Holmes D. Silastic sling for urethral incompetence in women. *Br J Obstet Gynaecol* 1985;92: 747–50.

237

22 Operations for prolapse of the uterus and vagina

Uterovaginal prolapse is a common gynaecological condition being associated with childbirth and older age. With increasing life expectancy and greater expectations of patients in recent years, those surgeons who have mastered the following operations will receive considerable gratitude from their patients. The basic principle of uterovaginal repair is to tailor the various procedures available to each individual case. Following improvements in anaesthetic techniques, the authors' views are that the need to resort to the use of vaginal pessaries to provide uterovaginal support should be occasional if at all.

Uterovaginal prolapse is often associated with urinary incontinence. When such conditions coexist, the reader is advised to follow the recommendations given in the preceding chapter.

Anterior colporrhaphy

The operation is performed for cystocele or a combination of cystocele and urethrocele. The principle of repair is to separate the vaginal skin from the underlying bladder, remove the redundant stretched skin, and support the prolapsed bladder by approximating the weakened pubocervical fascia which have been dislocated laterally with the use of buttress sutures. In the absence of genuine stress incontinence (GSI) the urethra should be left undisturbed, and if GSI is present, the incision and repair should extend just short of the urethral meatus, thereby elevating and supporting the bladder neck and proximal urethra.

Anaesthesia

The procedure is generally quick and straightforward and, as such, is ideally suited to regional anaesthesia.

Patient preparation

The normal lithotomy position is used with emphasis made on correctly placing the buttocks on the end of the table, ideally with a slight overhang. A minor degree of head-down tilt often helps to improve access to the anterior vaginal wall as well as allowing optimum direction of the operating light. Intraoperative antibiotics to cover *Bacteroides* organisms is advisable. Following vaginal and perineal cleansing, the bladder is emptied and a bimanual examination is performed.

Instruments

The gynaecological general set shown in Chapter 2 is used.

The operation

The incision
A volsellum is attached to the cervix, and the cervix is drawn downwards. Injection of a solution of 1% xylocaine with adrenaline 1 : 200 000 into the subepithelial space can be beneficial in delineating the tissue planes. A 1 cm transverse incision is made on the anterior aspect of the cervix. The superior flap is then seized with two Kocher's forceps and the subepithelial plane developed with the use of the Monaghan scissors. The vaginal skin at the mid-line is then incised in the direction of

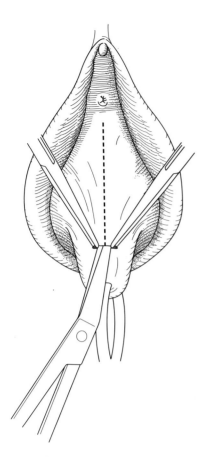

Fig. 22.1 Vaginal incision.

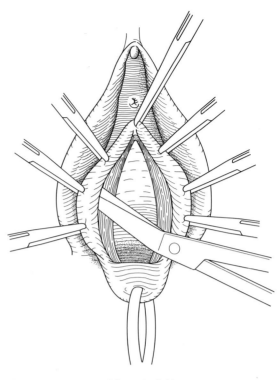

Fig. 22.2 Separation of the vaginal skin.

the urethral meatus (Fig. 22.1). The subepithelial plane is then developed further towards the urethral meatus, remaining in the mid-line whilst seizing the vaginal skin edges on either side with additional Kocher's forceps. The incision is continued until the superior aspect of the prolapsed area is reached, at which point another Kocher's forceps is applied.

Separation of the vaginal skin from the bladder and the pubocervical fascia

The assistant then applies traction to the superiorly applied Kocher's forceps upwards, and the additional Kocher's forceps on the right edge of the vaginal skin are pulled laterally, whilst maintaining traction on the Vulsellum applied to the cervix downwards. The dissection of the subepithelial plane is then continued laterally towards the patient's right side using a combination of sharp and blunt dissection (Fig. 22.2). This plane is relatively avascular, and bleeding will generally only occur if the correct plane is breached or if the patient has been subject to previous repair procedures. The dissection is continued until the lateral aspects of the prolapse have been reached. The procedure is repeated on the patient's left side. The cervicovesical ligaments are then incised on the anterior aspect of the cervix, and the bladder dissected off the cervix by a combination of sharp and blunt dissection (Fig. 22.3). The redundant vaginal skin with the attached lateral Kocher's forceps is then excised on both sides. A useful tip is to excise more than you think at the front when performing an anterior colporrhaphy, and less than you think from the back when performing a posterior colpoperineorrhaphy.

The repair

If GSI is present, a number of interrupted Kelly's sutures are then inserted at the area of the bladder neck approximating the pubourethral ligaments to provide

239

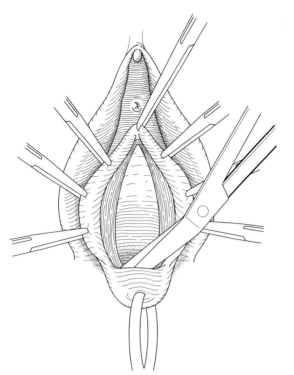

Fig. 22.3 Division of the cervicovesical fascia.

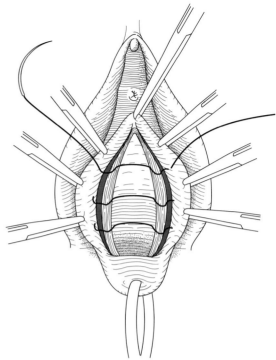

Fig. 22.4 Insertion of Kelly's buttress sutures.

additional elevation and support (Fig. 22.4). If GSI is not present, the vaginal skin edges are then approximated commencing at the cervical end, using a series of interrupted sutures or a continuous locking suture to prevent vaginal shortening (Fig. 22.5). The authors prefer interrupted sutures as these provide maximum support for the underlying bladder during the postoperative period, and also avoids the development of haematoma formation by allowing space between the sutures for any blood to escape. An indwelling transurethral urinary catheter is inserted if the bladder neck was not given additional support by the use of Kelly's sutures. Alternatively, a suprapubic urinary catheter, as described in the preceding chapter, should be inserted. A vaginal pack is not required.

Alternative techniques
A commonly used technique is to identify and excise the vaginal skin to be removed at the onset of the operation by demarcating the edges, and excising the redundant skin from the underlying pubocervical ligament and bladder, as shown in Fig. 22.6. Alternatively, the procedure can be commenced by incising a vertical incision between the urethral meatus and the cervix at the onset of the operation prior to the development of the subepithelial plane. The authors' preferred technique is the one described, as it ensures accurate entry and development of the subepithelial plane, crucial to the performance of an avascular operation, in addition to avoiding the error of removing too little or too much vaginal skin.

Posterior colpoperineorrhaphy

The operation is performed for a rectocele with or without an associated enterocele, and for a deficient perineum resulting in a gaping vaginal introitus. The principles are to excise redundant posterior vaginal skin, obliterate the enterocele sac, if present, and to reform the perineal body and perineum. Special care is required when performing this procedure, as poor

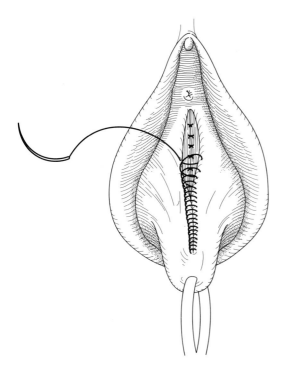

Fig. 22.5 Insertion of vaginal sutures.

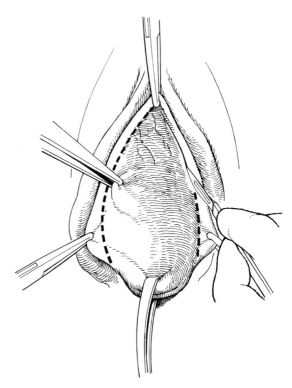

Fig. 22.6 Excising redundant vaginal skin.

surgical technique or surgical misjudgment can result in considerable dyspareunia and even apareunia, for the patient. The so-called 'registrar constriction ring' is seen to occur just as commonly after the operation has been performed by a consultant.

Anaesthesia, patient preparation and instruments

The comments made above should be noted, with the avoidance of a head-down tilt to the operating table. The instruments required are those in the gynaecological general set, shown in Chapter 2.

The operation

The incision

The apex of the rectocele is seized by applying a Kocher's forceps to the posterior vaginal wall; it is usually found that on drawing this point downwards it will reach the posterior margin of the introitus. The forceps is retracted upwards. Two Kocher's forceps mark the lateral points of the incision just internal to the junction of the vaginal and perineal skin and usually at the posi-

tion of the most posterior of the carunculae myrtiformes on each side. These two forceps are first approximated to confirm that the calibre of the new introitus will be adequate; they are then retracted laterally. A solution of 1% xylocaine with adrenaline 1:200 000 is now injected to raise the posterior vaginal wall off the underlying tissues. Drawing the two marginal Kocher's forceps laterally and towards the operator, the old scar is boldly excised with scissors (Fig. 22.7), the only exception being where the perineum is so deficient that the anus might be injured, in which case a transverse incision with the scalpel is to be preferred.

Separation of the rectum from vagina

The operator now retracts the distal vagina upwards with toothed forceps or a Kocher's forceps and his fingers; by dissecting against the fingers, the plane between rectum and vagina is found (Fig. 22.8). The open scissors are now inserted into this space laterally to separate the lower vagina from the superficial perineal muscles (Fig. 22.9). If the correct plane has been found, dissection of the rectum from the posterior vaginal wall

241

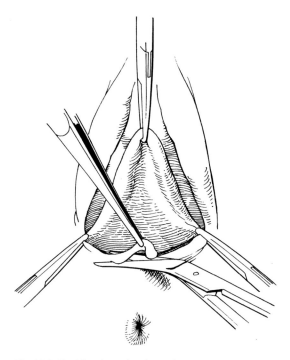

Fig. 22.7 Excising the perineal scar tissue.

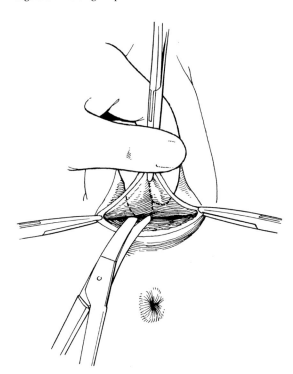

Fig. 22.8 Exposing the plane between vagina and rectum.

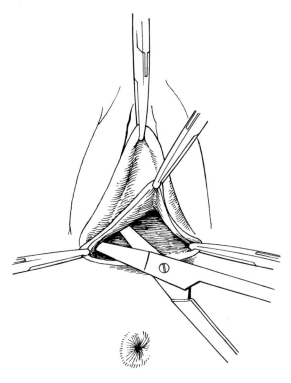

Fig. 22.9 Separation of superficial layers laterally.

and the margins of the divaricated levator ani muscles is easy with gauze dissection; this separation reaches the apical Kocher's forceps.

Excision of the skin
The redundant vaginal skin is now excised. Care must be taken to avoid a constriction at the junction of the upper third and lower two-thirds of the vagina; the anterior repair in the vault region tends to 'borrow' from the posterior vaginal wall, so that if too much vagina is excised in the upper part of the posterior repair there will be undue narrowing (Fig. 22.10). The closure of the posterior vaginal wall is now started using a continuous locking suture.

Reformation of the perineal body
After the first few stitches the muscle sutures are passed by retracting the vaginal suture upwards and holding the rectum back with the operator's left forefinger, which also stretches the puborectalis muscle. It is best to insert the highest stitch first; this is at levator ani level.

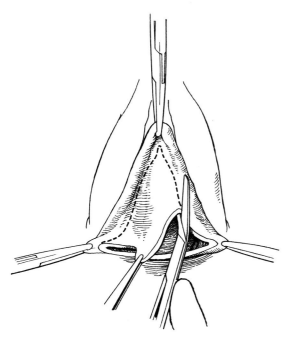

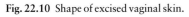

Fig. 22.10 Shape of excised vaginal skin.

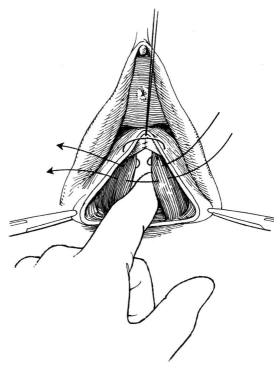

Fig. 22.11 Reformation of perineal body muscle sutures.

Taking a good bite of muscle on the right, the needle is taken through the vaginal wall into the canal and then back through the vagina to take a good bite of the left muscle (Fig. 22.11); this binds the vagina to the muscle and avoids dead space. The two ends of the suture are held in a Spencer Wells forceps which is pulled upwards and, with the rectum still being retracted posteriorly, another stitch is passed through the two muscles, omitting the vaginal wall this time. A third suture is usually required, placed in similar fashion. The Spencer Wells forceps are now allowed to hang downwards and the vaginal closure continues, each muscle stitch being tied as it is reached by the continuous vaginal suture. The continuous suture can pick up the conjoined muscles in the lower parts of the repair. On reaching the introital margin, the continuous suture is completed. The perineum is reconstituted by uniting the subcutaneous tissue and then the skin with fine suture material.

Where there is no need for perineorrhaphy, the rectocele can be dealt with similarly but a transverse incision with the scalpel is indicated. Alternatively, the vaginal wall can be excised first, the rectum separated, and the repair carried out in similar fashion to that already described.

Posterior colpoperineorrhaphy with enterocele repair

The previously described procedure is followed except the incision is continued to the vaginal vault, paying particular attention not to remove an excessive amount of vaginal skin. If the correct subepithelial plane is identified, the inferior and the anterior peritoneal margins of the enterocele sac will be encountered. After continuing the dissection of the peritoneum of the enterocele sac off the vaginal skin, the other attachments to the enterocele sac are then dissected using a combination of sharp and blunt dissection, until the enterocele sac is completely mobilized. The enterocele sac is then opened by incising the peritoneum, paying attention at this point to avoid injury to the small bowel, which may be lying within the sac. A minor degree of head-down tilt to the operating table can be particularly useful in emptying the sac. The remaining small bowel contents

243

are then pushed out of the enterocele sac by use of a small swab wrapped and held by a sponge holder. The redundant peritoneum is then excised up to the neck of the hernial sac, and the new peritoneal edges closed with a purse-string suture using Vicryl or Dexon. For severe, complex or recurrent cases, a culdoplasty stitch can be inserted to provide additional support. Closure of the vaginal skin is then continued as previously described, ensuring adequate obliteration of the space between the vaginal skin and the underlying fascia to provide additional support, and prevention of recurrence.

Postoperative care

If care is taken not to over-tighten the sutures at the perineum and the vaginal introitus, then pain is not a significant feature during the postoperative period. Routine urinary catheterization is therefore not essential on completion of the procedure. A vaginal pack is also not required.

Vaginal hysterectomy

Vaginal hysterectomy is frequently required for treatment of uterovaginal prolapse, usually but not always performed in conjunction with an anterior or posterior vaginal repair. The procedure is described in detail in Chapter 10. When all three procedures are required to deal adequately with the prolapse, the authors' preference is to perform the vaginal hysterectomy first, followed by the anterior repair and finally the posterior repair. The basis of the logic is that performing the posterior repair first can prevent adequate access to the upper vagina and the anterior vaginal wall; also, after dealing with the uterine and anterior vaginal wall prolapse, it often becomes apparent that it is unnecessary to perform the posterior repair for a satisfactory end result. As many women are post- or perimenopausal, the performance of a bilateral salpingo-oophorectomy should be performed at the time of the vaginal hysterectomy. If a bilateral salpingo-oophorectomy is not performed, then at the very least, the ovaries and tubes should be inspected for normality. When an anterior and posterior repair have been carried out, the authors' preference is to insert a bacterostatic soaked vaginal pack for up to 24 h in an attempt to avoid the development of vaginal adhesions between the anterior and posterior vaginal walls which normally lie in apposition. Separation of vaginal adhesions may still be required at the first postoperative clinic visit.

The Fothergill or Manchester repair

Although not recommended by the authors, some gynaecologists prefer this procedure for treatment of uterine prolapse in preference to vaginal hysterectomy; whilst it may be satisfactory for lesser degrees of uterine descent, it is not effective in uterine procidentia and is not satisfactory if an enterocele is present.

The principle of the procedure is to amputate the elongated cervix and approximate the cardinal ligaments anterior to the cervix to elevate and retract it backwards so that the uterus is both supported and anteverted. A curettage is performed at the onset of the operation to exclude the presence of intrauterine pathology.

The operation

The incision
This is as described for vaginal hysterectomy and repair. The vaginal skin is reflected from the cervix all round and the bladder reflected from the cervix.

Ligation of the ligaments and the descending cervical branch of the uterine artery
The ligaments are usually clamped on each side and the cervix then amputated (Fig. 22.12). The ligaments and vessels are ligated and the ligatures held.

Recovering the posterior cervix
A strong absorbable suture is passed through the skin of the posterior vaginal wall at the 7 o'clock position; the needle then passes through the wall of the cervix into the canal from where it is withdrawn to pick up the centre of the posterior vaginal wall, whence it returns into the canal and then out through the cervical wall at the 5 o'clock position and finally through the vaginal wall. When tied, the Sturmdorff suture covers the posterior half of the amputated cervix (Fig. 22.13).

The Fothergill stitch
This stitch covers the anterior half of the amputated cervix with vaginal skin and also approximates the ligaments in front of it. The needle passes through the

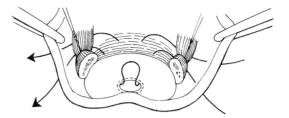

Fig. 22.14 The Fothergill stitch.

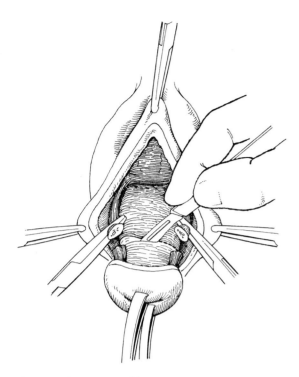

Fig. 22.12 Amputation of the cervix.

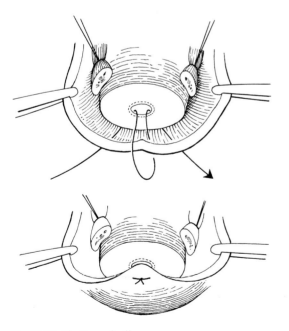

Fig. 22.13 The Sturmdorff suture.

vaginal skin under the marking lateral Kocher's forceps, under the supporting ligaments, and into the cervical canal from which it is withdrawn to be returned into the canal and out of the anterior wall to pick up the opposite ligament and through the vaginal wall. A second stitch, passing through vaginal skin, under the ligament, through the anterior cervical wall, under the opposite ligament and again through skin, supports the Fothergill stitch (Fig. 22.14). When the Fothergill stitch is tied, the Kocher's forceps on the angles of the vagina have their tips approximated and this allows the cervix to be covered. After tying the second stitch, the anterior colporrhaphy is completed.

Vault prolapse (enterocele following hysterectomy)

Vault prolapse can occur after abdominal or vaginal hysterectomy. The authors believe it is a myth that ligating the pedicles to the vaginal vault at the time of the hysterectomy significantly reduces the likelihood of a vault prolapse subsequently developing. Certainly, there is no strong evidence to support the practice.

Vault prolapses are often inadequately dealt with by the inexperienced gynaecologist. Attempts to deal with it by a combination of anterior or posterior repair, as is commonly practised, will do nothing to reduce the prolapse and will only shorten and constrict the vagina, making coitus virtually impossible and subsequent attempts to deal with the prolapse more difficult.

In fact, vault prolapses can be corrected very simply using reconstructive techniques that will impress the trainee surgeon, the patient and also many senior colleagues. Where vaginal access is satisfactory and there is also the need for a posterior colpoperineorrhaphy, a sacrospinous colpopexy is recommended performed by

245

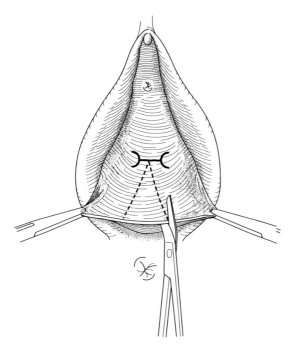

Fig. 22.15 Posterior vaginal wall incision up to vaginal vault.

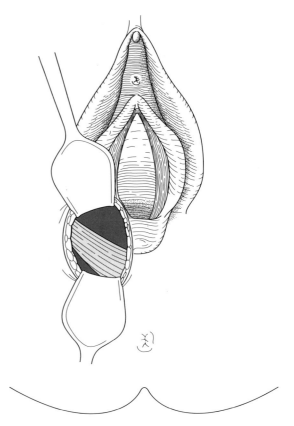

Fig. 22.16 Visualization of the sacrospinous ligament.

the vaginal route. For more complex, severe or repeat procedures, an abdominal sacral colpopexy is preferred. Both procedures will relieve symptoms and re-establish a coitally functional vagina and, with sufficient experience, can also be performed laparoscopically. In the authors' opinion, there is no place for the performance of obliterative procedures such as colpocleisis, and these will not be discussed further.

Sacrospinous colpopexy

Anaesthesia, patient preparation and instruments

The comments made above should be noted, with the avoidance of a head-down tilt to the operating table.

The operation

The incision
The posterior repair is commenced as described earlier, with the incision continued up to the vaginal vault (Fig. 22.15). The redundant vaginal skin is removed.

Identification and mobilization of the enterocele
The enterocele sac is encountered and dealt with as previously described.

Identification of the sacrospinous ligament and insertion of the sacrospinous stitch
The patient's right pararectal space is bluntly dissected in a posterolateral direction combined with regular palpation of the ischial spine, eventually allowing palpation and visualization of the sacrospinous ligament within the body of the coccygeus muscle (Fig. 22.16). The approach is aided by a large Sims' speculum placed in the posterior vagina with moderate traction in a downward direction by the assistant, to keep the rectum out of the operating field. A vaginal retractor placed along the right vaginal wall applying traction in an anterolateral direction also allows adequate displacement of the endopelvic fascia, easing access to the

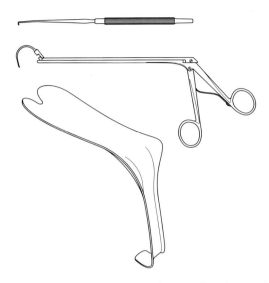

Fig. 22.17 The Miya notched speculum, needle and retrieval set.

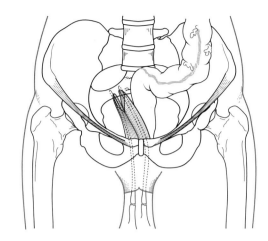

Fig. 22.18 Suspension of the vaginal vault to the sacrospinous ligament.

ischial spine and ligament. A fish-hook needle attached to a strong absorbable suture is then passed through the sacrospinous ligament about 2 cm away from the ischial spine, in a posteromedial direction. Knowledge that the pudendal vessels and nerve, and the sciatic nerve lie directly beneath the ischial spine should persuade most surgeons to keep well clear of this area. The application of firm traction to the suture length will test the correctness of its placement. Attention should also be made to insert the stitch through the ligament and not around it. Using a separate suture length, a second stitch is inserted for additional strength. Alternatively, an eyed needle can be used, or as is now becoming common practice, the use of a Miya notched speculum, needle and retrieval set (Fig. 22.17). The two sutures are then secured to the upper posterior aspect of the vaginal skin, allowing the vaginal vault to be drawn snugly on to the right sacrospinous ligament (Fig. 22.18). If necessary, the procedure can be repeated on the left side to provide the vaginal vault with additional support. However, in the editor's personal practice, to date, this has not been required.

Closure of the vaginal vault and completion of the posterior repair
The vaginal skin edges are then approximated as described earlier, in combination with the reformation of the perineal body and perineum. An indwelling transurethral urinary catheter and bacterostatic soaked vaginal pack are advisable.

Abdominal sacral colpopexy

Anaesthesia

The addition of an epidural or spinal anaesthesia to the general anaesthetic is helpful in reducing minor bleeding from the sacrum but is not essential.

Patient preparation

The patient is prepared as for any abdominal procedure. The authors' preference is also to insert a vaginal pack prior to commencing the operation to aid dissection of the rectum and bladder from the vaginal vault. Alternatively, an obturator can be inserted into the vagina and used to manipulate the vault during the procedure. An indwelling transurethral urinary catheter is also inserted.

Instruments

The gynaecological general set shown in Chapter 2 is used.

247

The operation

The incision

The procedure is ideally performed through a subumbilical mid-line incision for ease of access. Entry into the abdominal cavity is as described in Chapter 6.

Preparation of the vaginal vault

The firm pack within the vagina is easily palpated. The peritoneum overlying the vaginal vault is incised taking care to exclude the possibility that the bladder may be lying within the intervening space. Once the edges of the vaginal vault are identified and exposed, the plane between the posterior vaginal wall and rectum is developed as far as is necessary, this step having been made considerably easier by the insertion of a vaginal pack. The bladder base is then dissected off the superior aspects of the anterior vaginal wall. Sharp dissection is usually required as a result of the previous surgical intervention.

Preparation of the sacrum

With the sigmoid colon pushed over to the left side, the peritoneum overlying the sacral promontory and the upper three sacral vertebrae are then incised at the mid-line. The peritoneal incision is continued to the peritoneal incision overlying the vagina.

Placement of the mesh

A variety of synthetic and natural materials have been used including Marlex, Teflon, Goretex, Mersilene, rectus muscle fascia and dura mater. Using two Littlewood's forceps, traction is applied to the vaginal vault and the vaginal pack removed. In not removing the vaginal pack at this stage, the danger will be to suture the mesh to the pack in addition to the vagina. Although this may help support the vaginal vault, it is unlikely that you will be thanked by the patient. An adequate length of mesh should be made available, ideally 3×15 cm. Commencing at the lower aspects of the posterior vaginal wall and aiming towards the vault, the mesh is sutured to the vaginal tissues using full-thickness interrupted non-absorbable sutures. Attachment of the mesh to the vagina should continue sufficiently anteriorly also to deal with any cystocele which may be present. The mesh is then turned back on itself, aiming towards the vaginal vault and from there towards the sacrum, to which it is also secured by way of transversely placed non-absorbable interrupted su-

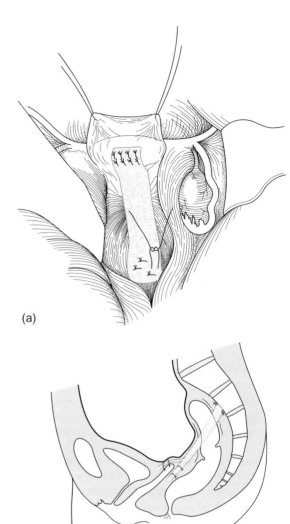

(a)

(b)

Fig. 22.19 Placement of the sacral colpoplexy mesh.

tures into the anterior longitudinal ligament or periosteum. The length of mesh used is gauged whereby it adequately holds the vagina in an elevated position, whilst lying within the hollow of the sacrum, free of any undue tension (Fig. 22.19). Any excess mesh length can now be excised and discarded. The area is then reperitonealized to avoid the development of adhesions, and combined with a Moschowitz or Halban's culdoplasty stitch if required (Fig. 22.20).

There is considerable doubt concerning the role of ventrosuspension procedures in the management of infertile patients. The positioning of the cervix and the lie of the uterus may not be of any significance in either the subfertile or the infertile.

When a ventrosuspension is performed there are a number of variations in technique, but as the indications are relatively few the authors will concentrate on the Gilliam's ventrosuspension with minor modifications.

Gilliam's ventrosuspension

Instruments
The gynaecological general set described in Chapter 2 will be required. The uterine packing forceps are the ideal instrument for burrowing subperitoneally along the round ligament.

The operation
Opening the abdominal cavity The low transverse or Pfannenstiel incision is very suitable for this procedure (see Chapter 6).

Elevating the uterus The uterus is raised by gently inserting the left hand into the pouch of Douglas and drawing the uterus forward. It is important to determine whether the retroversion is due to adhesions or the scarring consequent upon endometriosis. Occasionally, an extensive dissection is necessary in order to mobilize the uterus and to undo the retroflexion which can occur after endometriotic scarring. Great care should be taken to identify the ureter and keep it in full vision.

Plicating the round ligaments Once the uterus is mobilized, the round ligaments are identified and a plication stitch inserted as shown in Fig. 22.21; nylon may be used for this stitch. The suture should begin with a firm bite of the uterine musculature, taking care not to impinge on the entry point of the fallopian tube. The stitch is then carried along the length of the intra-abdominal portion of the round ligament, taking a zig-zag course. The two ends of the stitch are then drawn tight to concertina the round ligament and are tied.

This simple part of the procedure may be all that is required to elevate and antevert the uterus.

Passing the round ligament forceps The line of cleavage between the edge of the rectus muscle and the

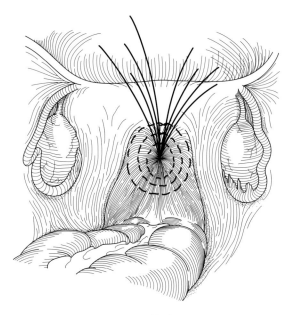

Fig. 22.20 The Moschowitz culdoplasty.

Closure of the abdominal wall
This is as described in Chapter 6.

Operations for the correction of axial displacement of the uterus

Indications

Operations to correct the position of the uterus have gone through periods of popularity, interspersed with equal periods of unpopularity. At the present time, there appear to be few sound indications for these operations. No longer should an uncomplicated retroversion of the uterus be regarded as pathological, nor should it be felt that it has any bearing on the ability to procreate.

The following indications for correction are agreed by most gynaecologists.

When a retroverted uterus is fixed in the pelvis by adhesions, endometriosis or infection and is causing dyspareunia, it is important that a cause for the dyspareunia is found, and laparoscopy is invaluable.

Occasionally, a prolapsed ovary causing dyspareunia may be preserved and elevated within the pelvis by a simple suspension procedure.

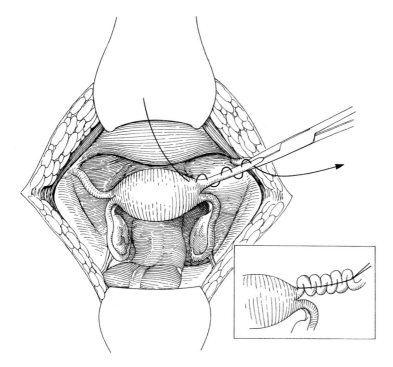

Fig. 22.21 Plicating the round ligaments.

aponeurosis is now identified at the edge of the wound. The packing forceps is gently insinuated between these layers, running in a lateral direction to the point at which the round ligament leaves the abdomen; the fingers of the left hand inside the abdominal wall help to guide the forceps. The ends of the forceps elevate the peritoneum, which can be incised; the long ends of the plication suture are then drawn along the track (Fig. 22.22). The suture must now be moved laterally to lie a short distance from the mid-line. This is done by cutting into the anterior layer of the rectus sheath and leading the long ends of the plication stitch out to the surface of the sheath (Fig. 22.23).

Final positioning of the uterus It is important not to tie the sutures too tight as this may cause the stitch to cut out of the uterine muscle; if too slack, the uterus will fall back into the pouch of Douglas. The correct tension is determined by observing the uterine position as the wound edges are brought together. In the authors' opinion, the low transverse incision has a clear advantage as the final position of the uterus is very accurately assessed, and does not alter as the abdomen is closed or

with abdominal wall movement in the postoperative period.

Closing the abdominal incision This is as described in Chapter 6.

Simple plication of the round ligaments

This procedure is carried out as described in sections 1–3 of the Gilliam's ventrosuspension (p. 249).

Complications
Pain is probably the commonest complication following this procedure, making what should be a relatively minor operation into a source of continuing irritation for the patient, emphasizing that the procedure should not be performed for trivial reasons. The cause of the pain is either that the sutures have been drawn too tight, or that damage to the round ligaments by the plication stitch have produced irritation. Occasionally, if the rectus sheath knot is not buried inside the sheath, the ends may be a source of pain and irritation.

Damage to the inferior epigastric artery and vein may

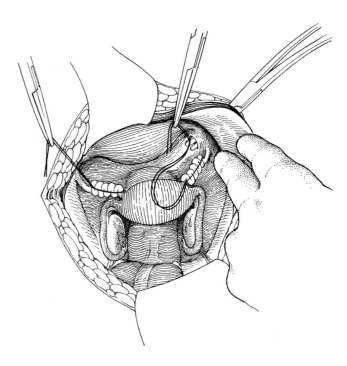

Fig. 22.22 Drawing the plicating suture through the abdominal wall.

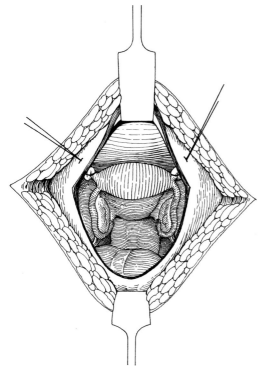

Fig. 22.23 The plication suture passing out of the rectus sheath.

occur during the burrowing under the sheath. Usually, the damage is immediately obvious and should be dealt with by exploration and ligation; occasionally, the damage manifests itself in the postoperative period; therefore, careful monitoring of these patients must be carried out. Intestinal obstruction may occur if the surgeon has left a small sulcus or passage between the round ligament and the abdominal wall; an internal hernia develops and shows itself as partial or total obstruction of the small bowel.

Damage to the fallopian tube may occur if the uterine suture is misplaced at the cornu. Great care is the only prescription.

Infection rarely occurs when dealing with the healthy pelvis; however, if it has been necessary to separate infected or damaged tubes, prophylactic antibiotics, especially those specific for anaerobic bacteria, should be prescribed. The use of a permanent suture material may exacerbate this risk of infection. Rarely, a sinus may develop at the abdominal wall over the site of the knot in the rectus sheath. If a haematoma has developed and has not been recognized or treated it may become infected, producing all the signs of a wound infection. It should be actively managed with antibiotics and may discharge spontaneously through the wound.

251

Variation in technique

It is now common practice to perform a similar procedure through the laparoscope; however, in the authors' experience there are pitfalls. The first is not to leave a space between the round ligament and the lateral abdominal wall, as the danger of small bowel herniation and obstruction is significant. The second is the risk of undiagnosed bleeding from the inferior epigastric vessels; this may produce considerable haemorrhage into the abdominal cavity, which may not be identified early in the postoperative period. The third is the occurrence of severe long-term pain from overtightening the ligaments during the course of the anteversion.

23 Operative procedures for therapeutic abortion

During the last three decades, there has developed a worldwide liberalization of therapeutic abortion with a consequent improvement in the techniques available. In those populations where it has become the most important method of birth control, serious thought should be given to the expansion of the preconceptual methods of population control.

It is now clearly understood that the earlier a therapeutic abortion can be performed, the safer it is for the patient. Therefore, any population must be informed of the need to report early in pregnancy so that, following proper examination and counselling, the procedure can be carried out at a time when the risks are minimal. If the termination is performed during the first 12 weeks of pregnancy (approximately 90% of all operations), the morbidity and mortality are extremely low.

The World Health Organization recommends an upper limit of 22 weeks' gestation, and many countries have adopted this limit.

Indications

There is considerable variation around the world as to the social, ethical and moral indications for termination of pregnancy; however, the medical indications are usually more clear:
1 Where there is significant danger to the mother if the pregnancy continues.
2 Where the pregnancy has to be sacrificed so that a life-threatening condition in the mother may be treated, e.g. cancer of the cervix.
3 Where the risk of delivery of an abnormal child is high or demonstrable using prenatal investigations.

The social indications are more contentious.

Timing and techniques

More than 90% of terminations are performed in the first trimester, usually by suction techniques. Of the remainder, the majority are performed early in the second trimester, often for genetic reasons, using some form of prostaglandin stimulation technique or by curettage of the cavity of the uterus. Rarely, abdominal, or, even more rarely, vaginal hysterotomy is performed.

First-trimester termination

All the techniques available are variations of simple evacuation of the contents of the uterus.

Menstrual induction and removal

This technique depends upon the patient attending for treatment within a few days or 1 or 2 weeks of the date of the last missed period. The abortion can be induced by inserting a prostaglandin pessary either into the upper vagina or into the uterus. A sequel to this technique has been the development of the 'morning after pill' which causes shedding of the endometrium and can be taken following an episode of unprotected intercourse.

Simple suction techniques using narrow suction cannulae such as the Vabra will quickly remove the endometrium with minimal morbidity to the patient.

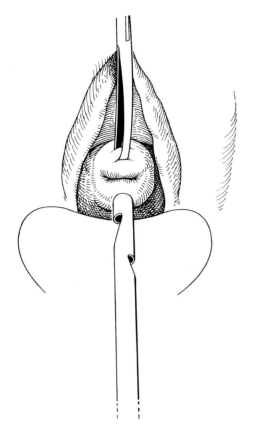

Fig. 23.1 The uterine suction curette.

Dilatation of the cervix and suction evacuation

This is the most widely used method of surgical termination; it involves slow dilatation of the cervix, usually to no more than 10 mm, followed by the evacuation of the contents of the uterus using a tube curette (Fig. 23.1) attached to a powerful suction machine. The procedure is performed as described in Chapter 5, taking the safeguards appropriate for a pregnant uterus. It is usual to give the patient an intravenous injection of Syntocinon 10 units immediately prior to the procedure; this reduces blood loss considerably. Bleeding will cease or become minimal once the cavity of the uterus is empty.

It may be necessary to augment the suction curettage with an exploration of the cavity of the uterus using blunt ring forceps so that the surgeon can be sure that the cavity is empty at the end of the operation.

Second-trimester termination

Although there are fewer second-trimester terminations, they are of great importance as the risks to the patient are so much higher than the first-trimester procedures.

The most frequently used middle-trimester termination technique is that of inserting into the uterus extra-amniotic prostaglandin (PG). The prostaglandins used are $PGF_{2\alpha}$ and PGE_2; they act by stimulating uterine contractions causing a 'mini labour'. The prostaglandins also soften the uterine cervix facilitating delivery of the fetus.

Curettage

It is generally accepted that middle-trimester sharp curettage has an unacceptably high complication rate and is not recommended as a technique. The hazards include the following:
1 Anaesthetic problems.
2 Inability to complete the procedure.
3 Uterine perforation.
4 Excessive bleeding.
5 Infection.
6 Cervical laceration.
7 Long-term effects, such as sterility, ectopic pregnancy, spontaneous first-trimester abortion.

Prostaglandin termination

Extra-amniotic technique
This method is the technique of choice for mid-trimester abortion, combining many of the advantages of other procedures and proving an extremely safe technique. It can be used for inducing abortion from 13 weeks onwards.
1 PGE_2 (dinoprostone) is supplied to be made up as a 50 ml solution containing 100 μg/ml.
2 The drug is administered using a syringe pump via a Foley catheter inserted through the cervix.
3 Before using prostaglandin, the surgeon should check that there is no contraindication for its use (i.e. asthma, glaucoma, mechanical obstruction to delivery, untreated pelvic infection).

The patient may have a light meal and may have fluids by mouth at least for the first 6 h of infusion.

A test dose of 100 μg of prostaglandin is given via a

Foley catheter; if there is no reaction within 15 min, infusion is started at a rate of 100 µg/h.

Unless there is a medical indication, there is no need for an intravenous infusion at this stage.

A strict fluid balance chart should be instituted, however, to avoid any possible fluid overload occurring.

4 A vaginal examination should be carried out every 6 h.

5 After 6 h:

(a) if contractions are established, consider setting up an intravenous infusion to combat dehydration or ketosis;

(b) if contractions are not established, increase the prostaglandin infusion to 200 µg/h.

6 After 9 h: if there are still no contractions in spite of the increased dose of prostaglandin, Syntocinon (oxytocin) should be added to the intravenous infusion at a maximum rate of 40 milliunits/min. Care should be exercised as regards fluid intake.

7 After 24 h: if abortion is not imminent, remove the Foley catheter and proceed to intra-amniotic injection. Where the pregnancy is less than 15 weeks' gestation, an intra-amniotic injection is difficult, and evacuation of the uterus per vaginam should be considered. Dilatation of the cervix should be easy or unnecessary.

Intra-amniotic technique

1 This approach is only suitable when the uterus is easily palpable in the abdomen. Either PGE_2 or $PGF_{2\alpha}$ may be used, but do note there is a difference in the equivalent dosages.

2 Using a transabdominal approach, a Touhy needle is inserted into the amniotic cavity and at least 20 ml (and preferably 50 ml) of liquor withdrawn. This is followed by the injection of 10 mg of PGE_2 (40 mg $PGF_{2\alpha}$), followed immediately by 200 ml of a freshly prepared 20% solution of urea.

3 Light meals or fluids by mouth are permissible for the first 6 h following the injection. There is no need for an intravenous infusion at this stage.

4 Once contractions are established, a vaginal examination should be carried out every 6 h.

5 After 12 h: if abortion is not imminent, give intravenous Syntocinon (oxytocin) at an infusion rate not exceeding 40 milliunits/min.

6 After 24 h: if the abortion is not imminent, give a second dose of prostaglandin into the amniotic sac.

7 Evacuation of the retained products should be carried out whenever there is any doubt about the completeness of the placenta. It is not necessary to do so in every case.

Variations in technique

In some centres intra-amniotic prostaglandins are used with or without intra-amniotic urea, saline or mannitol. Intravenous oxytocin may be used to supplement the intrauterine drugs if the patient is slow to begin contractions; water intoxication is a potential risk if large volumes of fluid are used.

Complications

These may occur and consist of diarrhoea, nausea and vomiting.

Hysterotomy

This procedure is now rarely performed because of the great improvements in uterine stimulation techniques.

The operation

This is best performed via a low transverse (Pfannenstiel) incision as described in Chapter 6.

1 *Opening the uterus.* As the abdominal cavity is entered the patient should be given 5 units of Syntocinon intravenously. The contracted uterus is now elevated and brought into the wound. The uterovesical fold of peritoneum is lifted by the assistant using toothed dissectors and the surgeon cuts through into the soft fascial space below. This allows the bladder to be pushed down easily, revealing the lower part of the anterior wall of the uterus. There is no true lower segment of the uterus at this stage in pregnancy; therefore, a short vertical incision is made as low down as possible.

2 *Emptying the uterus.* The membranes of the gestation sac now bulge through the incision; the surgeon should insert his index finger and carefully separate the sac from the inner surface of the uterine cavity. The entire sac is now free and can be expressed from the cavity. A gentle exploration of the cavity is made, removing small amounts of tissue with a gauze stretched over the finger.

3 *Closure of the uterine wound.* The incision in the uterus is now closed in two layers using continuous Vicryl suture in the same manner as the caesarean section wound. The peritoneum of the uterovesical fold is

now closed over the incision to protect it and reduce the risk of adhesions.

4 *Closure of the abdomen.* Before closure, peritoneal toilet should be performed and the uterus checked for haemostasis. The abdomen is closed as described in Chapter 6.

Variations in technique

When the risk of infection was very high, vaginal hysterotomy enjoyed a vogue but is now not performed.

Complications of termination of pregnancy

These are related to the type of procedure performed and to the extreme vascularity and softness of the uterus in pregnancy.

Haemorrhage may occur following and during any of the techniques; the most important contributory factor is the presence of retained products within the uterine cavity. At a later postoperative stage, bleeding may be related to the development of infection.

Damage to the cervix and *the uterus*, including perforation, may occur with any of the methods but is particularly likely to happen during overdilatation of the cervix, and exploration and curettage of the uterine cavity. When a hysterotomy has been performed, there is a long-term risk of rupture of the uterine scar in all future pregnancies.

Infection may develop after any of the methods but is most likely to occur if products of conception are retained. Endometritis may spread to affect the tubes producing long-term damage and infertility.

Infertility from infection, or the development of intrauterine adhesions (Asherman's syndrome), may also occur.

Psychological damage occurs rarely and often appears in a patient who had already shown evidence of mental instability.

Rhesus isoimmunization may occur; all patients must have their blood typed before the procedure and if the patient is rhesus-negative, she should be given anti-D immunoglobulin immediately following the termination before antibodies develop and jeopardize future pregnancies.

24 Caesarean section

Although Caesarean section is now regarded as a 'safe' procedure for both mother and child, it should not be forgotten that it was not until 1793 that James Barlow working in a Lancashire town managed to carry out the procedure with subsequent survival of the mother. However, until anaesthesia had developed sufficiently the procedure was no more than a heroic method of trying to terminate an obstructed and doomed labour.

It is extremely important that all obstetricians should carefully study the details of this procedure, particularly the features which can improve its safety, as Caesarean section remains an important cause of maternal morbidity and mortality. Despite dramatic reductions, one of the most common complications associated with caesarean section, mentioned in the 2001 Report on Confidential Enquiries into Maternal Deaths in the UK covering the period 1997–1999, is thrombosis.

A disastrous complication of pregnancy and post-caesarean section is the occurrence of a thromboembolic episode. This event may leave the patient with a severe postphlebitic syndrome, put her at very high risk of a similar episode in a future pregnancy, or at worst will result in rapid death. Emphasis on early mobilization should be made to all women following childbirth and especially following caesarean section, and for those patients at particular risk, appropriate prophylaxis should be mandatory during the perioperative period and until she is fully ambulant.

Clearly, many lessons have been learnt as the most recent confidential report has shown significant reductions in deaths following scheduled and elective procedures (12.8 and 38.5 fatalities per million maternities, respectively). However, one cannot be complacent, as the mortality following emergency procedures remains significantly high at 202.9 fatalities per million maternities.

Lower segment Caesarean section

This procedure is the standard method for the surgical removal of the fetus from the uterus. The lower segment of the uterus is that lower part of the anterior uterine wall which is covered by the loose peritoneum of the uterovesical sulcus or pouch.

The lower uterine segment incision has become accepted as the standard approach because it has certain distinct advantages over the classical operation:
1 The lower segment is less vascular than the upper part of the uterus.
2 The risk of rupture of the uterine scar in subsequent pregnancies is greatly reduced.
3 Postoperative complications such as ileus and peritonitis are much reduced.
4 The risk of adhesions and postoperative obstructions is greatly reduced.
5 As the incision is made in a relatively inactive part of the uterus, haemostasis is easily achieved and healing occurs readily.
6 In those cases where there is already infection present, the lower segment operation markedly reduces the risk of contamination for the remainder of the peritoneal cavity.

Instruments

The instruments included in the gynaecological general set described in Chapter 2 are required with the

257

addition of a Doyen curved retractor and four large Green-Armitage tissue forceps.

Patient preparation

Anaesthesia during delivery is potentially extremely dangerous; the risks of inhalation of gastric contents are significant. If this problem arises, the damage to lung tissue by the acid gastric fluid may result in Mendelson's syndrome, a potentially lethal pneumonitis. It is therefore vital if the patient is to have a general anaesthetic that steps are taken to reduce this risk. Two procedures may be effective: the first is to give antacids and H_2 receptor antagonists before induction; the second is that all patients must have endotracheal intubation.

It is now commonplace to use epidural analgesia in labour with an epidural catheter *in situ*, which can be 'topped up' as required. This technique has significant advantages as the patient is still conscious and retains her cough reflex, therefore reducing the risk of inhalation of vomit. The 'block' can also be rapidly and conveniently extended if an emergency caesarean section has to be performed.

Prophylactic antibiotics have also been shown significantly to reduce the risk of postoperative infective morbidity, and should be given immediately prior to the procedure commencing.

Anaesthesia

There is little doubt that the risks of general anaesthesia are far greater than that of local techniques, including epidural and spinal analgesia. The advantages of having a patient with her cough reflexes intact is considerable at a time of high risk of vomiting and inhalation problems.

The induction of a safe general anaesthetic in a pregnant woman at term, especially after a prolonged labour, can be a major test of skill for even the most experienced of anaesthetists. Intubation is often difficult and may be time consuming, whereas the risks of performing the procedure without intubation are enormous and of the severest gravity. Delay in performing the operation may also seriously jeopardize the fetus due to anoxia or complications arising from those indications that led to Caesarean section. Finally, a significant contributory factor to the problems which may occur during Caesarean section will be the relative inexperience of both the surgeon and the anaesthetist. It is thus of vital importance that the obstetrician is confident of his role in this procedure and allows the anaesthetist to perform his task without impedance or interference.

Syntocinon is traditionally given by the anaesthetist at the time of delivery of the fetal head. The syringe containing 5 units must be drawn up and available before the procedure is commenced.

The operation

Preparation and catheterization

The anaesthesia for the mother and fetus should be light and for as short a period as possible. To this end, the vulva and vagina should be cleansed and the bladder catheterized prior to induction of a general anaesthetic. The surgeon then completes his gowning while the patient is anaesthetized; he is then ready to begin the operation as soon as the patient enters theatre.

Opening the abdomen

The choice of incision is between a subumbilical midline and a Pfannenstiel low transverse. The decision should be based upon the speed of entry into the abdomen that is required.

For most Caesarean sections and probably for all elective procedures, the Pfannenstiel incision has considerable advantages. The wound heals rapidly, it is relatively comfortable in the postoperative period, it is not unsightly, the risk of ventral hernia is low and rupture is rare.

The subumbilical mid-line incision should not be totally dismissed. It is simple and quick, and is often the incision of choice when a placenta praevia is present or where the uterus has been the site of previous surgery, such as myomectomy or classical caesarean section.

The mid-line incision should not be extended too far into the hair-bearing area, as this does not improve access, may cause unnecessary bleeding and is often very uncomfortable when healing.

It is also important not to 'cross' incisions as the site of the crossing often heals badly due to damaged blood supply and may be the site of an irritating and persistent infection.

The length of the incision is usually from the line of the pubic hair to 1 cm below the umbilicus in the midline and 10–12 cm long for the Pfannenstiel.

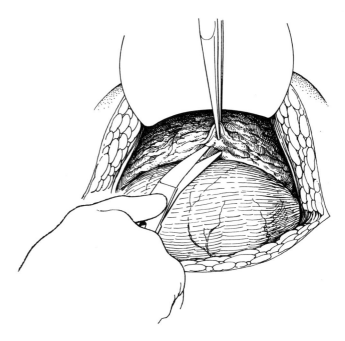

Fig. 24.1 Reflecting the peritoneum over the lower uterine segment.

The abdomen is opened as described in Chapter 6 with special care being taken to avoid the bladder when the mid-line incision is used as it may be drawn upwards by the growth of the uterus. The peritoneum should be incised in the upper part of the wound.

Packing around the uterus
In an emergency procedure, it is often found that packing off the bowel around the edge of the uterus can be dispensed with. In an elective procedure soiling of the abdominal cavity by liquor and blood can to a large extent be avoided if a large abdominal pack is inserted alongside the uterus. The pack must be marked with large forceps attached to the tapes which lead out from the abdomen. The insertion of the pack is recorded on the swab count board.

Reflecting the peritoneum over the lower segment
The curved Doyen retractor is now inserted into the lower end of the wound so that easy access is obtained to the lower segment (Fig. 24.1).

It is important not to pick up the peritoneum overlying the uterine segment too close to the uterine attachment as the peritoneum does not separate easily and troublesome bleeding will occur. If the peritoneum is picked up using toothed dissectors at the correct level,

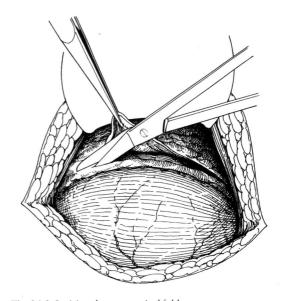

Fig. 24.2 Incising the uterovesical fold.

it will immediately begin to separate from the underlying lower segment (Fig. 24.2). The fold is incised and carried laterally towards the round ligaments on either side. The index fingers of each hand are then inserted

259

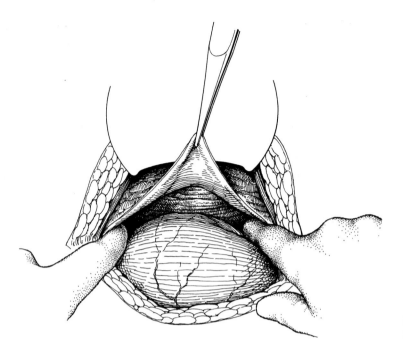

Fig. 24.3 Separating the bladder from the lower segment.

into the fascial plane, which is revealed, and the bladder is completely separated from the lower segment along this relatively avascular plane (Fig. 24.3). The ureterovesical angles are separated and dislocated laterally and downwards rendering the incision into the lower segment safe.

Incising the lower segment
The lower segment is now incised by stroking gently with the knife over a length of approximately 2–3 cm. The amniotic sac frequently bubbles through like an inner tube on a thin bicycle tyre if the membranes are still intact, or the hairs on the head of the fetus become visible as the lower segment thins.

The index fingers of each hand are inserted into the incision, which is extended laterally so that the presenting part can be delivered from the wound (Fig. 24.4). It is preferable to use the fingers for this separation rather than to cut the lower segment with scissors as the fingers push the uterine vessels to one side rather than cut them.

Delivery of the presenting part
When the incision in the lower segment is complete the Doyen retractor is removed and the presenting part delivered. If the head presents, the surgeon will insert

the hand below the head to disimpact it from the pelvis. Release of atmospheric pressure will ease this process; the assistant applies fundal pressure when the head is brought into the incision and the fetal head delivered.

Once the head is delivered, the respiratory passages are cleared of mucus, blood and liquor. It is at this stage that the anaesthetist gives the patient the Syntocinon (5 units) intravenously.

If the presentation is breech, the lower limbs are delivered and then the breech; the Syntocinon is then given. The arms may be delivered by the Lovset manoeuvre and the head then follows. Care should be taken to maintain flexion by jaw traction where necessary. The respiratory passages are aspirated while the child is held head downwards by the surgeon.

Fetal blood within the umbilical cord may be milked into the newborn if required and the cord is then clamped and cut, and the newborn passed to the paediatrician in attendance.

Removal of the placenta
The placenta and the membranes are now removed manually. If the uterus is contracting normally following injection of the Syntocinon, then traction on the cord together with fundal pressure will usually deliver the placenta from the wound. The membranes should

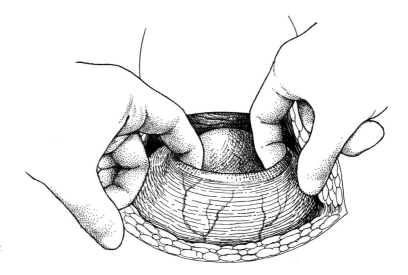

Fig. 24.4 Extending the lower segment incision.

be grasped with a sponge holder and gently drawn out, taking care not to tear them and leave fragments within the uterine cavity. If the uterus is soft and placental separation has not quickly occurred, then manual removal may be necessary but this should not become the preferred method of removal; if the surgeon exercises patience and deals with blood loss from the wound by applying the Green-Armitage forceps he will not run into many problems.

Controlling the bleeding

The abdominal wound is now held open by inserting a Balfour self-retaining retractor. Blood and clots mixed with liquor are now scooped out of the lower segment by the surgeon and his assistant, enabling the identification of the edges of the lower segment. The Green-Armitage forceps are then attached to the lateral edges of the lower segment incision anteriorly and posteriorly so as to occlude gently the most common and significant sites of haemorrhage (Fig. 24.5).

Suturing of the uterine wound

In previous editions it was recommended that the uterine cavity be explored and blood removed; this procedure was also accompanied by dilatation of the cervical os in elective sections so as to improve drainage. These procedures should be avoided as they increase the risk of infection with no benefit to the patient.

The Green-Armitage forceps are now gently elevated and the extreme corners of the wound clearly identified;

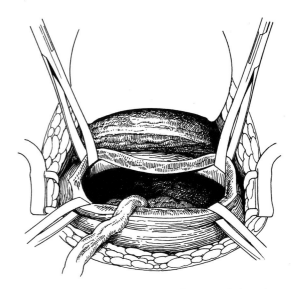

Fig. 24.5 Attaching Green-Armitage forceps to the lateral edges of the lower segment wound.

the uterine lower segment is now sutured in two layers using a continuous absorbable suture material. It is important to insert the first stitch a short distance lateral to the corner of the lower segment incision in order to be sure of achieving haemostasis at the angles. Although it is impossible to identify two separate layers, the surgeon should close the lower segment (Fig. 24.6a) and then oversew the line of sutures with a continuous

261

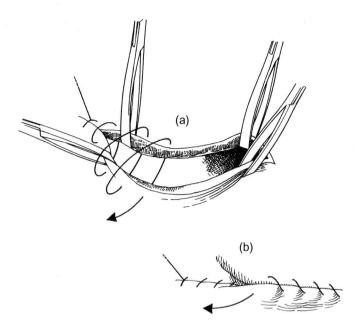

(a)

(b)

Fig. 24.6 Suturing the lower segment in two layers.

stitch (Fig. 24.6b). A small amount of ooze will often respond to pressure for a few minutes, or the application of a hot pack to the suture line.

Suturing the lower segment peritoneum
There would appear to be no value in suturing the lower segment peritoneum and it may therefore be left to heal spontaneously (Fig. 24.7).

Peritoneal toilet
The abdominal pack is now removed and the abdomen inspected to make sure that all clots and amniotic fluid have been removed. This procedure also allows for a full inspection of the pelvic and abdominal viscera, particularly the ovaries.

Closing the abdomen
The closure is performed as described in Chapter 6.

Cleansing the vagina
This procedure is as important following caesarean section as it is following hysterectomy; the surgeon must know that the vagina was empty at the end of the procedure in order that he can assess any blood loss that may occur in the postoperative period. The vagina should be mopped out using a swab either on a sponge

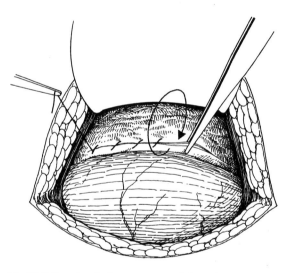

Fig. 24.7 Suturing the lower segment of the peritoneum.

holder or on the surgeon's finger. The uterine fundus should also be gently pressed to be certain that it is contracting and also to remove any retained clots, which are then cleared from the vagina.

Complications and dangers of lower segment caesarean section

Injury to the bladder

If the surgeon finds difficulty in identifying the uterovesical junction, then there is considerable danger of entering the bladder. The simplest safeguard that can be taken is to be certain that the bladder is emptied immediately before the operation and to follow the recommendations for identifying the loose uterovesical fold (see 'Reflecting the peritoneum over the lower segment', p. 259). Rarely, a part of the bladder may become loculated due to pressure of the presenting part obstructing proper drainage; this is unusual and should be recognized as the abdomen is opened.

Damaging the uterine artery and veins

If the lower segment incision is made too large and particularly if the incision is extended not with the fingers but with scissors, there is great danger of rupturing the uterine vessels producing heavy loss of blood. Experience and practice will allow the surgeon to judge the ideal length of incision for the average fetus; occasionally problems will arise if the presenting part is unusually large. In these circumstances, the surgeon must carefully extend the incision to an appropriate size.

Excessive haemorrhage

In most circumstances, a lower segment incision in labour will be virtually bloodless. However, occasionally haemorrhage can be torrential and life threatening. Even small amounts of bleeding can impede the surgeon's view and increase risks of damage to the surrounding viscera and the fetus. If the surgeon operates smoothly and rapidly, using broad haemostatic clamps such as the Green-Armitage and takes care not to damage large vessels by clumsy technique, haemorrhage can be kept to an acceptable level. If large, single bleeding vessels are isolated, the use of mattress sutures is recommended as these do not cut out and will be a more certain way of stopping haemorrhage than single sutures or attempted ties.

The most dangerous areas when dealing with haemorrhage are the angles of the incision; blind suturing at these points will greatly endanger the ureters. It is for this reason that the authors recommend early identification of the angles and clamping with the haemostatic Green-Armitage clamps.

Damage to the fetus

This usually takes the form of accidentally incising the skin of the scalp when the lower segment is opened; the surgeon must be cautious, cutting the lower segment over a short distance only and then extending the incision with the fingers.

Classical Caesarean section

There are few indications for the use of this technique; they include:

1 Transverse lie with the fetal back presenting over the pelvis.
2 As a preliminary to caesarean hysterectomy.
3 As a preliminary to treating carcinoma of the cervix, whether by surgery or radiotherapy.
4 Where there has been a previous classical section and the scar is dangerously thinned and would be best treated by resection of the scar and resuture.
5 Where a cervical fibroid obstructs access to the lower segment.
6 When the surgeon, is unhappy about coping with a placenta praevia with large lower segment vessels.

Preparation, anaesthesia, Syntocinon, instruments and position of the patient are as for the lower segment procedure. However, it may, depending on the circumstances, be sensible to have crossmatched blood arranged.

The operation

Opening the abdomen

A vertical mid-line subumbilical incision is used; care should be taken to avoid the bladder, which may frequently be drawn well up the abdominal wall. Opening the peritoneum in the upper part of the incision will avoid this problem.

The incision

The uterus is carefully checked to be certain that it is not rotated, a large gauze abdominal pack is inserted on either side and the tapes marked with a clip. An incision approximately 10 cm long is now made in the anterior surface of the uterus, which may extend into the lower segment. The incision should be made quickly as considerable haemorrhage may occur from the uterine muscle. However, care should also be exercised as the risk of cutting the fetus is greater in this procedure.

Bleeding may be further enhanced if the placental site lies beneath the incision; a careful estimate of the blood loss must be made and replaced if excessive.

Delivery of the fetus
The leg of the fetus is grasped and delivered, enabling the body and then the head to be delivered; the umbilical cord is clamped and cut between pressure forceps.

Extraction of the uterus
It is valuable to draw the uterus out of the abdomen to lie above the level of the abdominal wound. This is easily done by hooking the index finger into the cavity of the uterus and elevating it out of the wound. The packs placed alongside the uterus will control the bowel, although if the abdominal wound has been made an appropriate size it will fit snugly around the uterus.

Removal of the placenta
This is removed as described in the lower segment procedure.

Suturing the uterus
As the uterus has contracted down after delivery of the fetus and under the influence of the Syntocinon bleeding will have reduced, the uterine wound is now closed using a single layer of interrupted sutures followed by a layer of continuous suture using Dexon or Vicryl. Occasionally, oozing continues from the needle holes even when modern atraumatic needles are used; this problem is best dealt with by applying either pressure for a few minutes or a hot pack to the bleeding site.

Peritoneal toilet
The packs are removed and the uterus returned to the abdomen; any clots or amniotic fluid are carefully removed, and the abdomen inspected as described under lower segment caesarean section.

Closure of the abdomen
This is as described in Chapter 6.

Emptying the vagina
The vagina is carefully cleansed at the end of the procedure as described in the lower segment procedure.

General complications of Caesarean section

Haemorrhage

In general, haemorrhage is much reduced as soon as the uterine musculature begins to contract; thus, it is important to deliver the fetus expeditiously so that contraction of the uterine muscle may occur. Occasionally, bleeding will occur from the uterine wound as isolated spurting vessels; these should be underrun with single mattress sutures or lightly clamped with the Green-Armitage forceps until the edge can be sutured. Usually, suturing the wound is all that is required to control all haemorrhage.

If bleeding persists from the placental site, the uterus should be massaged and a second injection of Syntocinon (5 units) given.

Infection

There is always a risk of infection in any abdominal procedure; if the operation is performed under emergency circumstances, the risk increases. A further complicating factor is the length of time the patient has been in labour; it is not unusual for a caesarean section to be the culmination of a long and stressful labour. The tissues are congested and bruised, there have been many vaginal examinations, the bladder has been catheterized, and the membranes have been ruptured for a long period of time. Thus, it is not surprising that infectious morbidity is a common postoperative development.

Intraoperative prophylaxis and the use of broad-spectrum antibiotics should be mandatory in all caesarean sections.

The surgeon must also remember that in spite of the need for speed in an emergency, his attention should not be taken away from the need to observe the strictest aseptic techniques in both the preparation for and the carrying out of the procedure.

Rupture of a previous uterine scar

The patients who most frequently run into this rare complication are those who have had previous caesarean sections, but the surgeon must not forget those patients who have had hysterotomy, plastic procedures on the uterus or previous myomectomy.

There is no doubt that the risk is much greater

following a classical caesarean section, the relative rarity of this procedure accounting for the marked rarity of rupture at the present time.

Rupture may be acute and catastrophic, presenting with a moribund patient or a dead fetus, or, more commonly, may be relatively silent, being discovered at second or subsequent section as a 'windowing' of the previous scar with the membranes ballooning through the gap. The scar is usually avascular, so bleeding is often not a problem.

Pain during the pregnancy or in labour is an ominous sign and should not be ignored. Pain during labour, which is becoming resistant to a previously effective epidural anaesthetic, is particularly ominous and should warn the obstetrician that there may be danger in persisting for a vaginal delivery.

Further reading

Why Women Die 1997–1999: The fifth report of the confidential enquiries into maternal deaths in the United Kingdom. London: RCOG, 2001.

25 The management of cancers complicating pregnancy

It is a commonly held misconception that malignancies accelerate in their growth during a pregnancy; with the possible exception of malignant melanoma, this is not true. Cancers presenting during a pregnancy are fortunately rare, occurring approximately once every 1000 pregnancies. The problem, however, can raise some extraordinarily difficult questions and considerable heartache when decisions are made.

This chapter will concentrate on genital malignancies and breast carcinoma. It should be remembered that in the age group 15–35, the major childbearing years, the commonest cancers are central nervous system cancers followed by Hodgkin's disease and cervical carcinoma. In women over the age of 35, breast, colon and rectum, lung and skin cancers are all more common than any of the genital malignancies.

It is important to realize that pregnancy gives the clinician an unparalleled opportunity to perform a comprehensive examination of women who may never otherwise see a gynaecologist, and is possibly the first opportunity to carry out screening for precancers of the cervix.

Antenatal examination

Patients are encouraged to book early for delivery so that a comprehensive examination can be performed with minimal discomfort for the woman and little fear of disruption of the pregnancy. Examinations should consist of:

1 Full blood examination to include assessment for anaemia and a blood film which would pick up any of the haematological cancers.

2 Urine analysis not only to pick up metabolic disorders but also the presence of haematuria, which may be the first manifestation of urothelial cancers.

3 A bimanual pelvic examination should always follow visualization of the cervix and the taking of a cervical smear, when indicated. The clinician should be suspicious of any bleeding in early pregnancy because although this is most likely to be due to an obstetric cause, a carcinoma of the cervix must always be excluded.

The bimanual examination will allow the clinician to confirm the size of the pregnancy, the shape and consistency of the uterus, and also to detect cystic swellings of the ovary.

4 Breast examination should also be performed; although the pregnant breast is enlarged, this is a valuable procedure as masses can be identified and the patient can also be instructed in the correct method of breast examination and this valuable health habit inaugurated.

Breast carcinoma

Breast cancer is the commonest cancer in women and accounts for the most deaths; in women aged between 39 and 44, it is the leading cause of death.

As it is not uncommon for women to delay having their first child until they are in their thirties, the association of cancer of the breast and pregnancy is seen more frequently.

Often, the mass discovered in the pregnant breast is larger than those discovered in the non-pregnant state, possibly due to the enlarged breast masking the development of the disease until it is of a larger size. The progress of the disease and the speed of metastasis may also be influenced by the vascularity of the breast but this is not certain.

Management of the breast lump

When a mass is found in the breast at first examination, the most important step is to make a histological diagnosis. This may be achieved by excision biopsy, needle biopsy or fine-needle aspiration cytology.

The dilemma of mastectomy or conservative management

Currently there is a powerful change in opinion away from the more radical procedures involving removal of the breast towards those where the breast is preserved. The most favoured procedures are the 'lumpectomy' (segmental resection of breast), and wide local excision followed by radiotherapy to the entire breast, usually in the form of local implants and external beam irradiation.

Unfortunately, using these techniques there is no information available on the status of the regional lymph nodes; therefore, it is difficult to compare treatment methods in detail.

This pressure to perform less and less surgery has developed not only from within the medical profession but also from lay pressure groups. Because breast cancer has a prolonged lifecycle, there is no long-term information available as to the efficacy of these conservative techniques.

Should the pregnancy be terminated?

There is no necessity to carry out termination simply on the basis of the presence of the cancer; the surgery involved is relatively minor, and even if the patient is to have a full course of radiotherapy, it is not difficult to shield the pregnancy completely.

A problem arises if the patient is to be treated with chemotherapy, when it is advisable to terminate the pregnancy because of the theoretical risk of malformation or the induction of tumours in the fetus. If the pregnancy is advanced, there is no harm in delaying chemotherapy until the patient has delivered.

Breast feeding

This is usually discouraged on the grounds that the en-

gorgement and markedly increased stimulation of the breast may stimulate the development of field changes in the remaining breast tissue.

Subsequent pregnancy

The questions 'Is there a safe period following treatment when a pregnancy can be embarked upon?' and 'Does a future pregnancy alter the prospects for the patient?' are extremely difficult to answer. As this cancer has such a long natural progression interval, there may be no safe time when the patient may embark upon a pregnancy, and conversely there is no evidence that future pregnancies put the patient at higher risk of recurrence or the development of a new cancer.

Carcinoma of the cervix and cervical intraepithelial neoplasia (CIN)

The abnormal cervical smear in pregnancy will always present difficult management problems. It is now generally advocated that patients should be screened for CIN during the antenatal period if they have not attended routine screening.

Worries about difficulties in interpreting smears taken in pregnancy can be largely discounted; good cytology laboratories have little difficulty in differentiating pregnancy changes from those of CIN.

The general availability of colposcopy services has revolutionized the management of the abnormal cervical smear in pregnancy. Using this instrument it is possible to confidently differentiate those patients with an intraepithelial lesion and those with a possibly invasive lesion. The colposcopist is also able to identify the site of origin of the abnormal smear and to clearly delineate its full extent; his only limitations are those lesions which extend into the endocervical canal when the colposcopy is described as *unsatisfactory*.

The most important functions of colposcopy are to identify the site of origin of the abnormal smear and to enable the clinician to differentiate between non-invasive and possibly invasive lesions on the cervix. Having made this distinction, the management is straightforward.

1 The non-invasive lesion can be monitored during the remainder of the pregnancy using cytology and colposcopy. The patient is then reviewed 3 months following parturition and the cervix reassessed. It is at this

visit that the cervical lesion is biopsied and further management determined which, in the majority of cases, will take the form of some type of excisional procedure or local ablative therapy such as laser vaporization (see Chapter 4).

2 The possibly invasive lesion must be managed in such a way that the maximum information is obtained about its nature. This means that an adequate biopsy of the cervix must be made so that the pathologist may comment about the presence or absence of invasion, the depth of invasion and any involvement of endothelial-lined spaces in the stroma. All these factors will be taken into account when determining management.

Adequate biopsy

It is tempting to take a small colposcopically directed punch biopsy in the outpatient clinic. This is dangerous for two reasons: first, the punch biopsy is frequently too small for the pathologist to make an adequate comment about depth of invasion and vascular channel involvement; and secondly, the biopsy may be misdirected and not give a representative specimen of the area suspected of being invasive.

The authors have experienced the false sense of security engendered by a tiny biopsy taken in pregnancy, with tragic consequences as the patient presents with a metastasizing carcinoma in the postpartum period.

Cone, wedge or loop biopsy

This is the optimal type of biopsy, providing the pathologist with an adequate block of tissue upon which to base his comments, thus giving the clinician all the information required to organize the management of the patient.

The major problem associated with carrying out this procedure in the pregnant patient is the risk of bleeding and miscarriage.

Anaesthesia
Clearly, this is not a procedure to be performed under limited anaesthesia; therefore, it is usually recommended that a general anaesthetic is given.

Patient preparation
The patient is given a tocolytic if pregnancy is advanced, beginning a few days prior to the procedure. It is important that an adequate quantity of fresh blood is available for transfusion prior to the operation as there is a significant risk of haemorrhage both during and following the operation.

Special precautions to reduce bleeding
Various techniques have been advocated, including the Simmons cervical clamp, injection of vasopressin directly into the cervical tissue, and the placing of lateral haemostatic sutures as are used in a routine cone biopsy. Whichever the surgeon chooses, great gentleness is necessary when handling the cervix and sutures should not be pulled too tight or they will cut through the pregnant tissue and cause more haemorrhage. The authors advocate the use of a series of mattress sutures around the edge of the cone or wedge to control bleeding, but does not recommend the use of Sturmdorf sutures, or the prophylactic insertion of a McDonald suture to ward off abortion.

Management of the rest of pregnancy

CIN is not an indication for an elective Caesarean section. A vaginal delivery should be the method of choice. The patient who has had a cone biopsy performed during pregnancy is at higher risk of losing the fetus due to miscarriage or premature labour. Therefore, such patients must be carefully monitored for the rest of the pregnancy in a specialized unit capable of managing these problems. At delivery, the risk of cervical laceration or stenosis is also greatly increased.

Management of the CIN for the rest of the pregnancy

If the clinician is confident that he is not dealing with an invasive lesion, all that is required is that the patient should be reviewed at 3 monthly intervals for the rest of pregnancy using colposcopy and cytology. Close to term, colposcopy is difficult and uncomfortable for the patient, especially if the fetal head has descended into the pelvis; therefore, visits should be timed so that the patient is not called close to term. The cervix should be completely reassessed 3 months postpartum. This assessment must include colposcopic biopsies of any abnormal areas.

Dealing with a diagnosis of invasive disease

The method of management will depend entirely upon the pathologist's report. In it he must comment upon the limits of resection of the lesion, the depth of invasion, the width of the invasion, confluency and the presence of vascular channel involvement.

Depth of invasion

The depth of invasion which constitutes 'microinvasion' remains contentious. The generally accepted limit for relatively conservative management, where the risk of metastasis is minimal, is 3 mm. If the depth of invasion is less than this and the entire lesion has been removed in the biopsy, then it is not unreasonable to allow the pregnancy to continue to term.

At depths of invasion greater than 3 mm, the risks of lymphatic metastasis rises markedly; therefore the case should be treated more radically.

Limits of resection

Where the pathologist reports that the limits of resection cannot be confidently seen and the possibility of residual tumour arises, the patient must have further treatment. Except at the endocervical limit, it should be possible with the aid of the colposcope at operation to outline the entire limits of the lesion, thus eliminating a frustrating decision for the clinician.

Width of invasion

Not only is the depth of invasion important but also the width and possibly the volume of the disease. It is not practicable to measure the lesion in three dimensions, but it is reasonable to ask the pathologist to comment on the width as well as the depth.

Lesions up to 7 mm wide and 3 mm deep may be treated with conservative surgery (stage 1a$_1$).

Confluency

The question of whether a confluent or disparate lesion is more malignant remains unanswered; authorities have made conflicting statements.

Vascular channel involvement

Similarly, the finding of spaces filled with apparently embolizing tumour cells have led some to believe that this is an ominous sign but, to date, evidence is conflicting. It is the authors' view that where this occurs the patient should be treated radically.

It is important that a vaginal delivery should not be attempted in the presence of invasive disease.

It is now generally accepted that the pregnancy should be sacrificed so that the carcinoma may be treated. The main exceptions to this rule are when the pregnancy is close to term or where there is a possibility of producing a live fetus if a Caesarean section is performed. Prenatal assessment of fetal well-being, particularly ultrasound scan, should be performed. When fetal viability is borderline, improved lung function may be stimulated by the use of corticosteroids. It is possibly because of improvements in fetal medicine and in neonatal paediatrics, and the fact that many cancers of the cervix in pregnancy are diagnosed early, that caesarean section followed by a radical Wertheim's-type hysterectomy is the usual method of management.

Surgical treatment is the management method of choice in all young patients with stage Ib and IIa disease. This allows the ovaries to be conserved. In early pregnancy, the uterus is removed intact with the fetus *in situ*; in later pregnancy, the fetus is delivered to the paediatricians after Caesarean section.

The operation is usually easy to perform because tissue planes are easily found. However, this is often offset by engorgement of the pelvic vasculature; this is no place for the clumsy surgeon. The pregnant patient is at high risk of thromboembolic disease, infection from the necrotic carcinoma and haemorrhage from the engorged pelvic vessels. The prudent surgeon should take special precautions to obviate these risks.

Radiotherapeutic treatment is the best method of management for all later stage disease (stages IIb, IIIa, IIIb and the rare stage IV). If there is a viable fetus present, the radiotherapy should follow classical Caesarean section. If the pregnancy is deemed non-viable, radiotherapy should be given in the form of external irradiation which induces a spontaneous abortion followed by central boosting with an intrauterine source. There is a high risk of intrauterine infection.

Carcinoma of the cervix diagnosed during delivery

Unfortunately, this problem still arises. The optimum course of management is to deliver the fetus by emergency Caesarean section if the labour has not progressed. Where labour is advanced and delivery imminent, the best that can be made of the case is for the fetus to be delivered, any haemorrhage dealt with and treatment with radical surgery or radiotherapy organized.

The two areas of concern are the risk of dissemination of malignant cells from the cervix and the very significant risk of severe haemorrhage from the cancerous cervix. It may be necessary to perform an emergency radical hysterectomy if the haemorrhage cannot be controlled; the patient's life is at serious risk.

Carcinoma of the vulva

As this is predominantly a problem of the older woman, the mean age in the editor's series of over 270 cases being 68 years, it is rarely seen in pregnant women. The editor has seen one case developing in a 26-year-old woman and presenting at 20 weeks' gestation. This was successfully dealt with, utilizing the three-incision technique of radical vulvectomy and bilateral groin node dissection (see Chapter 13).

Pregnancy does not seem to have any bearing on the course of the disease.

The editor has experience of another patient in his series who has gone on after radical vulvectomy and groin node dissection to become pregnant twice and produce healthy children, albeit by Caesarean section. The obstetrician, unfortunately, had other indications for a surgical delivery. In general, there is no reason why a vaginal delivery should not be performed.

Carcinoma of the vagina

As with carcinoma of the vulva, this is predominantly a disease of women in later life, the mean age being 60 years. Rarely, the problem arises in young women and may be of the clear cell carcinoma type; the editor has experience of one such case presenting in a 20-year-old patient at 18 weeks' gestation. A radical hysterectomy and pelvic node dissection was performed, sacrificing the pregnancy; the carcinoma was lying in the posterior fornix of the vagina. The patient is alive and well years later.

Carcinoma of the ovary

The great majority of ovarian tumours complicating pregnancy are benign, usually being corpora lutea. Carcinoma of the ovary in pregnancy is very rare, occurring in 1 in 10 000 pregnancies.

As with ovarian masses in the non-pregnant state, the most important concern of the clinician is to make a diagnosis. This is suggested at bimanual examination,

provisionally made using ultrasound, and finally confirmed by the pathologist after removal at laparotomy.

The presence of the fetus merely complicates a well worked out diagnostic route.

Early pregnancy

As a general rule, unless there is considerable evidence of the presence of a malignancy, or the ovarian mass is undergoing some mechanical problem, surgery should be avoided in the first trimester. Most ovarian masses are corpora lutea; ultrasound should be used to determine whether there are solid or cystic areas present and to monitor changing size of the mass. However, the surgeon should remember that the corpora lutea may continue to grow to a large size under the influence of the gonadotropins.

Mid and late pregnancy

Once the pregnancy is maintaining itself independently of the ovaries, management of ovarian masses can safely be more aggressive. However, if there is a possibility at any time in gestation of a malignancy being present, a laparotomy should be performed.

If, when the abdomen is opened, there is evidence of a cancer of the ovaries the standard management of total abdominal hysterectomy, bilateral ovariotomy and omentectomy should be performed, the pregnancy sacrificed if non-viable or delivered by Caesarean section and handed to the paediatricians if viable. The surgical management should be followed by appropriate chemotherapy.

Mechanical obstruction is occasionally the method of presentation of an ovarian mass which, until removed, must be looked upon with suspicion. This problem usually arises later in pregnancy and is diagnosed in the course of investigating an unstable or unusual lie of the fetus. Ultrasound should be performed and the characteristics of the mass determined. If the fetus is viable an elective caesarean section should be performed, followed by appropriate treatment. When the cyst appears benign, it is removed and the remaining pelvic organs preserved. If there is a suspicion of malignancy, the procedure outlined above is performed.

Symptomatic presentation due to torsion, rupture or haemorrhage into the cystic mass will occur from time to time. This should be treated as an acute episode and, unless delivery is imminent, a laparotomy performed and the mass removed. If a diagnosis of carcinoma is made later, the patient should be re-explored after delivery and the standard surgical management performed (see Chapter 20).

Further reading

Textbooks

JS Shepherd, in Chapter 16 of *Clinical Gynaecological Oncology* (1985) Shepherd and Monaghan (eds), Blackwell Scientific, Oxford, has made a comprehensive review of the present state of the subject. He has carefully commented on the rare re-

lationship between the pregnancy and tumour growth, the rare involvement of the fetus, and methods of preserving reproductive capacity.

References

Many of the references available relate to single cases or collected cases from major institutions. The student should initially turn his attention to the major review articles, such as that in *Surgical Disease in Pregnancy*, Barber HRK, Graber EA (eds), Philadelphia: W.B. Saunders, pp. 310–35.

Also, Lutz MH, Underwood PB, Rozier JC, Putney JW. Genital malignancy in pregnancy. *Am J Obstet Gynecol* 1977;129:536–42.

26 Operations on the intestinal tract for the gynaecologist

It is rare for the gynaecological surgeon to be involved with bowel surgery as part of routine gynaecological surgery. However, he should be able to perform an appendicectomy, and repair occasional small injuries to the bowel created whilst separating adhesions. If he has any doubt or if the primary pathology is gastrointestinal, the general surgeon should be called.

Appendicectomy

The question of whether to remove the appendix at the time of laparotomy for pelvic disease remains contentious. In British practice, the appendix is not removed, except when it is found to be abnormal on inspection. The appendix should always be removed in cases of pseudomyxoma peritoneii as this condition is often associated with tumours of the appendix. The presence of faecoliths, mucoceles or any signs of inflammation warrants its removal, provided that the extra operating time does not hazard the patient. The major concern of the surgeon is the risk of contaminating the clean peritoneal cavity with the contents of the appendix. It is vitally important that a technique should be used which reduces this risk to zero and that the patient is given an appropriate prophylactic antibiotic.

Instruments

The general set described in Chapter 2 will be in use; the only addition which is required is a Babcock soft tissue forceps and a fine 2.0 Vicryl suture on a round-bodied atraumatic needle.

Patient preparation

No special preoperative preparation is required, although if the appendix is found to be inflamed at laparotomy or there is evidence of free pus, a Gram-negative-specific antibiotic should be given intravenously during the procedure.

Anaesthesia

No special requirement is necessary, except for general anaesthesia.

The operation

The incision
The appendix can be reached through most standard gynaecological incisions and therefore there is no special need to extend or alter the original wound. However, it is very important that the edges of the wound should not be soiled by contact with the appendix or the appendix stump when the appendix has been removed. The surgeon should take precautions to cover and screen the edges of the wound, and impress on the assistants the need to keep the appendix clear at all times.

Dividing the appendix mesentery
The appendix is elevated using the Babcock forceps, putting the appendiceal mesentery on the stretch. In thin patients, the small appendiceal artery can often be visualized. A short, straight tissue clamp is placed across the vessel with its tip close to the wall of the appendix (Fig. 26.1). Using scissors the mesentery is cut,

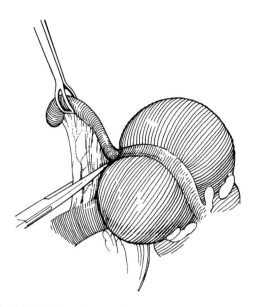

Fig. 26.1 Dividing the appendix mesentery.

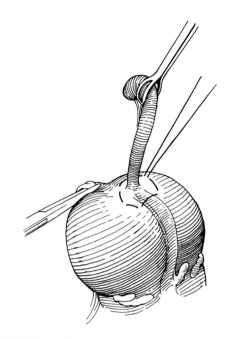

Fig. 26.2 Placing the purse-string suture.

leaving the appendix attached to the caecum solely by its base. When the appendix is long, more than one pedicle may be required.

Placing the purse-string suture
It is advantageous to place the purse-string suture around the base of the appendix before it is removed as this reduces the risk of contamination. The Vicryl suture is now inserted in a series of bites around the base of the appendix (Fig. 26.2), taking care not to place them too close as this makes inversion difficult.

Removing the appendix
The base of the appendix is now crushed using a straight clamp which is then replaced a short distance down the appendix; a Vicryl tie is now placed around the crushed part of the appendix and the ends left long and held in a forceps (Fig. 26.3). The surgeon now cuts across the appendix below the clamp and places it, and the knife which has been contaminated by the bowel contents, into a dish. (The scrub nurse removes this from the operative field.)

Inversion of the appendix stump
As the surgeon cuts through the appendix the assistant steadies the long tie in one hand and grasps the caecal

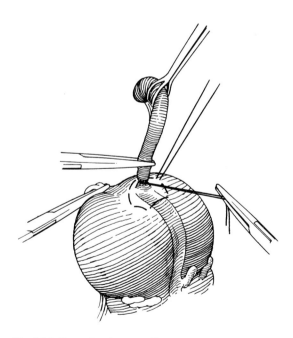

Fig. 26.3 Removing the appendix.

cut end of the appendix with a small forceps. Thus, as the surgeon begins to draw the purse-string suture tight, the assistant slips the end of the appendix below the surface produced by the invaginating edges of the caecum. The small forceps are then discarded.

Variations in technique

There are many minor variations of this procedure, including not burying the stump at all.

Retrograde appendicectomy may be necessary when the tip or part of the length of the organ is involved in adhesions or not readily accessible, such as in the retro-caecal position. The base is cleared around its circumference and clamped, tied, cut and invaginated as described above. The remainder of the appendix is then dissected free from all adhesions. If the surgeon stays close to the caecum there is a readily found tissue plane which is often very simply separated, reducing the risk of entering either the appendix or the caecum. Rarely, it may be necessary to remove the appendix piecemeal; this should be avoided as the risk of contamination of the abdominal cavity is considerable.

If the appendix is inflamed and pus is present in the peritoneal cavity, the surgeon should carry out peritoneal lavage with an antiseptic solution, having first taken bacteriology swabs for culture and drug sensitivity.

Management of operative injuries of the intestine

The majority of injuries to bowel are avoidable.

One of the commonest circumstances when bowel is damaged is when the peritoneum is opened. This may be due to adhesion of bowel to the parietal peritoneum or simply due to the fact that the surgeon has picked up an edge of bowel in the forceps when elevating the peritoneum prior to incision. The simple safeguard of running the fingers between the forceps will reduce this risk almost to nil.

Other causes include:
1 Lack of experience in handling bowel, particularly bowel damaged by irradiation or affected by disease such as carcinoma deposits.
2 An inadequate incision or poor light, which gives poor vision of the operative field and requires assistants to retract unnecessarily forcefully to gain access.
3 Unnecessary haste and carelessness in performing

the procedure, resulting in clamps being placed on bowel, or tears produced when adhesions are roughly separated.

The major pathological factors involved in the development of traumatic injuries to the bowel are:
1 Endometriosis, particularly the chronic disease with development of chocolate cysts of the ovary and multiple adhesions to tube uterus and bowel.
2 Pelvic inflammatory disease, particularly chronic disease, where multiple adhesions may have developed.
3 Malignant disease, particularly ovarian carcinoma.
4 Infective disease of the bowel, such as acute appendicitis, will also produce multiple adhesive problems for the gynaecologist as the infection commonly drains into the pelvis affecting tubes and ovaries as well as small bowel.
5 Radiotherapy damage and the recently reported adhesive peritonitis, which may develop after the combined use of radiotherapy and some chemotherapeutic agents.
6 Tuberculosis, which is now rarer than in former years but still occurs and presents grave management problems to the surgeon when the process of adhesive peritonitis has developed.

The operation

Closed trauma

If the damage to the bowel has not resulted in opening the lumen but has simply incised the serosa, allowing the mucosa to 'bubble' through, all that is required is for the serosa to be resutured over the defect using a single layer of continuous Vicryl on an atraumatic round-bodied needle.

Open damage

If the lumen has been entered, the surgeon must determine whether the bowel has been devitalized or not. If the damage is via a clean cut without crushing of the edges of the lesion, it may be possible to perform a primary repair. This should be performed in a single layer apposing the serosa using either a continuous or an interrupted suturing technique with Vicryl or Monocryl. It is important not to narrow the bowel lumen when repairing so the defect should be repaired transversely and sutures should not be drawn too tightly. The repaired bowel must be examined for patency by grasping the lumen under the repair between finger and thumb making allowances for the fact that postopera-

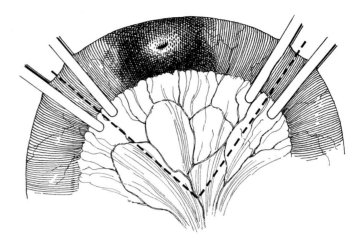

Fig. 26.4 Resection of a damaged segment of small bowel.

tive oedema may further reduce the diameter of the lumen.

Nasogastric tube
If the repair is in the proximal part of the small bowel it is a useful safeguard to ask the anaesthetist to insert a nasogastric tube during the anaesthetic and maintain it until satisfactory bowel action returns in the postoperative period.

Resection of a segment of bowel
If the traumatized length of bowel becomes dark due to loss of blood supply or where there has been extensive tearing or crushing of the edges, the surgeon must be prepared to resect the segment. This may be performed either in the traditional manner described here or using stapling techniques similar to those described in Chapter 28. The principles are identical.

Identifying the arterial arcade and resecting the affected segment If the segment of bowel containing the traumatized area is elevated and transilluminated, the arterial arcade can be identified. Soft, non-occluding bowel clamps are then applied so that an adequate vascular supply reaches the proposed resection lines (Fig. 26.4). 'Crushing' bowel clamps are then placed at either end of the segment to be removed and the segment is then resected by cutting along the 'crushing' clamps. The small vessels in the mesentery are tied with 2 or 3.0 Vicryl.

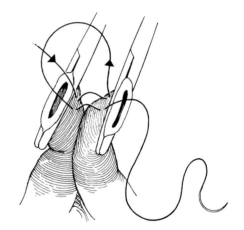

Fig. 26.5 Suturing the serosa of the bowel segments.

Suturing the bowel The two ends of the bowel are now drawn together and repaired in a single layer beginning at the posterior layer of serosa (Fig. 26.5) and continuing round (Fig. 26.6) to join the initial suture. The author uses a continuous suture of 2.0 Monocryl on a round-bodied atraumatic needle. Some authorities advocate interrupted sutures and others still recommend repair in two layers.

Suturing the mesentery The two edges of the mesentery are now apposed using interrupted Vicryl sutures. It is important to pick up the peritoneal edges on both

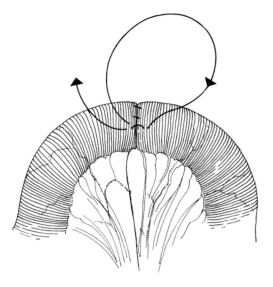

Fig. 26.6 Completing the serosal suture.

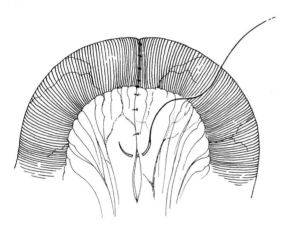

Fig. 26.7 Apposing the mesenteric edges.

surfaces of the mesentery and not to take bites which are so large as to damage the vasculature (Fig. 26.7).

The mesentery must be handled delicately at all times as it is very easy to traumatize the small vessels, producing a spreading haematoma which may further jeopardize the blood supply to the bowel.

This technique of resection of bowel can be applied to any length of bowel, both large and small.

The formation of a colostomy

In current practice it is unnecessary that a gynaecological surgeon know how to perform a colostomy, but it should be standard practice for a gynaecological oncologist. The indications for this procedure are various and include rectal involvement in ovarian carcinoma, the occurrence of gross radiotherapy damage in the pelvis, as part of the management of rectovaginal fistulae, certain cases of diverticulitis, and as a preliminary manoeuvre prior to an anovulvectomy.

Siting of the stoma

This is a skill which the gynaecological oncology surgeon should learn, but is normally performed by the stoma therapist who should visit the patient in the preoperative period if a stoma is planned or likely. For emergency colostomies the surgeon must rely on his own ability to site the stoma correctly.

Patient preparation

If the colostomy is a planned procedure, the patient should have the bowel as empty as possible and some authorities recommend the gut flora should be sterilized using a non-absorbable oral antibiotic.

The bowel should be emptied using a combination of an oral aperient with or without an enema. High colonic lavage and extreme purgation with agents such as magnesium sulphate is not acceptable and simply produces lassitude and demoralization in the patient.

Clearly, when the colostomy has to be made as an emergency procedure, bowel preparation cannot be carried out and the patient should be given intravenous antibiotics during and following the surgery.

The type of colostomy to be made will depend mainly on whether it is intended to be temporary or permanent.

Temporary colostomy

The position of the stoma will depend upon future surgical requirements. The colostomy should be sited away from areas where further intervention is considered. For most purposes, a mid-line upper abdominal site is suitable, the left iliac fossa site being used for a temporary colostomy only when no further surgery is envisaged in that area.

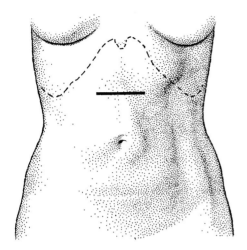

Fig. 26.8 The site of incision for a temporary transverse colostomy.

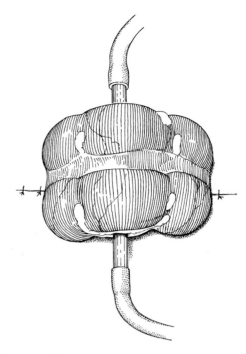

Fig. 26.9 Anchoring the loop of large bowel to the surface.

The operation
Opening the abdomen Frequently, the abdomen will be open when the decision to perform a temporary colostomy is made. However, if it is not, the site of choice is usually above the umbilicus in the mid-line (Fig. 26.8). The incision is made transversely, incising the rectus sheath and separating the muscles so that the peritoneum is entered in the mid-line.

Forming the loop colostomy The transverse colon is identified and drawn out of the wound; it is easy to identify the colon because of the taenia running longitudinally. The greater omentum is seen to extend from the inferior border of the colon and should be dissected from the colon over a distance of about 10 cm; small vessels are easily identified and ligated.

Anchoring the loop The cleared loop of colon is now drawn out of the wound and a small hole made in the mesentery through which a bridge is passed so as to anchor the loop above the surface (Fig. 26.9).

Closing the abdomen The fascia is now drawn together over the rectus muscles so as not to press too tightly upon the colon and the skin edges are sutured in a similar manner. It is not usually necessary to suture the colon to the edges of the stoma.

Opening the stoma The bowel is opened along its antemesenteric border through a taenia, as this area is relatively avascular. A stoma bag is immediately applied so that the patient leaves theatre with the colostomy completed and fitted with an appropriate appliance.

Removal of the bridge The stoma bridge can be removed as soon as serosal adhesions have formed, usually within 4–5 days.

Reversal of the colostomy The great advantage of the loop colostomy is the ease with which it can be reversed. All that is required is for the adhesions between the bowel wall and the abdominal wall to be carefully dissected free, the bowel closed using a single-layered closure (made transversely so as not to narrow the lumen) and the colon reinserted into the abdomen. The abdominal wall is then closed in layers as described in Chapter 6.

A permanent colostomy

It will be rare for the gynaecologist to have to make a

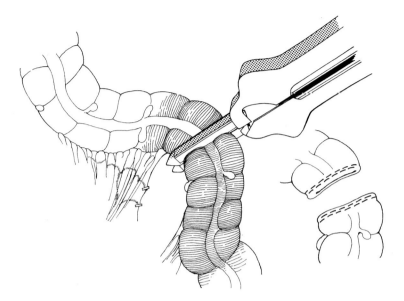

Fig. 26.10 Dividing large bowel using the GIA stapling device.

permanent stoma unless he is involved in gynaecological oncology. The optimum site for a permanent stoma is in the left iliac fossa, away from bony prominences and fatty folds. The site should be smooth, both when the patient stands and when she sits.

Patient preparation
The bowel should be prepared as described above.

The operation
Opening the abdomen The abdomen is frequently opened for another purpose but if not, a lower mid-line incision will give good access and allow the stoma appliances to be attached without impinging on the wound. Occasionally it may be adequate to make a small transverse incision at the site for the stoma and pull the sigmoid through it to form stoma.

Choosing the bowel segment The sigmoid colon is usually the site of bowel to be resected; the loop is elevated and transilluminated. If the sigmoid is not mobile it can be freed further by incising the avascular peritoneum lateral to the colon in the paracolic gutter; this releases and rotates the bowel medially.

Dividing the bowel The authors use the Gastro Intestinal Anastomosis (GIA) stapling device at all times for this procedure because of its great accuracy and cleanliness. When a suitable segment has been chosen, the small

vessels in the mesentery are divided and ligated so as to release a length of bowel which will reach to the stoma site without tension. The GIA stapling device is now placed over the loop at right angles to the lumen and fired (Fig. 26.10). This leaves the distal end of the bowel sealed with the staples which, having been checked for bleeding, is lowered into the pelvis.

Making the stoma The marked stoma site is now picked up with a Littlewood's forceps and by cutting transversely with the scalpel a perfect circle of skin is removed, approximatley 3 cm in diameter (Fig. 26.11). The peritoneum on the stoma side of the abdominal wound is grasped in a tissue forceps so that it is not drawn towards the stoma, distorting the intra-abdominal opening. The surgeon then places the first two fingers of his left hand under the stoma site (Fig. 26.12) and elevates the peritoneum and the abdominal aponeurosis, which he incises with a scalpel or diathermy, the assistant clipping the layers in turn as they are cut. The stoma so produced should comfortably admit the first two fingers of the hand.

Exteriorizing the bowel By passing a pair of Babcock's tissue forceps through the stoma, the stapled proximal end of the sigmoid loop is now drawn out of the orifice. The loop is checked for undue tension, and then the line of staples is cut off and the edge of the bowel sutured to the skin (Fig. 26.13). It is unnecessary to suture the edges of the aponeurosis and the peritoneum to the bowel.

Applying the colostomy appliance The stoma bag is applied in theatre making sure that it does not impinge on the mid-line incision.

Closing the abdomen The abdomen is now closed as described in Chapter 6.

The formation of a loop ileostomy

The authors are increasingly performing a temporary loop ileostomy in preference to a temporary colostomy. The reasons are numerous but include the fact that there is more mobility with the mesentery of the small bowel and the contents are more fluid, reducing the risk of anastomosis breakdown. The procedure is planned as a temporary stoma, but occasionally when formed for intestinal obstruction in ovarian cancer is never reversed. The technique is similar to that for a colostomy.

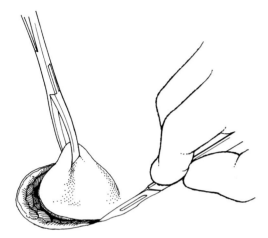

Fig. 26.11 Removing the skin disc at the stoma site.

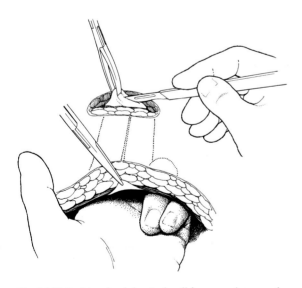

Fig. 26.12 Incising the abdominal wall fat, musculature and peritoneum.

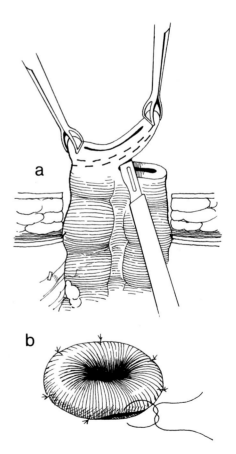

Fig. 26.13 Removing the staple line (a) and suturing the edge to the skin (b).

279

The operation

Opening the abdomen
The abdomen is usually open when the decision to make an ileostomy is made.

Making the stoma
This is prepared as for the permanent colostomy. All the authors' patients with advanced ovarian cancer are sited preoperatively for both a potential ileostomy and colostomy.

Forming the loop
The intended segment of terminal ileum is pulled through the stoma site using a Babcock's tissue forceps. A bridge can be inserted to keep the loop in place.

Opening the stoma
The bowel is opened transversely at the distal part of the loop and the incision is extended to about half the circumference (Fig. 26.14). A mucosa is inverted and a rose bud is formed, the greater prominence being the proximal segment of the loop (Fig. 26.15).

Removal of the bridge
This can be removed after 4–5 days.

Reversal of the ileostomy
This is similar to that for the temporary colostomy with the bowel repaired with a single layer closure.

Side-to-side anastomosis procedure

This technique of bypassing a segment of bowel which is obstructed or grossly damaged by tumour or irradiation is a valuable technique to learn.

Preoperative preparation

It may be difficult to achieve perfect preparation of the bowel if there is an element of obstruction. Therefore, the surgeon must be prepared to decompress the bowel if necessary prior to performing the procedure.

The operation

Opening the abdomen
The incision can be any which gives adequate access to

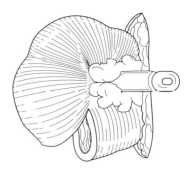

Fig. 26.14 Incising the ileum.

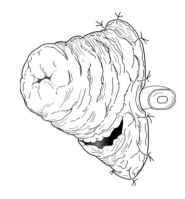

Fig. 26.15 Forming a 'rose bud'.

the entire abdomen, and is capable of being extended where necessary.

Identifying the site of obstruction
The surgeon must be prepared to spend some time in ascertaining the site of the obstruction and correctly identifying healthy bowel proximal and distal to the obstruction. It is particularly important that the bypass anastomosis should not be performed using irradiated bowel.

Stapling the bowel
One of the commonest techniques necessary is to bypass the distal small bowel and first part of the large bowel. The healthy ileum is drawn to the transverse colon and laid alongside it. The two lengths of bowel are lightly held using non-crushing clamps proximal to where the anastomosis is to be made (Fig. 26.16). A

small opening is made in each segment of bowel and the GIA instrument inserted and fired, producing a stapled communication between the two segments (Fig. 26.17). The device is withdrawn and the two small openings closed with a single layered closure using a Vicryl or Monocryl suture. The communication between the ileum and transverse colon will be approximately two fingers wide.

Producing a mucous fistula
If the reason for the bypass is gross radiation damage to distal small bowel, the area can be further managed by closing off the small bowel beyond the anastomosis and bringing out the free distal end to the skin surface as a mucous fistula.

Further reading

The recommendation which the main editor made in his earlier edition was 'to develop the habit of reading outside the subject is particularly apposite in relationship to this chapter. The gynaecologist must frequently pick up the latest ideas from his surgical colleagues and never be too proud to steal an idea or two'.

Within gynaecological texts I would recommend the 3rd edition of *Atlas of Gynecological Surgery including Breast Surgery and Related Urological and Intestinal Surgical Operations* edited by Hirsch HA, Hans A, Käser O, Ikle FA and Franz A; published by Thieme in 1997. This textbook includes

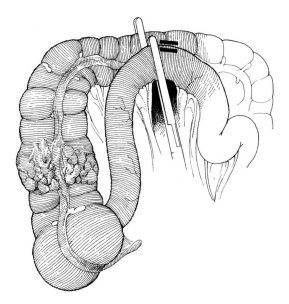

Fig. 26.16 Apposing the small and large bowel.

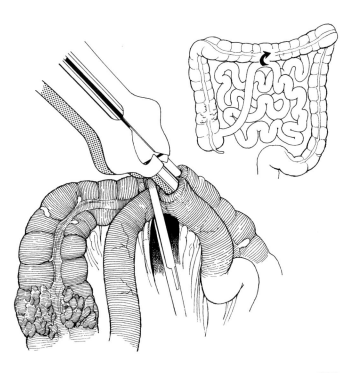

Fig. 26.17 Forming a stapled communication between large and small bowel.

two chapters describing intestinal surgical procedures related to gynaecological surgery.

Textbooks

Stapling is Surgery by Felicien Steichen and Mark Ravitch, published by Year Book Medical Publishing, Chicago, demonstrates the wide variety of techniques for managing both elective and emergency surgery of the bowel. The trainee gynaecologist should have a copy available.

References

There are many papers to which the reader should apply himself; one important paper dealing with a large experience of the use of the surgical stapler is that of Wheeless CR and Dorsey JH Use of the automatic surgical stapler for intestinal anastomosis associated with gynecologic malignancy: a review of 283 procedures. *Gynecol Oncol* 1981;11:1–7.

27 Presacral neurectomy

Occasionally, patients will present with intractable pelvic pain. This may be due to recurrent carcinoma, radiation damage to pelvic bones and nerves, chronic endometriosis and, very occasionally, chronic debilitating dysmenorrhoea. When all normal medical management methods have been tried and have failed, the patient may gain some relief from the performance of a presacral neurectomy. In general, the pain experienced in the pelvis due to the conditions above cannot be dealt with by resection of any single group of nerves; therefore, the surgeon must think very carefully before embarking on this procedure and must never offer the operation to the patient with extreme pain as a 'cure all'. The best results will be obtained if the pain is identifiable as originating from the uterus. Little if any improvement will be found if the pain is of more lateral origin.

The procedure consists of the excision of the presacral nerves as they pass over the first two segments of the sacrum. The nerves contained within these cords are of both sympathetic and parasympathetic origin. The nerves pass from the anterior surface of the lower aorta as a fenestrated cord to lie immediately below the peritoneum on the last lumbar and first two sacral vertebrae.

Instruments

The instruments in the gynaecological general set described in Chapter 2 are required.

The operation

Opening of the abdominal cavity
This is best performed using a subumbilical mid-line incision. Some authorities have advocated a paramedian incision extended above the umbilicus; this is only of value if the patient is excessively obese, when access will be difficult with any incision.

Packing off of the intestines
This is an important part of the procedure and is helped by using a steep Trendelenburg position. Access to the lower part of the abdominal aorta is required; this is easily achieved if the assistant holds the packed bowel with a broad-bladed short retractor such as the Morris or Pyrah.

Incising the peritoneum
The bifurcation of the aorta is identified and the peritoneum lying over it picked up lightly in toothed dissectors and incised. Care must be taken to cut the peritoneum only when its under-surface can be inspected. The surgeon must remember that the ureter is closely applied to the under-surface, only a short distance from the mid-line.

The peritoneal incision is extended longitudinally, the edges are gripped with tissue forceps and the area over the lower aorta exposed (Fig. 27.1).

Identifying and dividing the nerve trunks
The nerve bundle is easily picked up as it runs over the surface of the common iliac vessel. Having taken care to identify and if necessary isolate the ureters, the nerve trunks are picked up by under-running them with an

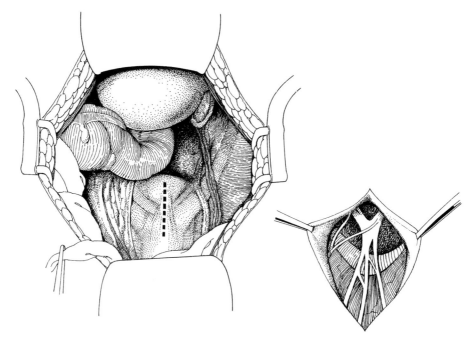

Fig. 27.1 The site of incision and exposing the presacral nerves.

aneurysm needle. The fenestrated bundle is now separated from the inferior mesenteric artery down to the first sacral vertebra and the nerve is clipped, cut and the segment removed. The segment should be sent for pathological examination, as a litigious flavour often pervades these cases.

Closing the peritoneum
The incision in the peritoneum is closed using an absorbable suture.

Closing the abdomen
This is performed as described in Chapter 6.

Complications

Most of the problems associated with this procedure are due to failure to identify properly all the structures in the operation field. If identification is meticulous, fears of dividing the ureters or the inferior mesenteric artery are groundless. Bleeding is rarely a problem but if small vessels ooze they may confuse the anatomy; small vessels should be dealt with using small metal artery clips (Auto sutures or liga clips).

The laparoscopic uterine nerve ablation procedure (LUNA)

Dysmenorrhoea is a major problem for many women during their menstrual lifetime.

Dysmenorrhoea will vary from the tolerable to the disabling. Many patients lose work and study time because of its effect and will have significant alterations in personal performance during the period of pain.

Surgery has been recommended in the past utilizing presacral neurectomy, but in recent years the division of the uterosacral ligament, whereby nerves passing to the uterus are resected, has achieved more prominent usage. The sensory parasympathetic and sympathetic nerve supply to the cervix and uterus pass under and around the attachments of the uterosacral ligament lying posterior to the cervix. The ligament is readily accessed laparoscopically and for those patients who have tried all standard medications for dysmenorrhoea and the problem has become chronic, this procedure should be considered. Unfortunately, the procedure cannot always be guaranteed to clear all pain, and patients should be advised that complete removal of dysmenorrhoea may or may not be achieved. The major aim is to reduce the discomfort of dysmenorrhoea rather than to guarantee to remove it completely.

Operative procedure

The standard laparoscopic equipment utilized in modern theatres will suffice. The procedure is carried out using a double puncture technique, usually utilizing the laser for the precise surgical destruction of tissue, although some others have used diathermy to transect the uterosacral ligaments.

Identification of the uterosacral ligaments

The assistant should antevert the uterus drawing the uterus over to one or other side in order to make the uterosacral ligaments stand out. This can usually be achieved by either simply inserting a Hegar dilator into the uterus or, more appropriately, a modern uterine manipulator. The ureters can be visualized through the peritoneum and large vessels associated with the ligaments noted and avoided.

Laser ablation of the uterosacral ligaments

The CO_2 laser may be transmitted down the central channel of the laparoscope or via the iliac fossa trochar. The double puncture technique allows better visualization and easier manipulation of the laser beam. The laser is set to a high power density of $10\,000$–$15\,000\,W/cm^2$ and the uterosacral ligaments are vaporized near the point of their attachment to the posterior aspect of the cervix. The concept of the procedure is to ablate the sensory nerve fibres completely. This is usually achieved by leaving a crater approximately 1 cm in diameter 5 mm deep over each uterosacral ligament. The safer side to vaporize is medially rather than laterally in order to avoid damage to major vessels which may lie alongside the uterosacral ligaments.

Care should be taken to make the ligaments stand out as prominently as possible as this will reduce the risk of vaporizing to too great a depth.

Other lasers including the Nd:YAG and the argon laser have also been employed.

If the laser is not available, electrodiathermy electrocoagulation may be used. Although it is rather more difficult to get an accurate depth of destruction, with experience this method can be found to be virtually as efficient as the laser technique.

Results

C Sutton working in Guildford has a major experience of the use of the LUNA technique and has achieved improvements in over 80% of patients in a large longitudinal series.

28 The formation of a urinary diversion

When it is inevitable that the bladder has to be removed during a surgical procedure, or when the bladder is so badly damaged that it will never function normally again, as occasionally happens after radical radiotherapy, then a urinary diversion must be considered. The production of a urinary conduit may also be part of a larger procedure such as an exenterative operation.

Various techniques have been used for urinary diversion, including:

1 Implantation of the ureters into the sigmoid colon (ureterosigmoidostomy).

2 The formation of a wet colostomy, combining bowel and urinary function into one stoma.

3 The formation of a rectal bladder and a left iliac fossa colostomy.

4 The production of a nephrostomy or ureterostomy bringing the ureters directly out to the surface ideally with cannulation. This latter technique continues to be commonly used as a means of the primary (emergency) management of renal obstruction until definitive procedures can be performed.

All these techniques have significant associated problems, especially of infection and electrolyte control in the longer term.

Once Bricker had demonstrated the ease with which an isolated loop of ileum could be used to function as an artificial bladder, variations of his procedure became the preponderant methods of diversion. Many different parts of the bowel may be used, including the ileum, sigmoid colon and, where there has been extensive pelvis and lower abdominal irradiation, the transverse colon.

There is also a variety of ways of joining the ureters to the isolated loop of bowel. In some centres the Leadbetter technique of implanting the ureters individ- ually into the bowel loop is used; however, the authors prefer the Wallace technique, which is described here.

Recently, more complex but aesthetically satisfying procedures have been developed, beginning with the Koch pouch and being extended and made more so- phisticated by a wide variety of eponymous procedures including the Miami pouch and the Mainz pouch, usu- ally taking the name of their originating centre.

All of these continent conduits rely on the use of a low-pressure artificial bladder being generated by den- ervation and expansion of the small bowel. The stomas are generally brought out through a tiny hole in the abdominal wall, sometimes the umbilicus, which the patient can self-catheterize as and when they wish to void. These low-pressure systems have many advan- tages over the relative lack of control of the Wallace diversion, but do have the major disadvantage of requiring considerable lengths of normal bowel, something which is not always available following extensive irradiation, frequently an indicator for this procedure.

Patient preparation

The patient must have the full impact of removal of the bladder explained to her. The advantages and disad- vantages must be fairly and honestly explained and the patient and her partner must realize the significance of the permanent alteration in function which will be generated. For many patients the alteration in voiding habit will bring a definite improvement, especially for those with postradiotherapeutic fistula or shrinkage fixity of the bladder. The translation from a complete lack of control of urinary production and the difficulties of maintaining cleanliness when translated into the wearing of a simple ostomy appliance are infinite, and the vast majority of patients have little difficulty in accepting this permanent change.

The patient should be encouraged to meet with other patients who have had diversionary procedures performed and be seen on a number of occasions by the stoma therapist. The surgeon and the stoma therapist should site the stoma and clearly mark the place on the day before operation. The bowel is prepared for resection by giving the patient a low residue diet for 2–3 days preoperatively, accompanied by a non-absorbent antibiotic such as neomycin or one of the sulphonomides. Bowel washouts are unnecessarily debilitating and should be avoided.

Instruments

The instruments required are those in the gynaecological general set augmented with the GIA and TA55 stapling devices. If the bowel is to be sutured, soft non-crushing bowel clamps will be needed. A variety of small (no. 6–10) soft rubber T tubes will be needed, the size depending on the size of the ureters identified at the operation.

Anaesthesia

No special anaesthetic will be required for the conduit to be made; however, an epidural or spinal anaesthetic is of great assistance for any exenterative procedure. The authors usually ask the anaesthetist to put in a nasogastric tube shortly after inducing anaesthesia in order to rest the bowel for a few days following the operation. Nowadays many surgeons do not use nasogastric tubes.

The operation

The incision

If the conduit is the sole procedure to be performed a mid-line or paramedian incision lying alongside the umbilicus will give adequate access. The authors find that a high transverse interspinous incision used for exenterations (Maylard) will give perfect access to the lower para-aortic region where the conduit can be constructed.

Opening the abdomen

The incision should be designed so that the lower part of the para-aortic area is accessible at the level of the inferior mesenteric artery. When the operation is performed as part of an exenteration, the conduit should lie well above the pelvis out of the irradiated field. Once the abdomen is opened, the bowel is carefully packed away from the operation site while the ureters are identified and divided.

Identifying and isolating the ureters

It is usually easiest to pick out the ureters as they cross the pelvic brim. They can often be seen shining through the peritoneum exhibiting movement. The peritoneum close to them is picked up and carefully incised. This incision is extended with scissors and the ureters identified on either side. Occasionally, one ureter will be found to be disproportionately larger than the other ureter. This is not a contraindication to the use of the Wallace technique and the ureter should be identified, raised and separated gently from the peritoneum and structures around. The ureters are usually divided at or about the level of the pelvic brim. It is particularly important on the left side not to cut the ureter too high as the ureter has to be drawn across through the mesentery of the large bowel in order to meet with the right-sided ureter over the right side of the aorta and the inferior vena cava. Once the ureters have been identified and divided, the distal ends are tied with Vicryl sutures unless they are to be removed with the pelvic specimen during an exenterative procedure. At this time the proximal end of the ureters are allowed to lie free and the relatively small amounts of urine which are exuded can be removed easily at the end of the procedure.

Bringing the ureters to an intraperitoneal position

A point is now chosen on the right side of the posterior abdominal wall approximately 5 cm above the pelvic brim and 5 cm to the right of the mid point of the aorta. The peritoneum is elevated and incised, usually a continuation with the initial incision for identification of the ureters, and using a blunt forceps or the index finger a tunnel is developed so that the divided right ureter can be brought out through the space. The left ureter is a little more difficult to transpose as it has to negotiate the sigmoid colon mesentery. The authors find the easiest way of performing this transposition is to burrow under the mesentery with the fingers of the left hand,

287

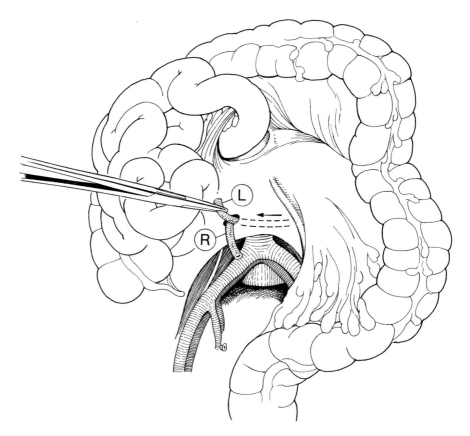

Fig. 28.1 Bringing the ureters into an intraperitoneal position.

taking care to identify and avoid the inferior mesenteric artery. This gentle burrowing separates the peritoneum allowing a blunt forceps to be passed from the hole on the right side, across the aorta, through the mesentery, to pick up the ureter on the left and draw it gently out of the hole on the right side of the mesentery (Fig. 28.1).

Preparing the segment of bowel
If the small bowel has not been irradiated then a segment of distal ileum may be chosen for the conduit. If extensive pelvic irradiation has been used, it may be prudent to utilize a segment of the transverse colon for the conduit as an alternative. The principles involved are identical and therefore only the ileal segment procedure will be described here.

A segment of ileum lying approximately 20–25 cm from the ileal caecal valve is chosen. The bowel is elevated and transilluminated to outline the arterial arcades. Ideally, the segment should contain at least two separate major arcade vessels. It should be approximately 10–12 cm in length and be fully mobile. The segment is elevated by the surgeon and his assistant, and the line of separation identified by incising the two leaves of the mesentery, taking care to either avoid or ligate small vessels which are present (Fig. 28.2). Individual small vessels can be ligated using either clips and ties or small metal clips which are easy to apply as the dissection develops.

Division of the bowel
This is most elegantly done using the GIA stapling device (Fig. 28.3) producing a sealed isolated segment of ileum. This segment is laid down on a dampened pack below the divided bowel.

Recently, the authors have changed their pattern of working to simply divide the bowel using soft non-

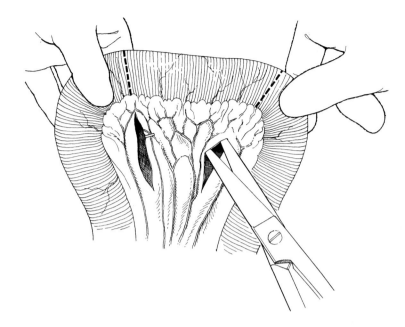

Fig. 28.2 Choosing an ileal segment with a broad-based arterial arcade.

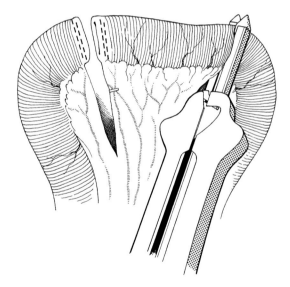

Fig. 28.3 Resecting the bowel segment with GIA stapling device.

crushing clamps so that the bowel is then immediately ready for repair and reconstitution.

Reconstituting the bowel
The two divided ends of the bowel are now elevated so that a functional side-to-side anastomosis can be made.

The two ends are held side to side with Babcock's tissue forceps so that a small incision can be made alongside each of the staple lines (Fig. 28.4) or, if the open ends of the bowel are present as is modern practice, the GIA stapler can now be introduced down into the bowel lumen and fired. The GIA stapler cuts a communication between the two limbs of the bowel and surrounds this communication with an intact staple line. Thus, a functional side-to-side anastomosis is formed which is completed by repairing the upper part of the anastomosis using a TA55 stapler (Fig. 28.5), or a further GIA stapler, to simply close the segment (Fig. 28.6). The space between the mesentery of the small bowel is now closed using three or four interrupted fine Vicryl sutures (Fig. 28.7). It is important not to make this repair too tight, and it is also important to draw together the individual layers of peritoneum rather than make deep bites into the mesentery.

Formation of the ureteric platform
Having brought the two ureters together intraperitoneally, the terminal 1 cm is incised with scissors so as to splay out the ends. These splayed out ends are then sutured to each other (Fig. 28.8) to produce a platform. The central suture is left long so that the T tube, which is now inserted into each ureter, can be anchored on to the base plate.

289

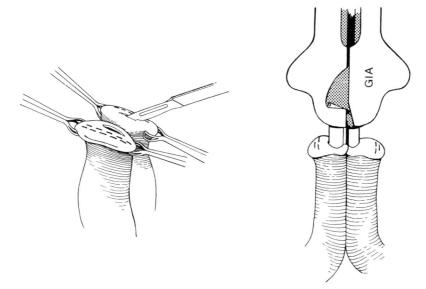

Fig. 28.4 Reconstituting bowel continuity using the GIA stapling device.

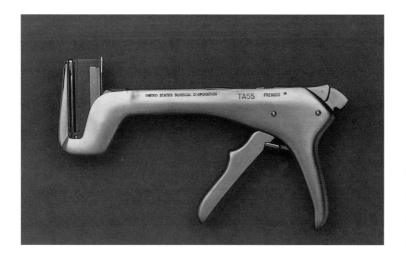

Fig. 28.5 TA55 stapler (this artwork was originally prepared for the United States Surgical Corporation's General Atlas and for publications by Professors Mark Ravitch MD and Felicien Steichen MD, ©USSC 1981).

Suturing the ileal segment to the ureters

The staples on each side of the ileal segment are now removed or, as in modern practice, the isolated ileal segment can now be lifted up. The long arm of the T tube is threaded through the segment. This is ideally done by passing a soft bowel clamp down the length of the segment, grasping the tube and drawing it gently through. It is important to make sure that the tube passes in the direction of peristaltic flow, and as the T tube is threaded through the segment (Fig. 28.9) the edges of the platform can then be carefully sutured to

the edges of the bowel using a series of interrupted Vicryl sutures. The conduit base is now attached to the posterior abdominal wall peritoneum with two or three individual sutures of Vicryl. This is important so there is no tension on the ureters themselves, and the conduit does not prolapse into the pelvis.

Formation of the stoma

A circle is cut in the skin at the site marked by the stoma therapist. This incision is carried down to the aponeurosis, which is cut and the edges clipped. The surgeon

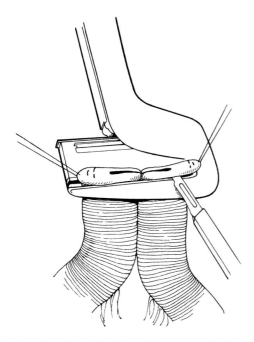

Fig. 28.6 Completing the side-to-side anastomosis using the TA55 stapler and removing redundant tissue.

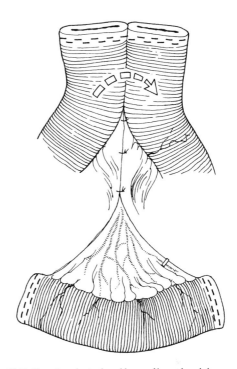

Fig. 28.7 Showing the isolated loop of bowel and the completed reanastomosed small bowel.

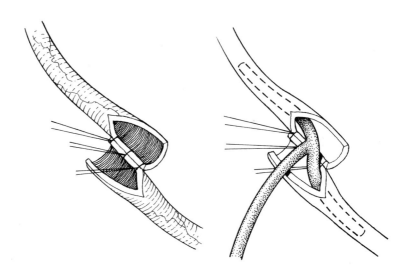

Fig. 28.8 Joining the splayed out ends of the ureter and inserting a T tube.

now places his left hand in the abdomen and elevates the abdominal wall under this incision. With his right hand he continues to cut down through the peritoneum, producing a hole through which the index finger can be easily passed.

A Babcock forcep is now passed through the hole and the distal end of the conduit with the T tube is gently drawn through. The conduit should be inspected to make sure that it is lying comfortably without undue tension or torsion. The edges of the peritoneum and the

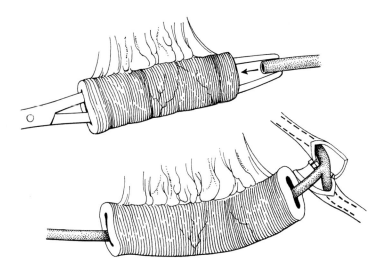

Fig. 28.9 Drawing the long arm of the T tube down the segment of bowel.

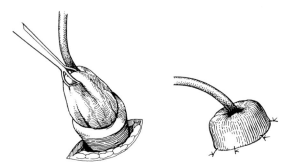

Fig. 28.10 Forming the 'rose bud' stoma.

aponeurosis in the stoma hole are now sutured to the bowel to fix it in position. The position and fixity of the bowel should be at a short distance from the open end of the conduit. The Babcock forcep is now inserted a short distance into the stoma and used to grasp the mucosa (Fig. 28.10). This process everts the end of the bowel, and the edge of the bowel which is now rolled back on itself is sutured first to the serosa and then to the skin edge so that a rosebud stoma is formed. The stoma appliance is put in place feeding the shortened T tube down into the back.

Closing the abdomen

This is carried out as described in Chapter 6. It is prudent to place a drain close to the anastomosis site, but

this is usually removed within 24 h of the end of the procedure.

Variations in technique

Recently, the authors have performed all the stapling with the GIA stapling device. This simplifies the operation, allows one instrument with replaceable cartridges to be used throughout, and improves the speed and cleanliness of the procedure.

Postoperative care

It has been the authors' practice to maintain the nasogastric tube for 3–4 days. It is then removed and the patient allowed free fluids and light diet by mouth. Many surgeons now do not use nasogastric tubes but the evidence base appears to be low. The T tube is kept in place for approximately 10 days and is then gently pulled to see if it can be removed. If it does not easily release, further attempts should be made on the next 2 days, but then the patient can be allowed home with the T tube in place, and it is usually found after a short period of time that the conduit naturally discharges the T tube into the ileostomy bag. The patient will require intensive training in the maintenance of the ileostomy appliance. This is performed by the stoma therapist once the patient is mobile and confidence is developed at this time. It has been the authors' practice to maintain prophylactic antibiotics, not only during the operation but for some days after the procedure, until good urinary flow is developed.

It is important to maintain good hydration so that a fast flow of urine can be maintained in the postoperative period. This will reduce the risk of clot formation blocking the ureters or the conduit itself.

Further reading

Textbooks

Stapling in Surgery by Felicien Steichen and Mark Ravitch, published by Year Book Medical Publishing, Chicago (pp. 298–301), demonstrates another way in which stapling techniques can be used for the formation of conduit and reanastomosing bowel segments.

Buchsbaum and Schmidt's *Gynecologic and Obstetric Urology*, 2nd edition, published by W.B. Saunders, Philadelphia, in 1982, pp. 168–188, contains a complete review of the major techniques for urinary diversion. They clearly cover the indications and the wide variety of methods available to the surgeon for making a diversion.

29 The management of injuries to the urinary tract

There has been little need for major changes to this chapter since the last edition. Although injury to the urinary tract is one of the major concerns of the gynaecological surgeon during routine gynaecological procedures, actual injury is rare. The surgeon should know the whereabouts of the ureters and bladder during any procedure to avoid being 'a urinary tract neurotic' and taking ridiculous precautions to avoid the ureters and bladder. These structures should be treated with care but not with the type of respect which results in never handling them.

Anatomical relationship

The source of the gynaecologist's concern is the close relationship of the ureters to the cervix and the uterine arteries, and the retroperitoneal course of the ureter in the pelvis and its close contiguity with the infundibulopelvic ligament at the pelvic brim. The attachment of the bladder to the anterior part of the uterus and the necessity to separate the two structures often places the bladder in considerable danger of damage.

Predisposing factors

These are summarized in Table 29.1.

Traditionally, injuries to the urinary tract have been classified into those recognized at the time of operation and those which manifest themselves later in the postoperative period.

Damage recognized at the time of operation

Bladder injuries

The most common circumstance for damage to the bladder is when the bladder is being separated from the anterior surface of the lower uterus and cervix during hysterectomy or caesarean section. If the surgeon is unsure about the possibility of an injury he should insert diluted methylene blue into the bladder through a urethral catheter and look for any leakage into the peritoneal cavity.

Damage to the muscularis
If the bladder is not entered but a 'bubble' of mucosa can be seen pushing through from the muscularis, all that is required is that the area should be oversewn with an interrupted or continuous Vicryl suture and as a precaution the bladder drained with a Foley catheter for 7 days following the procedure.

Breaching of the bladder wall
If the bladder has obviously been entered, the area should be clearly identified by placing Allis's tissue forceps on the edge of the defect. The mucosa and muscularis can be sutured separately in two layers with a continuous suture followed by an interrupted layer using a Vicryl suture. However, if trauma is minimal, the repair can be in a single layer to the muscularis coat with a continuous or interrupted suture technique.

It is vital to identify the ureteric orifices if the damage has occurred close to the trigone or the site of entry of the ureters into the bladder wall. In these

Table 29.1 Predisposing factors leading to urinary tract injury in gynaecological procedures

Congenital anomalies, including duplex ureters and ectopic kidneys
Endometriosis
Chronic pelvic inflammatory disease
Retroperitoneal masses such as broad ligament fibroids and large ovarian cysts
Previous pelvic surgery
Radiotherapy with scarring and compromised blood supply

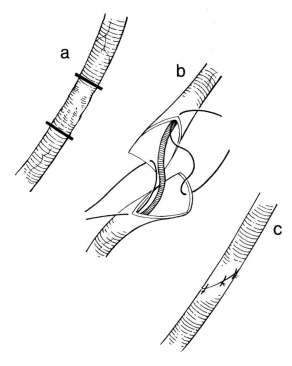

Fig. 29.1 Anastomosis of the ureter after either transection or resection of a short length of damaged ureter.

circumstances, the gynaecologist would do well to call upon the assistance of a urological colleague to perform the repair.

If it is necessary to carry out a repair without assistance, the gynaecologist should open the bladder at its upper part, identify the ureteric orifices, catheterize them and proceed with the repair under direct vision.

Where the damage to the bladder has occurred following irradiation, there is a significant risk of failure of healing and subsequent fistula formation. The interposition of an omental flap may improve the blood supply to the area and reduce the risk of necrosis.

Ureteric injuries

Where it is suspected that the ureter has been damaged at operation, whether this be by cutting, crushing or inclusion in a suture, then the ureter should be widely exposed so that a full inspection can be carried out. This is best done by separating the pelvic peritoneum from the pelvic side wall and exposing the full length of the pelvic part of the ureter. It is not necessary to separate the ureter from the peritoneum for its full length as this would merely jeopardize its blood supply. An immediate repair of the damaged ureter gives a very good prospect of complete recovery without the need for further surgery.

Injuries to the pelvic ureter

Crushing injuries

These may be caused by crushing or nipping by tissue forceps or by inadvertent ligation. The management should be to resect the crushed area and anastomose the two ends (Fig. 29.1).

Incision of the ureter

It is rare to partially resect the ureter; more commonly, it is completely resected. In these circumstances the management is to anastomose the cleanly divided ends of the ureter, having first made the ends spatulate (Fig. 29.1).

The operation

Identifying the site of damage The area affected is exposed and the damaged area resected.

Making the anastomosis The clean ends of the ureter are spatulated (see Fig. 29.1), and sutured using 4.0 Vicryl over a ureteric stent.

Management of the stent The commonest stent used is the 'pigtail' Silastic stent (Fig. 29.2), which can remain in the ureter for considerable periods of time. The upper end of the stent is inserted into the renal pelvis and the lower end into the bladder. If a pigtail is used, no fixation is required as the 'memory' of the catheter will

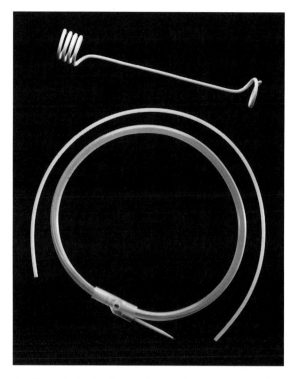

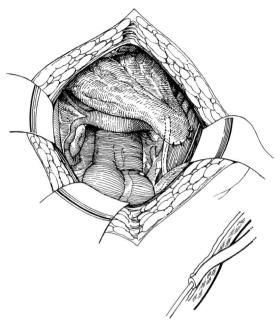

Fig. 29.3 The psoas hitch.

Fig. 29.2 The Bard coil stent, showing the Silastic stent and the coiled introduction wire. Photograph kindly supplied by Bard Urology Division, Bard Limited, Sunderland, Tyne and Wear, UK.

unwind the terminal few centimetres and provide adequate fixation (see Fig. 29.2).

Extraperitoneal drainage The operative area should be drained to monitor for leakage of urine during the first few days.

Injuries to the distal ureter

This type of injury tends to occur in association with gynaecological surgery. It differs from injuries higher up the ureter in that it is often difficult to mobilize the ureter sufficiently to anastomose it without tension. In this situation the method most used to deal with this problem is to produce a new point of entry into the bladder; the damaged distal portion remaining can be either ligated or resected. The ureter should be implanted using an antireflux mechanism which will require the bladder to be opened.

The operation

Preparation of the ureter The damaged distal end of the ureter must be 'freshened' by removing any necrosed or traumatized tissue. A short length of ureter is mobilized and the distal end drawn towards the bladder.

Assessing ureteric tension and bladder mobilization If there is any tension, then the bladder should be mobilized by separating it from the symphysis pubis, gently lifting the bladder towards the ureter (the psoas hitch), or by developing a 'Boari–Ockerblad flap'.

The psoas hitch This simple technique involves suturing the bladder wall to the iliopsoas muscle on the pelvic side wall, thus elevating the bladder and shortening the distance between the bladder and the ureter to be anastomosed (Fig. 29.3).

The Boari–Ockerblad flap Where there has been significant loss of the distal ureter, this technique allows the gap to be bridged by bladder tissue and a satisfactory anastomosis to be achieved without tension.

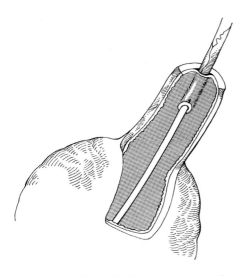

Fig. 29.4 The Boari–Ockerblad flap: developing the flap from the bladder wall.

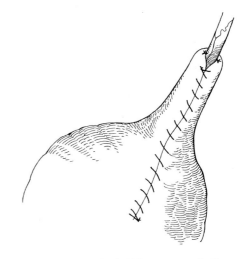

Fig. 29.5 The Boari–Ockerbald flap: suturing the flap to form a tube over the antireflux anastomosis.

The most important point to be considered when fashioning the flap (Fig. 29.4), is to be careful not to make the flap too narrow. It is extraordinarily easy to forget the relationship between the width of the flap and the tube which it must become. The flap is more readily performed with a full bladder and it may be worth filling the bladder before the incision. An oblique U-shaped incision is then made in the bladder wall and the distal end of the ureter is either sutured directly to the end or is tunnelled submucosally. Figures 29.4 and 29.5 show the technique for producing a flap with an antireflux anastomosis.

Direct implantation of the ureter into the bladder Once the end of the ureter is clean and it has been decided that it is possible to implant it into the bladder, the first step is to open the bladder and confirm the site of anastomosis. Again, this is more readily performed with a full bladder. An oblique opening is then made in the bladder and the distal end of the ureter is drawn through it using two stay-sutures attached to its edges (Fig. 29.6). The edges are then sutured to the mucosa and two further stitches are placed to fasten the side of the ureter to the outer surface of the bladder in order to anchor it and counter any tendency to retraction. The ureter is stented and the coiled end left to lie in the bladder to be retrieved later using a cystoscope.

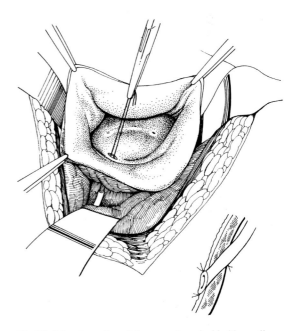

Fig. 29.6 Implantation of the ureter into the bladder wall.

Bladder closure and drainage The bladder is drained with an indwelling catheter and the extraperitoneal space is drained with a suction drain.

297

Postoperative care

Prophylactic antibiotics specific for bacteria affecting the urinary tract should be used. The ureteric catheter should be maintained for at least 7 days, preferably longer.

An intravenous urogram with special views of the lower ureter will confirm the security of the anastomosis.

Ureteroureteral anastomosis This may be necessary if it is impossible to bridge the gap between the end of the damaged ureter and the bladder. The damaged ureter is cleaned and mobilized; it is then brought across the mid-line without tension and directly anastomosed into the side of the remaining ureter. Ureteric stents should be used to support the anastomosis until healing has occurred.

Ileal conduit In the rare circumstances where both ureters are damaged and reimplantation into the bladder cannot be achieved, it is preferable to produce a urinary diversion such as an ileal conduit rather than make a skin ureterostomy.

Management of the delayed diagnosis of urinary tract damage

The management of the late diagnosed urinary tract damage is mainly the area of expertise of the experienced urologist; the gynaecologist should not delay in calling for his colleague's advice as further delay will seriously risk the function of the kidney.

The diagnosis of urinary tract damage may be made following the development of symptoms such as urine leakage if a fistula has occurred or loin or ureteric pain where obstruction to the outflow develops.

The management of urinary fistulae is dealt with in Chapter 15.

The management of obstructive damage to the ureters can be divided into two phases: drainage and repair. *Drainage* of the obstructed renal tract is best performed by radiologically guided percutaneous nephrostomy. Ureteric catheters can sometimes be passed beyond the point of obstruction, especially when the blockage is due to extrinsic pressure.

Repair of the damage to the ureter needs to be carried out if the obstruction could not be relieved by a stent.

Frequently, it is not possible to bridge the obstructed or damaged length of ureter and more extensive procedures are necessary. These are entirely in the province of the urologist and will merely be listed here.

(a) Ureteroileoneocystostomy, or the use of an isolated segment of ileum to bridge the damaged length of ureter to the bladder.

(b) Transureteroureterostomy may be used if it is not possible to reanastomose the damaged ureter with the bladder or the urologist feels that the long-term problems of using a segment of intestine are not justified.

(c) Nephrectomy may be necessary if renal function is markedly impaired.

Radiotherapy damage

Where the patient has had irradiation to the ureter which is damaged, great care and skill is called for when deciding on the optimal method of repair. It is also important to remember that the irradiation may have also compromised the blood supply of organs close to the ureter, particularly bowel; consequently, if conduits are to be produced, a segment of bowel outside the irradiation field should be chosen.

The gynaecologist must not be slow or too proud to ask for advice and assistance from his urological colleagues; early recognition and management of damage to the urinary tract is in the patient's best interests.

Further reading

Textbooks

Buchsbaum and Schmidt's *Gynecologic and Obstetric Urology*, 2nd edn, published by W.B. Saunders, Philadelphia, in 1982, is a valuable source of information on many urological problems found in obstetrics and gynaecology. The sections on the various traumas to the urinary tract are well hidden in the text but are worth searching for, drawing the reader's attention to many valuable diagnostic and management principles.

References

WF Hendry, in a review in *Progress in Obstetrics and Gynaecology*, vol. V, John Studd (ed.), published by Churchill Livingstone, has summarized many thoughts on the subject.

He has also used his own wide experience to demonstrate the methods of diagnosis and management of a variety of obstructive problems of the ureter in patients with gynaecological disease.

The 2nd edition of *Atlas of Urologic Surgery*, by Frank Hinman, published by W.B. Saunders (1998) is an excellent book with full descriptions and useful illustrations of the relevant urological procedures.

Index

Page numbers in *italic* refer to figures and **bold** refer to tables